Reading Birth and Death

Reading Birth and Death
A History of Obstetric Thinking

Jo Murphy-Lawless

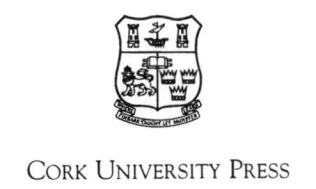

CORK UNIVERSITY PRESS

First published in 1998 by
Cork University Press
Cork
Ireland

© Jo Murphy-Lawless 1998

All rights reserved. No part of this book may be reprinted or reproduced or utilized in any electronic, mechanical or other means, now known or hereafter invented, including photocopying and recording or otherwise, without either the prior written permission of the Publishers or a licence permitting restricted copying in Ireland issued by the Irish Copyright Licensing Agency Ltd, Irish Writers' Centre, 19 Parnell Square, Dublin 1.

British Library Cataloguing in Publication Data
A CIP catalogue record for this book is available from the British Library.

ISBN 1 85918 176 7 hardback
ISBN 1 85918 177 5 paperback

Typeset by Elaine Shiels, Bantry, Co. Cork
Printed in the UK by Redwood Books

Contents

Acknowledgements vii

Introduction 1

1. Women, Power and Obstetric Rationality 17
2. Obstetric Pairings and Knowledge Formation 62
3. Body, Power, Death: The Problem of Puerperal Fever 105
4. Calculating Life and Death: The Risk–Death Pairing 158
5. The Production of Norms in Labour: Active Management 197
6. Reading Birth and Death 229

Notes and References 265
Bibliography 319
Index 333

For Oisín
For the future

Acknowledgements

How can the act of writing, which is done in isolation, be such a communal act at the same time? Everyone got dragged in, including a group of eight remarkable cats. I want to thank: Denise Arnold, Cecily Begley, Clare Brady, Ciaran Byrne, Therese Byrne, Michael Cooke, Peter Corrigan, Emer Coveney, Adam Danby-Smith, Anne Davis, Maria Davison, Nicole Harper, Dara Higgins, Dominick Jenkins, Patricia Kennedy, Ruth Kenny, Tom Kilgallen, Bridget McAdam-O'Connell, Frances McDonnell, Philip McNab, John Matthews, Robert Mills, Dervla Murphy, Oisín Murphy-Lawless, Kathleen Murray, Nexus Research Cooperative, Laury Oaks, Brenda O'Brien, Marie O'Connor, Máire O'Regan, Joseph Owen O'Reilly, Nellie O'Reilly, Eilish Pearce, Ciarán Power, David Redmond, Astrid Schmelzer, Sheila Sheridan, Gill Smith, Mary Smyth, Gerry Sullivan, Eleanor Taaffe, Cassandra Torrico, Maryann Valiulis, Marsden Wagner, Linda Weldon, Caroline Williams, and an anonymous reader for unstinting help, encouragement and critical reading. Without them, there would be no book.

I also want to thank the hundreds of women and midwives who have talked with me about childbirth since I first became involved with childbirth support groups more than twenty-five years ago; and the women whom I have been privileged to teach in the Centre for Women's Studies, Trinity College over the last eight years, whose engagement with and passionate responses to the issue of gender and medical science have helped me clarify so much.

Jo Murphy-Lawless

An earlier version of Chapter 5 appeared in *Canadian Journal of Irish Studies*, vol. 18, no. 1, 1992 as 'Reading birth and death through obstetric practice'.

Introduction

The daylight quickly strips itself from the Andean sky. Although it was only late afternoon, the sun was already gone from the near mountains while we talked. I was sitting on a stone slab with my two colleagues, a linguist and a health educator or *promotora* both working, like me, on a project about contemporary childbirth practices in Bolivia in rural and urban settings. We were in a small inner courtyard, walled by stone, with doorways leading to the main house behind us, where parents and young children usually sleep, and two outhouses, one where chickens shelter and one where water is stored. The small homestead itself was torn from the side of a rock-strewn hill, and beyond the stone corrals for the few animals lay a steady challenging descent; in sum, a demanding and isolated way of life which is a half-day's motor transport away from the nearest tiny *pueblo*, if you can find any.

The young woman whom we were visiting had already described at length her experiences of childbirth to one of my colleagues. In the Quechua language of this tiny community, the young woman spoke with special intensity about the threat of *sajt'ay*, a Quechua word that describes an affliction which is greatly feared and believed to be nearly always fatal.[1] With *sajt'ay*, a woman's blood becomes the focus for a deadly attack by pernicious spirits in the immediate aftermath of birth when her body is weakened by labour. Because of the threat of *sajt'ay*, the woman must not be left on her own by her family, even for a moment, in the days following birth, in spite of the fact that she might have given birth while unattended. When the blood from the birth is cleaned up, it must not be put outside the door. Otherwise it might attract these spirits to the woman in her vulnerable state. A thong of cowhide and cow's horn are also used to frighten away the spirits, as is the grain *quinoa* which is sprinkled round the entranceway to the home where people gather to eat. The grain is meant to indicate a large household, too numerous for the spirits to attack. A mirror representing slippery rocks (*lusk'a qaqa* in Quechua), which the spirits cannot cross, is put in place to further protect the woman as is a comb (*sajra's*), made from strong stubble, which represents brush cover in the open country that these spirits cannot penetrate. Her family will also make smoke with pig's hair mixed together with medicinal substances to protect her. Without these defences, the perception is that a woman can go to her death.[2]

This is an important complex of beliefs in the high *puna*, where appreciable numbers of women die in childbirth. One current estimate is 591 deaths for every 100,000 births.[3] Records for Northern Chayanta Province in the Department of Potosí, which includes the community where we were that afternoon, indicate that 66 women died as a result of complications in birth in the twelve months between October 1993 and 1994.[4] The precautions, that I have described, that women take to protect themselves from *sajt'ay*, are seen as a practical response to a perceptible threat of maternal mortality. However, there is another way to view these deaths which demands our attention.

Those of us raised in the shadow of scientific thinking in the West attribute such deaths to closely defined physiological processes of blood loss and infection that have done irreversible damage. Because we have been taught these definitions of post-partum haemorrhage and puerperal sepsis, we accept their relevance as the two most common causes of maternal deaths, accounting for 40 per cent of the 510,000 to 585,000 women worldwide who are estimated to die each year as a consequence of childbearing.[5] There is a radical difference between these two explanations of causality – between *sajt'ay* as a result of a successful onslaught by pernicious spirits, and the clinical description of death as a result of too severe a loss of blood, leading to cardiopulmonary failure or the overwhelming invasion of bacteria in the circulatory system or pelvic connective tissue. The radical nature of this difference suggests the outline of one set of problems I seek to examine in the course of this book. How has obstetric science acquired its knowledges of the female body in pregnancy and birth? On the basis of what conceptual models? And how has obstetric science successfully argued a higher order of rationality as a result of its knowledges? Perhaps most importantly, how have women dealt with the impact of a science whose greatest claim is to have rescued them from death in childbirth?

I have found the responses and actions of women who are not yet totally subject to this science a valuable focus in framing these questions. The fact that women in more remote areas of the Bolivian Andes do not view pregnancy and birth as necessarily dangerous events in themselves forces one to think more rigorously about obstetrics. These women are wary of poor birth outcomes, even apprehensive, but unlike many of their sisters from the developed countries of the North Atlantic, they are not riven with an all-pervasive disquiet throughout pregnancy. Rather, there is a precise ethnotaxonomy of women's bodies which is used to identify who will give birth easily and who may find birth difficult. For example, women who labour quickly are thought to have hot interiors, predisposing them to easy labours. They may have wombs which give them beneficial 'pathways' for birth, like a 'vicuña pathway', named after the llama-like animal with the silky wool coat. This 'pathway' is said to be an attribute especially of women who give birth easily and alone, often while doing their herding work in the hills. Concerns and fears are about specific problems, few in number and concrete, like the position of the baby in the uterus. If a woman thinks her baby is not well positioned, she commonly seeks help from a *partera*, a traditional midwife, who will work with a sophisticated system of massage, first feeling out the alignment of a woman's internal organs with her spine and from that reference point, repositioning the baby to avoid the outcome of an obstructed labour.[6] But it is the woman's decision to consult the *partera*, to seek her help and advice, or even to seek help from the *sanitario*, the state medical officer who may live nearby in the health station or *posta*.[7] Her decisions about her pregnancy are based on her sense of her body and she determines her priorities for herself. She has what we term agency.

Andean women grow into this level of competence. It is usual in the course of a first pregnancy to attend a *partera* as a kind of apprenticeship to learn the local knowledge and ways of thinking about childbearing. It is usually during a first birth that a young woman has attendants throughout labour to help her, most probably older women family members. For subsequent births she knows the ropes, the ways of doing things and takes control of the birth process herself. Once a woman is practised in giving birth, assistance during labour may amount to no more than help with cooking and other domestic chores. In the actual moment of birth, the woman may well be alone by choice. After the baby is born, her husband comes to pick up the baby, to cut the umbilical cord and to perform another important custom, to tie around her waist a belt, the *cintura*, specially woven for this moment.[8]

Just because a woman might have had a previous difficult pregnancy, where she was in pain and the *partera* worked to correct a malpresentation, or a labour where there were difficulties and help was sought from the *partera*, it does not follow that a woman will want the constant presence and assistance of someone else in a subsequent pregnancy and labour. On the contrary, women consistently self-diagnose and even if they have a malpresentation, they often choose not to consult the *partera* unless or until their own resources have proved insufficient. If the *partera* is called during labour, she will do what is required of her and withdraw, leaving the woman to give birth on her own.[9]

This sense of purpose on the part of the birthing woman raises more than the issue of differing systems of explanation about the body in childbirth. It is so striking to my eye precisely because Andean women have knowledges and skills whereby they can judge their situation for themselves. That act of judgement is valued in its own right and it points to a second broad theme with which this book is concerned, the problem of agency for childbearing women in contemporary Western society (and Western-affected societies). Of course there are limits to the control that rural Andean women can exercise, limits on their capacity to act independently of the social systems of which they are a part. But not only do they read their pregnant bodies as experts, they also tend their bodies, using their acquired interpretative skills. This exercise of personal agency stands in sharp contrast to the lack of knowledge which women in North Atlantic countries now accept as their lot. In the latter, in a social domain where there is no comparable apprenticeship system, the exercise of personal agency is a political struggle for each woman against a dominant institutional voice which argues that her compliance with its norms must frame the outer limit of her actions during pregnancy. By and large, North Atlantic women have come to accept their incapacity to judge and to take action, an incapacity which is linked directly to the way obstetric medicine has organised itself. Continuing efforts by activists and midwives, feminists and non-feminists alike, to resist and contest that image of incapacity over the last four decades have not dislodged obstetric medicine from its position as the principal authority on the birth process.

Susan Sherwin has argued that Western biomedicine defines itself as a 'good science' because it pursues the goal of protecting health. In turn, women in the West have come to accept the argument that biomedicine is the 'best instrument' for achieving and maintaining health. Within this frame of reference, especially when it concerns women's bodies as reproducing entities, women are actively discouraged from self-help and certainly from making judgements about the welfare of their bodies.[10] When it comes to what is seen as the major issue, what is best for the baby, women's role in their health care is limited for the most part to carrying out what Sherwin terms the 'negative injunctions' medicine places on women. We are told what we must not do while what we are permitted to do is limited in all but the most minor of ailments to the message that we should seek professional advice. This is a remarkable exercise of power on the part of biomedicine. Specifically in relation to obstetrics, it has to do with the development of specialised knowledge which works to preclude and exclude any interpretation of the female body which lies outside its area of expertise.

In train with its remit to oversee the management of birth, obstetric science has demolished other ways of handling birth with apparent ease. How it has accomplished this can be seen quickly enough when looking at the medical response to practices that pre-date obstetric science or that still fall outside its ambit. Although these practices may be considered valuable in developing a more thorough historical and cultural understanding of a people or epoch, they are most often characterised by obstetric medicine as superstitious beliefs that contribute nothing intrinsically helpful to a woman giving birth. At best, they are viewed as forming an interim stage on the way to establishing superior biomedical methods. More often, they are viewed as practices which endanger the woman and her baby and therefore need either eradication or reform to come closer to the obstetric model which is assumed to be the universally proven model that provides the best outcome.[11]

From this perspective, Andean teaching and traditions are seen as both quaint and dangerous, the problem of the placenta or afterbirth providing a useful example. Certainly, both traditional and modern systems of childbirth management are alert to the danger for women in the period after the baby's birth, waiting for the placenta. The issue is how best to deliver the placenta in order to minimise danger. We will see in a later chapter how obstetric science has a history of uncertainty and confusion about delivery of the placenta and the associated problem of post-partum haemorrhage, yet is nevertheless critical of methods of management used outside its domain, including methods linked to traditional or pre-scientific cultures. Andean culture gives us one such example of a different scheme of management. Amongst the many practices which Andean women learn to employ to counteract threats or problems in childbirth is skill in handling the placenta. Within their tradition, the idealised placenta is integral to the process of agricultural production. It is believed that when the placenta of the celestial black llama, which holds the young llama at its centre, falls to the horizon, the black llama releases her amniotic fluids so that rain and the rainy season begin. Placentas in human births are treated with care for they too have their own destiny.

Thus the placenta of each child is often buried in a hole at the entranceway to the house, with some salt, to rot.[12] But care must also be taken to ensure that the placenta is completely expelled from the mother's body. Women believe that the placenta must be prevented from rising up in the mother's body after the baby is born, for otherwise it will kill her. This accounts for why, after the birth of the baby and as soon as the umbilical cord has been cut, her husband sits behind her and ties her *cintura* around her waist to prevent the placenta from rising and to ensure that it is expelled. It is also common to tie the cut end of the umbilical cord with a thread of wool which is then tied to the woman's big toe. The woman can tug gently with her toe to coax the placenta out while massaging her stomach and sides at the same time.[13]

Similar beliefs about the need to tether the umbilical cord are not so many generations gone from the Irish countryside. In 1849, Sir William Wilde wrote that one of the popular practices of midwifery 'amongst the lower orders in the remote districts' was to either tie the cord to the thigh of the woman giving birth or for her birth attendant to hold fast to the cord:

> I remember having been sent for to a case of this description in a distant part of the country; I found the midwife on her knees at the bed side with a firm grip of the funis in her hand, which she exultingly displayed to me, observing, 'Doctor I never let it out these five hours.' It is a popular belief that if the funis was let go, it might slip back into the uterus and be for ever lost sight of. I have known more than one instance in which eversion of the uterus was produced by the midwife forcibly dragging on the funis.[14]

Predictably, Wilde presents this as a quaint anecdote to illustrate the untutored nature and dangerous practices of non-professional people in an article, the purpose of which is to document customs and practices which were fast disappearing beneath the tide of modern medical thinking. But Wilde's presumption that the midwife's worry was based on ignorance is not quite right. Her concern was not that the *funis* (umbilical cord) would vanish, so much as the realisation, similar to that of Andean women, that a woman dies if the placenta does not come out. The cord vanishing 'forever', the uterus flying up into the chest, are metaphors which reveal how in both these practices and sets of reactions there is a clear sense that death strikes at women after birth because of the failure to deliver the placenta.

Wilde's dismissal of the local midwife's action as a 'popular belief' masks the fact that medical practitioners themselves were committed to similar procedures with the umbilical cord, with similarly disastrous outcomes of inverted uteruses and haemorrhage. But of course their arguments about their practices were conducted as a debate within a scientific frame of reference (I will explore this particular debate in Chapter 4). I want to show that while medical doctors put forward their actions as part of a science with a provable logical basis, they also put in place a number of damaging limitations. Their history reveals that their theoretical concerns were focused on the structure of the supine female body, whether on the delivery table or the autopsy table. Stemming from this singular focus, their descriptions of pregnancy and birth, and the definitions of how the female body worked, limited the scope of who might intervene to help a woman and how. They became the sole experts and, in their pursuit of the power accruing to experts, they routed all other birth attendants: family members, traditional handywomen and traditional midwives. Because they argued that they could describe, explain and even predict death within their scheme of things, the order of their knowledge appeared a more certain hedge against the dangers of childbirth. In effect they argued that they would handle death. However, the price women paid for this claim to more certain knowledge was a severe limitation of their agency and an absolute diminution of their own knowledge base and skills. Paradoxically, given its focus on defeating death, obstetrics also came to severely limit the discussion of death and the possible range of metaphors whereby people could deal with outcomes which might lead to death. I think it can be shown how this has done harm over time, not least because we have accepted the rhetoric of progressive scientific advances which in reality have so often been a practice of disempowerment for the individual woman, leaving her unprepared for a less than perfect outcome (this dilemma is examined in Chapter 5).

In the pre-obstetric period which was just ending when Wilde wrote his piece, rural Irish women still had recourse to a labour girdle, similar to the *cintura*, worn during labour to ensure a safe delivery. The girdle was made of ribbon, a band or a scarf and had a charm set on it on St Brigid's Day to achieve protective power. Thus it was known as *Brat Brighde* or St Brigid's Garment and was thought to be special help for a woman's well-being if any manual intervention were needed in her labour. (Interestingly, Wilde reports this latter form of use as common for women from the 'middle ranks' implying that they more frequently had manual intervention, though whether by doctor or midwife is not made clear.) He relates that round ovoid stones, still at that time often found in graveyards, ruined churches or by the sides of holy wells, were thought to have 'obstetric virtues' and were often carried a great distance to be put in the bed of a woman in labour to ensure a quick and safe delivery. Another way of expressing help was to unlock any locks, to loosen all knots, unbar doors and windows, even to set free the cows from their shed, the very act of loosening a way of encouraging the woman in labour to dilate expeditiously, to unloose the 'knot of childbirth'.[15]

In 'popular beliefs' such as these or with the Andean practices to protect a woman from *sajt'ay*, the sense of what must be done to hold off or challenge a threat during birth seems to me to be clearly and vividly stated. With fewer channels of expression and with curiously limited accounts of causality despite its commitment to scientific method, obstetric medicine is somehow muddier. In the instance of post-partum haemorrhage, for example, it has failed to establish a taxonomic system that works in setting out when haemorrhage will occur as well as how it occurs. Although contemporary obstetric texts list a wide-ranging number of predisposing factors or 'risk' factors that may lead to post-partum haemorrhage, and can produce percentages on the incidence of occurrence in relation to these factors, and can argue that post-partum haemorrhage is frequently predictable, it has not been able to establish a watertight predictive train of events that will definitively end in post-partum haemorrhage. We are led to expect precise predictive schemes by the fact that obstetrics is a science, its practices grounded in a scientific method.[16] Instead we find that obstetrics limps home with the strange conclusion that all women must receive prophylactic treatment as they give birth on the grounds that haemorrhage *might* occur. We must conclude that in reality obstetrics is powerless to predict its incidence. How different a belief is the obstetric reaction to reach for prophylactic drugs to the belief of Andean women about the need to protect against the possible event of *sajt'ay*? I will argue that this reaction of obstetrics to the possibility of post-partum haemorrhage, despite its many declarations of intent that careful observation is the cornerstone of its scientific method, is directly linked to its poor conceptual models, based on a supine non-dynamic body. In turn, this reaction sets up for practitioners still greater tensions around the issue of the possibility of death. For when they argue that they have had greatest success in overcoming death, it is their belief that their science constitutes a higher order of rational knowledge. In effect, they have created a foe they must always be seen to be able to overcome in order to justify their position. But has obstetric science not been significantly aided in its work by a host of socio-economic factors outside its control which it is very reluctant to acknowledge because it is then compromised in its hegemony? This too urgently requires investigation for it is crucial to the issue of women regaining agency in childbirth.

Post-partum haemorrhage and its management provide an excellent, if troubling, example of the problem obstetrics has created for itself and, ultimately, for women – the all-encompassing anxiety of obstetrics that pregnancy and birth cannot be judged as normal until after birth, that all manner of things commonly malfunction, colour how women view pregnancy and birth. How did obstetric science come to the extraordinary conclusion that no birth is normal except in retrospect? I suspect this is linked to an account of normality that is derived in part from an abstract female body rather than on the multiple possibilities of individual women's bodies.

By contrast with this global anxiety, the Andean taxonomy of bodies appears to be far more concerned with quite specific difficulties that can arise. And of course that taxonomy rests on skills being known and deployed by quite a wide range of people, not simply *parteras*. In a slow labour, for example, when the slowness is linked to a malpresentation, a birth technology called a *manteo* is used. The woman is placed on a blanket which is then held securely at its four corners by her husband and three others and she is gently rolled back and forth in the blanket, a movement which frees the baby in the pelvis and so enables it to turn spontaneously or be turned by a *partera* to a more advantageous position for birth.[17] Technologies like the *manteo* to assist women in birth are common to all cultures and they extend to techniques of psychological-physical interaction. Lévi-Strauss writes of an example of a birth technology, where psychological representation is employed to correct physiological disturbance.[18] The song of Muu, from the Cuna Indians in the Panama Republic, describes how the shaman is consulted by the midwife when the mother appears to be losing blood before the birth and is too weak to push the baby out. Muu, the force which is responsible for the baby-to-be, has captured the soul of the mother, which has resulted in her loss of vital physical strength, as the mother explains it to the shaman. The shaman sets out to contest the power of Muu who has overstepped her function. Employing richly allegorical images of the expedition he leads against Muu, the shaman recaptures the mother's soul. And, with her soul restored, her strength returns and she is able to deliver her baby without further mishap. In our Western terms, psychological manipulation is employed to help the woman recover herself, to 'release' and 'reorganise' a physiological process which has gone wrong, to right it, so that the woman can complete her labour successfully.

Compare these two kinds of birth technologies with, for example, the decision of an obstetrician to intervene in a breech birth by using a Caesarean section to deliver the baby. The signal difference is that both the *manteo* and the song of Muu enable women to maximise their own capacities and resources to deal with birth while the Caesarean overrides the woman's body. The former are technologies which are problematic for obstetrics precisely because their aim is to permit the woman to retain control and judgement over her own labour.[19] What is up for debate here is not the rights or wrongs of these techniques but the completeness of the conceptual packages of birth management and the claims that go with them. The pre-obstetric modes appear to be more modest in what reassurance they give to women, stating that death may be an outcome, while still leaving the woman as the central agent in determining birth management. They are arguably more complete in emotional and spiritual terms. Practical skills like the *manteo*, psychological devices like the song of Muu; beliefs that midwives can transfer the pains of labour onto a hapless deserving male (a practice reported by both Wilde and by Lady Gregory) or that wearing a cuckold's hat will bring an overly long labour to a conclusion are palpable responses to the struggle of work that childbirth is. In the same way, the elaborate customs for safeguarding a woman, for marking her passage through birth, are intelligible expressions of concern about the problem of death.

By contrast, obstetrics is not modest. Its lack of modesty is tied to the assertion it makes about its capacity to deliver the hard scientific facts. It argues that its account of birth is the most definitive and its route the most certain way to avoid death. One critical result of that assertion is the obstetric position that care of the emotions and spiritual matters during birth are not its remit. But most importantly, in enforcing its account obstetrics has usurped any sense of agency on the part of the birthing woman. In effect the science tells women, 'You can escape death if you follow us. But you must hand over to us your role as the central player in childbirth.' Examining the history of obstetric thinking has led me to conclude that we need to interrogate the obstetric demand that it should remain the single arbiter about childbirth management because – it contends – its practices have brought to an end danger in childbirth for the vast majority of women and their babies in the West. This demand with its accompanying rationale is, I believe, at the heart of our dilemma with obstetric science. We should be demanding of obstetrics that it acknowledge the limits of its actions, that it has been but one element, and one with contradictory effects, in a complex picture of the changing lives of women in the modern period. We also urgently need to question whether obstetrics as a clinical science is sufficiently flexible in the ways it organises itself and in its forms of cognition to understand and respond to the multiple connections and complexities which make up the reality of each woman who becomes pregnant. Both these propositions, however, pose a threat to the position that obstetrics has carved out. Obstetrics cannot easily acknowledge that its ways of thinking and modes of practice have as frequently contributed to women's deaths as not in its bid to build its science which, as Ann Oakley has observed, had more to do with establishing a new domain than with women's lives and needs.[20]

The difficulty women have experienced with this domain has stemmed from the impact of what Foucault terms 'the effects of the centralising powers of an organised scientific discourse'.[21] Obstetric science, at the same time as it has closed off our agency, has dragged us with it into an altogether different space. We no longer want to consider death or a difficult outcome as a possibility and choose to believe that with obstetric management we need not consider those issues. Yet we are not offered any truly satisfactory alternative to counting nine articles of men's clothing over a woman during each of her labour pains, or knotting and untying ribbons to achieve our safety.[22] And, on the other hand, we are troubled by the notion of a science of norms. If anything, it seems to have created a consuming sense of unease for we recognise, however dimly, that we cannot individually meet these norms, or become these norms, because they are abstracted concepts. But we still try to do so. For after all, stones, ribbons and cuckolds' hats are superstitions, we know that. However, we also sense, as Kierkegaard phrased it in *Sickness Unto Death*, that the 'disinterested scientific approach' which presents itself as a 'superior heroism' is actually a form of cowardice, a distancing, a kind of human untruth, far removed from the heroism of the woman who on becoming pregnant must engage immediately with the possibility of profound loss, because there can never be guaranteed outcomes.

I am not an anthropologist and it is not my intention to compare traditional bodies of knowledge, like the Andean system of ethnophysiology, or the practices in the Irish countryside 150 years ago, with obstetric science, in order to view each one of them as distinctive sets of cultural beliefs. However, I am profoundly interested in the confidence with which obstetric science argues that its discoveries have superseded all other knowledge bases about the female body. I want to know how this confidence has been made possible, how it relates to the history of obstetric reflections about the female body, how obstetrics has theorised about that body.

I am a feminist sociologist who has been involved in the childbirth issue for a quarter of a century and, in asking questions like this, I am aware that obstetrics has gradually come to speak like the other physical and social sciences of modernity. The two critical notions, with which all these sciences work and which have slipped effortlessly into our everyday discourse are the notions of norm and risk. They are reassuring anchors for us at many levels, for they suggest – and their proponents claim about them – that if they are used accurately, they produce a fail-safe reading of what is going right and what might go wrong. If one of the hallmarks of modernity is the security of a stable predictable order, as Weber argued, then these two, norms and risk, are the *modus operandi* for maintaining that order.[23]

These notions have impacted deeply on the way women as childbearers think about birth. We accept that within science normal is related to a norm which implies a measurable level of functioning. So for example, in the commonplace setting of the antenatal clinic, women have their blood pressure monitored, amongst other routine tests, and come away to tell family and friends that everything is 'normal'. We do not question how an average reading of blood pressure is derived, whether the range of normality at thirty-six weeks gestation takes into account the woman who has a low pre-pregnant blood pressure of 100 mmHg over 60 mmHG. If there is a dividing line between normality and abnormality, a systolic pressure of over 140 mmHg and a diastolic pressure of over 90 mmHg, we are told that it is not our concern how that particular boundary is determined. Rather we tend to accept that science can measure the way the body functions in order to quantify what is normal. In any case, we may recognise that we are not in a position to influence debate or disagreement about what constitutes hypertension and when to include or discount labile hypertension (high blood pressure that is very temporary in the course of a day and subsides).

It may be clear to a woman visiting a crowded antenatal clinic, where the staff changes frequently and the throughput of women is rapid and impersonal, that even the thought of going along to stand in the queue makes her heart race unpleasantly. She may also fear that the routine check will reveal her as having abnormally high blood pressure, because her heart is racing, and that the discovery will increase surveillance of her pregnancy, perhaps putting her under pressure to go into hospital for bed rest or treatment. She may perfectly well see the connection between the two events and seek a strategy to avoid dealing with the stress of antenatal check-ups. If she does so and skips her check-ups she will be held culpable, and informed that her actions are those of a negligent mother. What will not occur to her is that the reading itself should be contested, that she can question what 'normal' means.

In fact, the boundaries between what is 'normal' and 'abnormal' are constantly shifting. If we say of our birth experiences, that birth was a 'normal' straightforward delivery, we are confident that what we say can be borne out by a physiological explanation of labour, one that is derived from obstetric medicine. However, if birth experiences are broken down into their component parts, it soon emerges that what is normal for one woman, a hospital birth with epidural analgesia and an episiotomy, is emphatically rejected by another woman, who defines normal birth as one without any medical intervention at all. Yet both women desire a birth outcome where the baby is born without mishap and, now in Western societies, where it is taken as given, that the woman's life is not under threat as a consequence of birth.

Ultimately we want those reassurances both for woman and baby, that all will be well because we recognise, again too dimly, that there are unexpected and unwelcome outcomes even if we have the goal of a 'normal and natural birth'.

The notion of risk is how, in modern society, we have come to deal with, to cushion ourselves against the possibility of outcomes which may entail loss, damage and death. What lies behind our use of the everyday expressions 'taking chances' or 'taking a risk' is what we trust to be an objective mathematical measurement of all the factors involved in launching a new business with a fixed sum of borrowed capital to achieve a certain return over a given period of time or having a heart bypass operation to replace a faulty valve, where the risk of major surgery is judged to be less great than the risk of having a damaged valve which might otherwise lead to a heart attack. This process whereby variables can be identified, weighed and added up to enable us to reach rational decisions is integral to modernity, to everyday living. However, risk-production and risk assessment also become sources of deep worry, even threat. Large numbers of women who are using a contraceptive pill are regularly reported as having panic-stricken reactions in the wake of the latest press release about a possible link between the Pill and breast cancer, abandoning any form of contraception which itself leads to higher numbers of abortions in the fullness of time.

So we accept at some level that using risk schedules is a complex business, that there are different weightings of risk, even that experts disagree. Thus, for instance, the factors which doctors argue are indicators of who is at high risk of developing breast cancer have entered into popular health strictures for women, in spite of their contradictory nature. Witness the argument, based on statistics, that bearing children protects women from breast cancer, but equally the argument, also based on statistics, that women bearing their first child over the age of thirty-five are more at risk than women who remain childless.[24] Is the argument about the protective effect of childbearing still valid? The isolation of two of the genes thought to be involved in breast cancer has led to the marketing of a genetic test for these genes and the claim that doctors can predict a woman's risk of contracting this cancer, if she carries them.[25] But we are still dealing with a notion of risk, not a reality. For all its scientificity, a prediction about the risks of these genes, BRCA1 and BRCA2, is still only a prediction. And there is still the necessity of making a judgement based on that prediction about how one lives one's life. Yet we are perhaps less equipped than ever to make that judgement, not least because we are so saturated with the idea that because risk is a scientifically generated concept, it is a reliable basis on which to structure our judgements.

As with the problem of norms, we find it difficult to question the process of constructing risk itself, only challenging applications of the process in particular instances. We are not prepared to jettison the notion of risk. On the other hand, we do acknowledge that there are hierarchies of risk and risk-taking. In general, taking a risk on a business venture is culturally weighted as far less significant than taking a risk on life. Some forms of risk-taking, like mountain climbing, have a cachet attached to them and are marked out as permissible even when loss of life results. Some are simply impermissible. The cultural weighting in modern society against a pregnant woman taking a risk with her baby in labour and birth is vast. The opprobrium women can face on this matter has been consistently reinforced by the production of increasingly prolific risk schedules within obstetrics which have hugely affected us as childbearers.

The assertion of obstetrics, that it has conquered death, making childbirth safe for women, requires careful examination because the medicalisation of childbirth has not been an unqualified success and has not given to women all the benefits it claims to have done. This intensive process of medicalisation has entailed a continuum of technological interventions which have required the hospitalising of most women for childbirth. An entire system of obstetric intervention has evolved, from routine artificial rupture of membranes to its possibly most sophisticated variant, the 'active management of labour', which is accomplished with the use of oxytocic drugs. Over the last three decades women activists from the childbirth movement, the women's health care movement, childbirth educators and midwives have submitted the system to criticism and scrutiny, knowing that the obstetric system is often dehumanising and alienating and always expensive. The reply is that this is but a small price to pay if death is held at bay. But what exactly does that mean? Is the effort to convince us that it does possess certain knowledge not a kind of hard rhetoric to justify its capital-intensive operations, its quest for power, its desire for control?

Obstetrics seeks to make birth 'safer' and this is the reason we are surrounded by these complex injunctions about what we can and cannot do during pregnancy and birth, injunctions which are backed up by arguments about risk. Women face palpable disapproval and censure if we try to undertake a course of action which is perceived as being risk-laden and we will be told of the statistical risks we are running, for instance, if we choose to give birth at home. In many situations, we are not able to exercise any control over decisions. If a woman is carrying a breech baby, the obstetric decision to give her a Caesarean section, rather than to allow her to give birth vaginally, will be argued on the grounds of least risk to the baby. The risks to the mother of Caesarean section will not be discussed. Nor will it be discussed that it is an unproven assumption that, owing to damage during vaginal birth, there can be poorer perinatal outcomes and a higher perinatal mortality rate.[26] Observations about what is safe and unsafe in labour and delivery are in any case made in relation to observations based on medicalised birth techniques. So, as Wagner has pointed out, it is impossible to determine what the true rate of vaginal tears is when the tissues are regularly cut which leads to tearing, and the same stumbling block exists for virtually every issue in childbirth management.[27] In other words, what is measured is often meaningless, but without measurement, there is no science.

In a situation in developed North Atlantic countries, where maternal mortality rates have ceased to be a significant element in annual statistical returns (in 1994, there were two maternal deaths in Ireland amongst the 47,929 births) and neonatal mortality rates are lower each year (4.0 per 1,000 births in Ireland in 1994), the problem of death, the challenge of death continues to hover over birth and the debates about birth management.[28] But whose problem is this? Is a continuing challenge to defeat death part of that inhuman heroism that Kierkegaard locates at the heart of science? Do women have a different position in relation to death, compared with doctors?[29] I think this is very probable. The anguish and aching physical loss experienced by the woman whose baby has died, an anguish so terrible because she alone has known that baby, is an entirely separate order of meaning to the hospital which must record one more perinatal death. The former has to do with a wholly subjective experience in being pregnant and giving birth which always brings a woman close to the possibility of death, her own or her baby's. The latter has to do with theories, strategies, birth-management policies, with the making and breaking of medical reputations: it has to do with a way power has been expressed within modernity.

Obstetrics uses norms and risks to argue the efficacy of its scheme of things whereby exposure to death will be reduced. Women most often hear only the first part of that statement however, that its approach must be adopted to avoid difficulties. However, obstetrics is extraordinarily reluctant to discuss the possibility of death with the individual woman except in the most covert terms, which make it her responsibility, not theirs. Its watchword that a normal birth is one which exhibits no pathological symptoms (and therefore can only be judged to be so retrospectively) is a cloaked way of saying that death does occur. I think obstetrics cloaks this message because of the concern with its reputation; in a stark sense, with the ambition of exercising power over life which is so characteristic of science and which a death jeopardises. What a peculiar position it is that death is considered an abnormality, a deviation. Unexpected, unsought, a source of profound grief but a deviation from the human condition? It is pure hubris to reach such a conclusion. And yet as childbearers, we accept, far more than we recognise, that obstetrics seeks to rationalise its practices on the basis that it can control exposure to death. It cannot, as it happens, but we have gone along with those beliefs and they have gradually divested us of our experiential knowledge and skill in giving birth. And, as the dominant scientific voice about birth, obstetrics will do so in turn to women still outside its sphere of influence, like women from the Bolivian Andes.

To return here briefly to the problem of the placenta and post-partum haemorrhage (and in greater detail in Chapter 4), obstetrics finally struck lucky on this one, not in its explanatory schema of how the placenta separates and therefore how it should be managed, but in its use of pharmacological agents which undercut the female body in giving birth, and thus bypass it. This is the most frequently repeated pattern in obstetric science which has sought to minimise the potential of the female body in labour and birth while maximising its control of that body.

In this book I want to examine the obstetric reading of the female body, reading those scientific processes which have silted up during the last two hundred years and more, to be clear at least that their lens is nowhere near as clear and predictable as the word science suggests to us. I want to see how obstetrics has utilised and contributed to this generalised fear, this nameless globalised anxiety around childbirth which has so disempowered us. I think we need to recognise and maintain our awareness of our proximity to death in the sense that there are never guaranteed outcomes. If we reclaim the awareness that there are no guaranteed outcomes, we can deal critically with obstetrics' strategies of risk, its categories of normalcy. We have the potential to be as astute in our judgements of these biomedically interpreted bodies of ours as the young Quechua woman who can speak cogently and authoritatively about childbirth. But we must review comprehensively the range of women's experiential resources during labour and birth and then work to encourage the restoration of those resources in order to contest the obstetric view of our bodies and the obstetric position that it alone can set the rules of engagement with us. In this way, we can relocate ourselves once more as subjects when we give birth.

1

Women, Power and Obstetric Rationality

Modern Beliefs, Rational Practices

Obstetric science has organised itself as a rational practice. It argues that its beliefs about how to manage women in childbirth are the sum of its cumulative experiences and are provable in scientific terms. Like other 'normal' sciences, to use Thomas Kuhn's phrase, obstetrics seeks to establish that its proofs reflect the world as it is. In this case, the particular concern is an objective verifiable reading of the female body. So, like other sciences, it presents itself to the larger non-scientific community as a superior model of rationality when compared with alternative non-scientific or pre-scientific accounts of childbirth. It argues that when improvements to its key theories and shifts in its practices take place, these reflect the careful and closely reasoned approach of its practitioners to the work of refining and improving its observations. It does not present itself to the larger community as a human activity that is as much subject to competing local agendas, irate concerns, and a desire to control as other human undertakings. Rather obstetrics argues that its power to determine what ought to be done in childbirth is founded on its authority as a form of scientific rationality and it is not amenable to accepting as expert any voice from outside that community (and dismisses the dissident voice within).

Women see the issue of obstetric power differently and question what we experience as an overt exercise of power, one that is often expressed in distinctly irrational practices and language. This irrational response emerges pretty rapidly whenever we query obstetrics and it always turns on the same issue, the risk of death in childbirth whether for woman or baby. Despite the fact that we have become increasingly incisive in the way we challenge obstetrics, its reaction to us, that we do not sufficiently comprehend the threat of death which hangs over us, remains unchanged. I want to recount two incidents, separated by fourteen years and different locations, that nonetheless permit us to examine the irrationality of obstetrics when pushed to account for its way of doing things. They also illustrate how obstetrics uses 'shroud-waving', and attempts to frighten us with 'what if' accounts of possible damage and loss, to discourage us from voicing our criticisms.[1]

In April 1982 the Royal Free Hospital in London was the site for a mass protest which its organisers called the '*Birthrights Rally*'. Thousands of women, dozens of midwives, childbirth educators and other professionals involved in the childbirth movement along with their petition signed by an estimated 100,000 people, focused on the deeply controversial issue of control in childbirth. Two models of birth management had developed in the Royal Free over the previous few years, one an 'active birth' approach under the obstetrician, Yehudi Gordon, where women were encouraged to exercise elements of choice in their labours; the other, a more clearly medicalised approach, favoured by the head of the obstetrics department, Professor Ian Craft, who considered the first a rogue strand of birth management. The immediate flashpoint for the rally was an incident in the Royal Free where a woman declared to medical staff that she wanted to remain mobile during labour and to use an upright position for the moment of birth. Her resolve about the conduct of her labour resulted in the withdrawal of all medical assistance to her, including midwifery help, until she complied with Craft's regime.

The protest rally banners captured some of the metaphors and rhetorical slogans through which women were politicising experiences like this which they had come to see as unacceptable: 'Choice in Childbirth', 'Save Natural Birth from Extinction', 'Ban Battery Births', 'Stand Up for Natural Childbirth'. Sheila Kitzinger, the acknowledged authority of the British childbirth movement, declared that a 'tidal wave' of women in Western countries was demanding 'a woman's right to natural childbirth'. She spoke of 'the succulent newborn baby', of how the incident in the Royal Free was a goad to political action to challenge the 'male dominated model of childbirth, of the need to topple the autocratic control of a profession directed towards the treatment of pathological conditions'.[2] This stance on birth was incomprehensible to Professor Craft, who favoured interventions like routine 'lift-out' forceps deliveries, arguing that these were kinder to women and babies alike. He stated his unequivocal opposition to not intervening in birth as a matter of course: 'Childbirth is as much a natural event as is death, but whether it should be allowed to be so is a different matter.'[3]

At the heart of the row over the Royal Free was Craft's insistence that because a baby's life was potentially 'at risk' during labour, it was the decision of the expert obstetrician about any and all actions taken in labour to deal with that potential risk. The woman (then and now commonly referred to as the 'mother' by obstetricians, as if her work in life was solely limited to childbearing and domesticity) had no role in active decision-making.

The second incident began with a discussion on Irish radio in June 1996 about the reasons why women want to give birth at home. The possibility that a woman might exercise this kind of choice impelled a Limerick obstetrician, Dr Donal O'Sullivan, to declare in Irish on Raidió na Gaeltachta that a husband, faced with his wife's insistence on a home birth, must use a bridle – a *ceannrach* – on his wife, driving her before him to hospital to give birth there. On this and other programmes, and in the press in the following days and weeks, outraged women and birth activists contested his depiction of a woman as an unruly animal that must be brought under control. O'Sullivan's response to the public anger was that he believed a husband must 'act as head of the household if his wife intended to put her life and that of her baby at risk' and that any means were justified to get her to hospital.[4]

The two incidents share the same anxious response on the part of obstetrics, when faced with the possibility that a woman might seek to control her own delivery. Is there a genuine basis for the fear that a woman or her baby might come to harm in a hospital setting if she is upright in labour and, if so, why actually withdraw services from her? Does the healthy woman who elects to give birth at home actually endanger herself and her baby? I suggest that in both instances, what the practitioners fear is losing control over childbirth and part of their response is to try to frighten women by raising the possibility of death. Obstetric science believes profoundly that there is a remit to reduce women's exposure to death, to rescue women from death, a remit which belongs entirely and exclusively to itself, and not to women as those principally affected. While both Craft and O'Sullivan might concede that birth is a 'natural' event, insofar as it is a biological event, they cannot concede that birth can be easily accomplished. What Craft argues is that birth is inherently uncertain, and therefore to reduce that uncertainty, it must be brought under complete control. This is the obstetric ambition. I will argue that it is unachievable.

In historical terms, the ambition to achieve total knowledge and thus to be able to claim to reduce or eliminate uncertainty is part of modernity and when it speaks this way, obstetrics is revealed as a modern science. It is also notable that in incidents like these, where obstetricians are forced into more public and explicit statements about their thinking, death takes on a resonance of an event which should properly be at a great distance from birth, coming at the end of a productive life, not cutting that life short as occurs with infant mortality. This too is a belief of modern society which has conceptualised time as a resource that contributes to productivity. Therefore an early or untimely death disrupts possible productivity.[5] Being able to think this way about the timing of death is in part a result of our modern perception that death no longer appears beyond our control as it did in the pre-modern period. We believe that death no longer strikes in a random manner in modern societies, as it once did through phenomena like famines and epidemics, nor that death is any longer an arbitrary event at the whim of the most powerful, as it was with a kingly edict to put someone to death. Instead death now appears orderly and predictable. Tables of life expectancy, the machinery of laws and judges, economic projections, weather forecasts, antibiotics, all these modern practices give rise to the belief that we can control the untoward, that death is predictable and in the normal course of events, a long way away from birth.[6]

This seeming predictability is not without its own price. The writer and philosopher, Michel Foucault, links our shift in perceptions to the way power works in modern society. The sorts of practices described above, which are now part of everyday living, have also created sources of power, and specifically, the growth of power to 'foster' life. The king's power to take life away has been replaced by a plethora of practices which express a different capacity and ambition to permit life, to secure it, to administer it, for 'it is over life, throughout its unfolding, that power establishes its dominion'.[7] This ambition is one that is firmly anchored in the project of the Enlightenment of which obstetric science is a part. Over the last 250 years, the desire to administer and control life has been embedded in obstetric medicine at least as much as in other sciences.

With its project to create a definitive account of the female body, obstetric medicine has imposed a complex series of relationships and effects on us as childbearing women. At a concrete level, the story of the protest at the Royal Free and the reactions to the statement that women should be bridled and driven to hospital like cattle, are reactions to the way medical power works, which power has invoked a fundamental disquiet from women in contemporary Western society despite its perceived advantages of rescuing us from death. Emily Martin, in her study of how women feel about their bodies in relation to reproductive medicine, has argued that women 'represent themselves as fragmented, lacking a sense of autonomy in the world and feeling carried along by forces beyond their control'.[8] This sense of fragmentation, of losing our bodies to the way obstetrics sees us, is precisely what those thousands of women sought to challenge in the Birthrights Rally. Their demands for active engagement in their labours are concerned with the problem of male power over the body, our female bodies, and of the corresponding diminution of our sense of autonomy and control, of what can be termed our personal agency.

These are issues which have been central themes in the evolving women's movement over the last thirty years, where contesting patriarchy has meant asserting our claims to physical and emotional integrity. But the validity of physical integrity takes on specific meaning in a situation where a woman has no way to guarantee that she will not be subjected to painful and disruptive medical techniques, whether she wishes them or not, whether they are necessary or not, except by completely removing herself from medical supervision while giving birth. However, in most Western countries, including Ireland and England, modern legislation has declared it illegal for a person unqualified in either medicine or midwifery to intentionally assist a woman to give birth alone unless it is an emergency situation. This is an indication of how wide-reaching the scope of medical power is.

This brings us to another dimension of the Royal Free controversy, which Craft alluded to but which was avoided by the demonstrators. This is the problem of death and our relationship to it as we undertake pregnancy and birth. For despite the modern presentation of death as a predictable factor, the reality of birth is that there is always the possibility of unexpected and unwanted outcomes, including death. The problem is how that reality affects practices. Obstetrics deals with it through schemes of risk management. For example, Craft was talking about risks to the foetus, risks which he could measure. The question of risk has been a constant reference point for obstetrics whenever there has been a controversy over who should control the birth process, women or medicine. For example, if hospital birth, where doctors are in charge, is compared with home births, which are most commonly attended by midwives, they are usually discussed in terms of the comparability of safety for mother and baby, safety that means a measurable reduction of the risk of handicap and death.[9] But when protagonists of home birth argue against the obstetric establishment, they do so on the grounds that home is 'safer' than hospital, often without recognising that the notion of risk, with its attendant statistical frequencies, is a category that medicine has used to justify its claim that it can diminish the occurrence of adverse outcomes, including death.

That claim that obstetrics can measure and respond to risk factors needs to be carefully examined by women. For despite what obstetrics says about its ability to predict, control and diminish death, outcomes in childbirth can never be guaranteed. Marsden Wagner, one of obstetrics' sharpest critics (himself a medical doctor) points out that the argument around risk, of something going wrong, of death, is a 'bludgeon' used to scare women, even though there is absolutely no uniformity in defining risk. The reason for this lack of uniformity is that the complications of pregnancy and birth have consistently escaped the systems of risk prediction which obstetrics has set up. The tendency has therefore increasingly been to define every aspect of pregnancy and birth in terms of risk in a mistaken attempt to cover all possible eventualities. In this sense, the entire female body has become risk-laden, as the possibilities for something 'going wrong' proliferate. Of course this is an impossible undertaking because obstetrics cannot predict all the possibilities but on the other hand, the thinking behind the risk systems has helped sustain the near total control obstetrics has over birth.[10]

Recognition of the role that risk and death have played in decision-making is only gradually emerging in the work of feminists, often in relation to foetal damage, miscarriage and loss.[11] One of the few people from the childbirth movement to have written about this aspect is the midwife, Ina May Gaskin, who says that birth is always an instance of 'life and death tripping'.[12] Gaskin sees women as properly at the centre of this event, fully capable of dealing with their proximity to the possibility of death whereas obstetrics sees itself as the central actor, acting on the woman's body to prevent death. This suggests that the problem of unexpected outcomes is a crucial element that we need to reflect on to enable us to better articulate our complex relationship as women with obstetric medicine.

Understanding Our Disempowerment

In this book, I want to push still further the critique of obstetric science which has been substantially developed since the 1970s from a number of standpoints: feminism, the childbirth movement, academic sociology, anthropology and history, and women's health care activism.[13] Despite these diverse origins, writers have converged around the convincing thesis that male medical control of childbirth has disempowered women as mothers and as care-givers, principally through its argument that childbirth is full of risks and danger, that it is pathological and thus requires the medical expert to oversee the event. Ann Oakley lays out the consequences in her Transition to Motherhood study: the disempowerment women experience as a result of this medical approach to birth reinforces the widespread perception that we are the victims of our uncontrollable reproductive systems which in turn increases our sense of helplessness.[14] In a masculinist culture, it is exceptionally difficult to escape these effects. It is even more difficult to come to terms with the way in which obstetrics turns this sense of learned helplessness against us, demanding that we take responsibility for our psychological 'well-being' within this perverse organisation of our reproductive care where our bodies are only incidentally our own. Paula Treichler argues that the masculinist bundle of discourses about childbirth, medical, psychological, and economic, is intensifying and exploiting women who are already trapped by confusing representations of the self, multiplying the contradictions around what we are and what we do with childbearing.[15] It is no surprise that contemporary accounts of medicalised birth reinforce that sense of acute fragmentation the women describe in Martin's study, explaining why to feel in pieces is a rational, if self-defeating, response. Meanwhile, the possibilities for further fragmentation abound. One recent example comes from the British Medical Association annual conference in July 1994 where there was a lengthy debate on 'donated ovarian material' and the lower age limit at which young women might be allowed to carry ovary donation cards so that in case of accidental death, their 'creation potential' might be shared by infertile couples. In medical eyes, where the essence of our subjectivity has long been defined as synonymous with our reproductive role, we are not now even the sum of our reproductive parts but merely a source from which they can be 'harvested', the latest vogue phrase to tie the body to nature.[16]

What I propose to do in the succeeding chapters of this book is to analyse our relations with obstetric science by examining how obstetric discourse has constructed its organising principles. What I want to show is how our reproductive bodies have been constructed within it and how this has contributed to the medical practices we must deal with when giving birth. My concern is to identify the building blocks and conceptual tools which were useful in the creation of a science of childbirth; how obstetrics saw itself as a science; and the way that scientific process functions in current obstetric thinking. This requires delving into the conceptual origins of obstetrics and its ways of organising itself so I will be making use of its own texts as primary material.

There is a dual gain in doing this. Firstly, these texts enable readers to see close up the basis on which obstetrics claims that what it says and does is scientific truth. Weedon has put it well when she writes about the problem of truth that 'discourses demonstrate their inevitable conservatism, their investment in particular versions of meaning and their hostility to change'.[17] We need to develop our ability to identify the truth claims of obstetrics for what they are and for what they seek to resist or deny about women. Of course there is a problem of truth claims with all expert discourses but it is a special problem with medicine which has had the capacity to convince us of its absolute distinctiveness from other social practices, a capacity which is linked to the core argument that medicine has the power to deal with death, if not to hold off death entirely.[18] Penetrating what Foucault has described as medicine's solid scientific armature is an especially critical skill for women because the truth claims of obstetrics have such enormous cultural and social power to define our lives. Once we begin to menstruate, we are told by obstetric medicine that we forever teeter on the edge of pathology because of our faulty reproductive system and hence our bodies are subject to continuing medical surveillance, with the emphasis on our potential to malfunction, not on our inherent well-being. The intensity of this surveillance and its scope are now extending even beyond the menopause, with the creation of the post-menopausal woman who continues to require medical treatment because of her reproductive system and its legacy of malfunction. This is the message that is bundled up with the prescription for HRT, as it has formerly been bundled up with those prescriptions for PMT, postnatal depression, nausea and possible miscarriage in pregnancy (these latter two led to the disasters of thalidomide and DES, diethylstilbestrol-linked cancers), to name but a few of the syndromes that obstetric medicine has identified in connection with the female body. Through a detailed examination we can see the ways in which these medical readings of the female body take peculiar twists and have unpredictable effects. This confusion belies the authority with which medical discourse is presented in the consulting rooms, antenatal clinics and delivery wards, where women are confronted with a pathological account of themselves of apparently unimpeachable scientificity which is linked to the concomitant argument that medicine must retain control at all times.[19]

This male discourse (the history of medicine shows how male dominated the science has been) has distanced itself from any reality of our bodies other than its own creations and yet we have absorbed its definitions of how we work. Often we have engaged with obstetric medicine reluctantly, often without thinking, often even wholeheartedly, because we are not skilled in confronting its truth claims or because we are convinced of its 'shroud-waving' and therefore fearful or because we cannot see alternatives.

The second gain that I think can come from dealing with primary texts is a vitally necessary clarity about the way we engage with these medical rationalities in our daily lives. Emily Martin, Ludie Jordanova, and Alexandra Todd have all argued that we should be aware of the extent to which the conceptual framework of the biomedical sciences is shared by doctors and women alike.[20] Unless we can see what the basis is for this shared frame of reference, what it is that we accept from obstetric ideologies about us, we cannot create a politically coherent opposition that is sustainable and we will continue to be fragmented within its field of operations. We need to be absolutely clear about what we want when we engage with obstetric medicine and this will mean our confronting our own fears and ambivalence also. Examining medical discourse at first hand will at least enable us to determine how their ambivalences and fears have become ours.

For women in Ireland, the book has perhaps a special resonance because of the pre-eminent role played by Irish obstetricians since the outset of the new science. Dublin's Rotunda Lying-in Hospital can trace its history back to a charity in George's Lane where, late in the evening of the 15 March 1745, Judith Rochford became the first woman to give birth in a hospital specially designated for lying-in women in Britain and Ireland.[21]

The Lying-in Hospital for Poor Women, so called by its founder, Bartholomew Mosse, moved to a new building in Great Britain Street, equipped with a Royal Charter in 1756 and from there, the Rotunda, as it came to be called, established a reputation throughout Europe and the United States as an outstanding teaching hospital. In the nineteenth century, the Dublin School of Midwifery in obstetric writing was synonymous with the Rotunda. Thus when the head of the Vienna Lying-in Hospital, Professor D.F.H. Arneth, came to visit the Rotunda in the middle of the nineteenth century, he wrote: 'one of the chief attractions of the Dublin School is the great Lying-in Hospital. The Dublin School of Midwifery is properly speaking the only one of importance in Great Britain.'[22]

From the Rotunda's inception in 1745 down to the current promotion of 'active management of labour', a system of hospitalised birth which has been fostered by the National Maternity Hospital and exported world-wide, hundreds of textbooks and thousands of articles have marked out a distinctive Irish contribution to obstetrics, a contribution which has implicated hundreds of thousands of Irish women. We retained a high rate of fertility compared with other western European countries throughout the nineteenth and twentieth centuries, and in that sense our contribution to the science of obstetrics has been vast. When we are reading the clinical records, textbooks and debates, the assertions and contentions of Irish obstetrics, we are reading our own history as Irish women of institutionalised childbirth.[23]

Agency and Death, Then and Now

In her meditation on being a woman poet, Eavan Boland writes of the death of her grandmother. In 1909, pregnant with a sixth child, after five children were born at home in Drogheda, Boland's grandmother travelled to Dublin by train to give birth in the National Maternity Hospital, and died there from puerperal fever or peritonitis, as it was often listed. Boland wonders what her grandmother thought, saw and thought about as she travelled alone to what would be her death. Something unusual, something out of the ordinary had brought her there, Boland writes.[24] For me, the account suggests a decision, a series of reflections about which we know little in women's history. Until the middle of this century, a woman's death in childbirth was frequent enough an occurrence to require some thought each time a woman became pregnant, if not some discussion with her immediate family about what would happen to her children, should this be her fate. Sometimes women in childbirth were acutely aware that they faced the crisis of death and were able to state what they wanted done. Frederick Jebb, who became fourth Master of the Rotunda Hospital, recorded such a case in 1772 when an upper-class woman died as a result of a retained placenta.[25] Women must often have known, hoping that the worst could be avoided. But how they thought about it, how they came to terms with it, remains almost entirely closed to us.

Yet the point I think we should consider is that the greater part of our history as childbearers has involved our dealing directly with death. We have made our decisions about childbirth, if not about getting pregnant, with that factor being one possibility amongst others. Now as it happens, women in the West (at least) no longer need consider their own deaths as a likely consequence of birth. In Ireland, for example, maternal mortality has fallen from hundreds a year at the beginning of this century to fewer than a handful in any one year. In place of maternal death, the possible death of the foetus or newborn baby has now become the most constant determinant of obstetric medicine's actions, although such an outcome is infrequently spoken of in any direct or open way to women. More commonly, it is part of 'shroud-waving'.

However, what has been broken is the explicit link between our thinking through that possibility of death and our ability to make decisions about such outcomes, between agency and death. We can define agency as being the capacity to act, as well as to form a judgement about the meanings of one's action: agency involves reflections, decisions and actions taken together. Londoño has argued that to achieve authenticity as a woman, each of us must do so through the choices, decisions and actions which come from our female self, from our female specificity. This is how agency has become a primary demand in the feminist agenda for reproductive freedom, especially when the issue of abortion has been to the forefront of debate about reproductive freedom. The concept of bodily integrity and bodily self-determination that has been central to the pro-choice movement recognises the biological and social realities of women as reproducers and the incontrovertible fact that women 'are the only persons who can be inhabited by another being, not in the metaphorical sense, but in the real, emotional, biological sense'.[26] This is why we require control of our bodies and this is precisely how we have argued the need for safe abortion on demand. Relatively speaking, feminism has been more successful here than it has been in arguing the need for autonomy and control in childbirth.[27] The demand for control during birth is simply unacceptable to obstetrics.

Both sides, women and medics, in this immensely intricate arena of social relations, draw on complex arguments about the meaning and realities of women as reproducers and about birth as a natural biological event. It might be arguable, and some (notably Edward Shorter) have argued that for feminism to articulate its agendas about agency and control, the scientific advances of obstetrics have been necessary preconditions, securing us from the risk of death by making reproduction safe.[28] In this scenario, our 'natural bodies' have placed us in peril until medicine was able to resolve the threats posed by our bodies which are inherently dysfunctional.

It has not been easy to argue in favour of or against women's dependency on medicine because of the ways medical discourse operates. Even if we have no intention of being placed in the position of unending gratitude to obstetrics that Shorter argues is appropriate, medicine nevertheless confronts us with seemingly irreducible physical categories, of which death is the most definitive, about which it says there can be no debate or equivocation. Fortunately, we have been able to sift through many of these categories, producing hilariously effective deconstructions, like those of Ehrenreich and English, of how medicine has invented our minor ills and supposed feminine weaknesses for us.[29] But when it comes to major issues: continuing or discontinuing the pregnancy with a foetus which has tested positive for severe disability,[30] responding to the problem of repeated miscarriages for a childless woman,[31] dealing with a pregnancy where the rhesus-negative mother has already been isoimmunised,[32] we are co-opted by a medical agenda that tells us we or our babies are at risk but that simultaneously saddles us with its ideologies about the female body. The issue then becomes how we can retain what Anne Finger states is 'our absolute and essential right to have control over our bodies'[33] within a science which says so much about us that is patently not 'true'. There are many traps in this one which demand our thoughtful analysis, not least the problem of restoring judgement to us as a right and a responsibility for each woman.

However, contrary to what male writers like Shorter argue, the demand for autonomy over our bodies is not a recent development. In fact, the argument for women's agency runs parallel to the establishment and growth of obstetric science. The call for autonomy was the basis for the treatise that the English midwife, Elisabeth Nihell, wrote in 1760 in which she attacked the growth of male midwifery (which we now know as the beginning of obstetric science). Entitled *A Treatise on the Art of Midwifery: Setting Forth Various Abuses Therein, Especially as to the Practice of Instruments*, the treatise sets out the problem of women's agency in the management of childbirth, both as mothers and as women midwives. And although specific techniques of birth management have changed, changing also the content of the arguments between women and doctors, the problem of agency remains unresolved close to 250 years after Nihell composed her attack. Consider the following extract where Nihell urges parents to reach their own conclusions on the claims of men midwives to make the passage through labour and birth safe. In a prefatory dedication I find particularly wonderful for its robust quality, she addresses 'all Fathers, Mothers and likely soon to be Either' to compare the claims of men midwives with the needs of pregnant women before reaching a decision about who is competent to help a woman through birth:

> Nature would have such just reproaches to make to you, for cruelty to yourselves, if you was indolently to determine yourselves without either examination or on a blind implicit confidence in others. Happily, then for you, in a matter of such common concernment to human-kind, Nature has not been so unjust nor so unprovident as to place a competent notion of it out of the reach of common sense. Deign then for your own sakes, to examine it by that light of Reason, the spring of which is forever in yourselves. In virtue of such your own fair examination, the decision will no longer be dangerously and precariously that of others for you, no longer be nothing better than a lightly adopted prejudice, but become truly and meritoriously the genuine result of your own judgement.[34]

This is a voice of the Enlightenment, speaking with confident optimism about the capacity of the autonomous subject to construe the truth of the matter for herself. Nihell proclaims the ability of laypeople to understand and interpret what medicine is saying, to make judgements, to exercise agency. Nihell's treatise is one of two texts written by a woman in Britain or Ireland in the eighteenth century on the practice of midwifery and one of the few written by women midwives anywhere in the seventeenth and eighteenth centuries.[35] Just as Nihell published her book, obstetric discourse was reaching a point of critical mass, transferring the main location of its work from private homes to the institution of the lying-in hospital. Nihell had trained at the famous Hôtel-Dieu in Paris, the hospital which began to take in women midwifery pupils in 1631. She returned from Paris to London at a point when men midwives were rapidly expanding their ranks, so much so that Nihell's principal target for attack, William Smellie, claimed to have personally trained 900 pupils in the new science in the space of ten years. Nihell rips apart their rationales and training, their encroachment into an area traditionally dominated by women practitioners. As the title indicates, she specifically attacks the notion that male midwives, aided by the forceps and legally sanctioned to use them as experts, can possibly provide better midwifery than that available from women midwives (who were forbidden by law to carry out instrumental deliveries).

The *Treatise* is in two parts, the second part being a discussion on resolving problems in labour with skilled midwifery. In the first part, Nihell reviews all the claims that men midwives have made about the superiority of their new science, including their knowledge of anatomy, their arguments about greater safety for the mother and child, the necessity of using instruments in labour, and the objections they have expressed to the practice of women as midwives.[36] She also examines the role 'fashion' has played in boosting the popularity of men midwives, a notion she says that first caught on in the upper classes of society and which the lower classes then followed.[37] Nihell declares that the public have been 'duped' by the claims of men midwives that where a man midwife is in attendance with his forceps, birth is far safer than when attended by women midwives. She argues exactly the reverse, that instruments used in childbirth mean greater numbers of women and children dying. Men midwives have argued in favour of their methods by 'forging the phantom of incapacity' in women, in other words, that women midwives are incapable of handling births. Their arguments to the public have been laden with 'scientific jargon' and a

> cloud of hard words ... a cloud which is oftener the cover shape of ignorance than the vehicle of true knowledge, and perhaps oftener yet the mask of mercenary quackery than a proof of medical ability ... .[38]

It is a gripping polemic, all the more delightful for its being written by a professional woman midwife. We might now be rightly wary of the notion of a 'true' knowledge about childbirth that all women possess, that there is a single self-evident essence of truth about the female body. But Nihell uses that position of essentialism, her belief in an intuitive knowledge grounded in women's experiences of birth, to contest the obstetric texts which are claiming very different truths about that same female body.

Of course the most significant aspect of obstetric texts then and now is that these texts have created truths about the female body. Obstetrics legitimated its standing as a science by making 'truth claims' about women in two broad areas. Firstly, it invented the 'poor suffering woman' in labour. Initially, in the seventeenth and early eighteenth centuries, men midwives attended births only in upper-class homes because they argued that upper-class women were physically more delicate and needed expert help to get them through childbirth. Once there was scope to extend the professional reach of men midwives through the establishment of lying-in hospitals, their argument about female feebleness and delicacy spread rapidly down the class ladder. Every pregnant woman became a 'poor' woman who was at the mercy of innumerable dangers, the ultimate one being death.[39]

In addition to the argument about the essential weakness of women's bodies in birth, the second broad truth claim obstetrics employed was its argument about women midwives as ignorant 'Females meddling in science',[40] who were incapable of providing skilled assistance and who contributed to women's deaths through their incompetence and inaction. It was argued that even 'in the most favourable labours poor women endure as much pain as mortals are well able to undergo',[41] so it was vital to have expert male medical assistance at the birth, not women midwives.

This dual theory of female incompetence, the fragile and unreliable body of the poor suffering woman, of which we will be seeing a great deal in the chapters to follow, and the unreliable knowledge of the woman midwife, was used to account for the necessary presence of the male midwife, for why obstetrics was a necessary science. In later chapters, we will discover that the traces of this initial argument have remained a central fixture in obstetric thinking. A young, healthy, well-nourished woman, pregnant for the first time, is still viewed as a potentially unreliable entity, both physically and emotionally.

It is much less easy to account for women's reliance on and relationship to obstetric medicine. The nature of this reliance has changed over time and has grown stronger as women in the West have been drawn into obstetric categories and ways of thinking. This appears to be an inescapable process, as inescapable as modernity itself. Its totality comes across in a newspaper interview given in Dublin in 1988, just after a High Court case in which a judgment against the National Maternity Hospital resulted in an award for one million pounds in compensation to the parents of William Dunne, who had been born a quadraplegic.[42]

The heart of the plaintiffs' case was that the hospital and the private obstetrician, who was not in the hospital during the whole of Mrs Dunne's labour, had been negligent in the management of her labour, resulting in a tragic outcome. When Catherine Dunne, the child's mother, was asked by the press what she would do differently if she had to live over again the day she went into labour with William, she replied that she would have wanted her obstetrician by her side because she believed he would have listened to her:

> I'd look for Dr Jackson the minute I went in and get him to check the babies. I wouldn't send messages second or third hand; if I couldn't get up to walk to the phone, I'd have a phone brought to the bed. I'd also ask that no-one should take a woman in labour lightly: to humour her if that's all it takes for just a few minutes and if it turns out to be mistaken, then there's no harm done. They should listen to a mother.[43]

The distance between Catherine Dunne's abject belief in obstetrics, and the energy of Nihell's assertions about women reaching their own decisions about their care in labour, warrants serious consideration as a marker for this problem of agency. Dunne's reactions are based on an acceptance that a reasoned judgement cannot be hers, that she must rely on what is scientific to prove what is happening in her body. Nihell's confidence at the beginning of scientific childbirth management illuminates an entirely different mental frame, where the woman still has scope to exercise her own judgement about scientific claims. That capacity is the basis for Nihell's argument that the operation of reason will triumph. Of course Nihell cannot see the hubris and confusion that will emerge from this Enlightenment position for, ultimately, Reason does not triumph, not least because there are many forms of rationalities, not just one. But the ground stretching away between these two women has to do with what Foucault would term the constitution of the subject, how the individual comes into being under certain historical conditions; in this instance, how the individual comes to be the subject of obstetric discourse, and the price that is paid for that. Catherine Dunne's comments indicate that she has a definition of herself as a woman and as a pregnant subject, who welcomes the necessity of her doctor's presence, although she eventually must go to court to force that doctor to account for his actions. In spite of this, she accepts the logic of obstetrics, which although it may be one of several or even many ways of construing pregnancy and birth, of reading the female body as a reproductive entity, it is by far the most powerful in Western society.

I hope to show how that process of constituting the pregnant woman as a special subject has been made possible by obstetric science and at what price.[44]

Constructing What Appears 'Normal and Natural'

As feminist theory has developed over the last twenty-five years, one of the most frequent points of discussion has been the issue of how patriarchal structures have silenced women. Dorothy Smith argues that male writing and speech have been the basis for constructing the authority of modern social structures and institutions, which we have learned to take for granted because they are so integral to the way we live. But women have not taken part in building that authority. Although women have been at work in the making of modern bourgeois society in the arenas of family, childbearing and caring, the latter often turned into a subordinated semi-professional task, the arena from which we have been consistently excluded is the one where authority is shaped, the arena which produces the mainstream forms of knowledge, culture and ideology. Smith refers to this as a 'peculiar eclipsing' of women.[45]

I encountered that 'peculiar eclipsing' when I first began to examine the growth of modern forms of childbirth management, and I wrote about my frustrations in trying to get through what seemed to be a vast silence from women themselves about these new forms. There were thousands of pages of clinical records from lying-in hospitals but few published firsthand accounts of hospitalised childbirth from women themselves (and very few outside hospital) up to the emergence of the childbirth movement in the 1960s. I could not make sense of that silence until I realised how it was mediated, until I was able to identify that the history of childbirth in modern society begins with the obstetrician and his texts, not with our experiences.[46] Another way to state this is that our experiences are constructed by obstetrics and both their theories and practices. Therefore reading their texts tells us why our experiences are what they are for us. When we give birth with our legs cantilevered upwards and held in place by stirrups, our experience of birth necessarily includes a practice which is imposed on us by obstetric science and the way it theorises about our bodies in birth, whether we assent to its theories or not. To give birth under these constraints changes the way we think of ourselves and our bodies. Even though we have no purchase on either the theory or the practice, the obstetric viewpoint becomes part of our experience. And the real dilemma for us is how that process is made to appear ordinary and normal. The weight of our disturbing and uncomfortable personal experiences within this dominant male institution pulls at us to challenge that appearance of normality but we are very often left without effective tools to do so.

This brings me back to Smith's comment about the dominance of male forms of thought in the production of our social institutions. She pinpoints a critical feminist endeavour; the analysis of male texts has been the point of departure for many feminists in the task of elucidating how our everyday world has been mediated for us and this has helped us to begin to account for the problem of our silence, our 'eclipsing' in Smith's words. The strategy to achieve our silence is composed of several distinct parts, both exclusion from speaking altogether (or a refusal to hear us), and a way of speaking which is only considered legitimate if it uses male terms of reference. This is how women's voices are shaped by dominant discourses. Deborah Cameron comments that the way language is regulated, using what might be termed discursive practices, is integral to the success with which male-dominant institutions exclude us or include us by speaking exclusively in their own terms which is, of course, a male language.[47]

Nothing is more masculinist in our culture than science and scientific language is rife with metaphors of conquest, domination and subjection. At the same time, that language of conquest can be made to sound like a rigorous language of discovery that reveals previously unknown facts, which is seen as an honourable achievement, the apogee of human endeavour, a natural form of progress.[48] Obstetrics is a scientific discourse which speaks exactly like this, a dominant discourse which argues that it is making steady scientific progress, steadily revealing more of the 'natural facts' about the female body in pregnancy and birth. But the facts it presents in its discourses are not so much discovered as produced.

Obstetrics is a medical specialism and, even though it has an exclusive focus on the female body, it has strategies of knowledge production and organisation similar to other branches of medical science. Similar to the rest of Western biomedicine, obstetrics presents specific social realities as a 'natural given', bundling them into what is then presented as a scientifically proven basis for its practices.[49] The way in which observations on the restricted physical way of life led by many upper-class women were used as the basis for the natural fact about the feebleness of the female body in childbirth is a case in point.

Obstetric science has most often spoken of the female body as a unitary essence or a natural domain. Thus in the model where the natural world is explored or discovered, there is a set of facts waiting to be retrieved which is the *raison d'être* of that natural domain. And, somehow, women and their bodies are always closer to the natural world than the rationalist male body. This problem of our association with the natural domain and with 'natural facts' which are distinctively gendered has been the focus of Ludie Jordanova's work.[50] Her discussion of the work *Systeme physique et moral de la femme* written in 1777 by the French physiologist, Pierre Roussel, provides an interesting example of the production of a 'natural fact'. When speaking of a woman's 'soft parts' (the phrase obstetrics used for a long time to describe women's reproductive organs) Roussel states that their 'functions' are bound up with 'the passive state to which nature has destined her'. For Jordanova, this is representative of how the biomedical sciences set about articulating a system of beliefs about women. Our problem is that these beliefs are presented as 'facts' and, as Jordanova argues, the themes, metaphors and images we encounter in biomedical writing like Roussel's, about women's physiology, have enormous cultural force. In a similar vein, Barbara Duden argues that the body that has been constructed by the sciences of anatomy and physiology has also been imbued by these sciences with the appearance of being a natural phenomenon. Yet at the same time, the social process whereby this natural body was created has been made invisible, while concepts about it have become part of our world view.[51]

The eighteenth-century identification of women with the natural realm had specific meanings within obstetric science, and produced specific tensions. It created a natural maternal body, but birth as an unmediated natural event was fraught with danger. If women were passive, as Roussel and others contended, their bodies were also feeble and weak. So, in line with the Enlightenment scientific project to reason about nature and to act on it, there was a drive to rescue women from a natural world which was capricious and dangerous and which they were incapable of withstanding on their own. This is one of the enduring metaphors of obstetrics which itself is the essence of a male science, bent on penetration and conquering.

With the exception of Elisabeth Nihell's work, all the older midwifery and obstetric texts that I will be referring to are written by men. Most of them are Irish, reflecting the prominence of Irish obstetric practitioners in establishing the theory and practice of obstetric medicine in the last two centuries and, incidentally, raising the issue of how Irish women's bodies were colonised twice over. The manufacture of facts that appear natural and unquestioned emerges in three significant areas of discussion in obstetric texts: in relation to the body, to death and to power. All are presented in a self-evident manner that we must de-centre, if we are to understand better the process of theory construction.

Manufacturing the Natural Female Body

The problems that surround the body, especially the female body, have received enormous attention within recent Western feminism, where the body has been targeted as a concrete site for political action. The title of the book that is arguably the vade-mecum of the women's movement in the West, *Our Bodies, Ourselves*, captures perfectly this political thrust and, from its first edition in 1971, the Boston Women's Health Collective, the original editors, urged us to assume greater control over all aspects of our bodily being in society, including pregnancy and birth. Yet despite its intentions, there is often a political *naïveté* in *Our Bodies, Ourselves*, an acceptance that medical information about our bodies can exist as transparent facts. The introduction to the first edition spoke of how the women in the collective realised 'more and more that we were really capable of collecting, understanding and evaluating medical information',[52] as if facts about the female body were objective and incontrovertible and therefore unproblematic, as if medical information itself did not represent and incorporate ideologies about women, about our role within the social scheme of things which considerably circumscribed us.

Of course the 'facts' are extremely problematic, not least because of medicine's belief that visibility itself can reveal the 'facts'. The move to achieve total visibility, which dramatically shifts the parameters of medical thinking, is what Foucault describes in *Birth of the Clinic*. The opening passage is from an eighteenth-century medical text by the French physician Pomme, on his theories and descriptions of the treatment for (female) hysteria, which becomes a 'language of fantasy' for doctors by the beginning of the nineteenth century.[53] Pomme's mode of reasoning about nervous pathology loses meaning because a different mode of seeing comes into play for clinical medicine at the end of the eighteenth century, which shifts the medical claim to authority on the concrete nature of its knowledge. This knowledge is above all a 'seen' knowledge, acquired by 'opening up a few corpses' so that to go beneath the surface, where the individual body slides into illness and pathology, enables the doctor to grasp the essence of that pathology and hence the essence of death.

It will be no surprise then that in dealing with obstetrics, this principle of visibility, whereby facts can be ordered and verified about the body, can be found in constant operation, whether we read a late eighteenth-century text on puerperal fever, a mid-nineteenth-century text on rates of maternal mortality or a current article on the management of the third stage of labour. What is most striking is that medicine assumes the authority to speak, based on its empiricism and positivism. Even though at some level, medicine itself is well aware of its internal fissures and its errors and disagreements, it wants us to hear only the authoritative whole. What then appears as a 'universal truth of the body'[54] or a 'vision' of the body[55] is as difficult to question for disciplines as it is for individuals. Thus, for instance, David Armstrong argues that the assumptions which underwrite the sciences of human biology, physiology and anatomy held an unquestioning sway over sociology for a very long time.[56]

However, coming from the politics of the women's movement, feminism has gradually carved out an alternative remit about medicine, and critical feminist analysis has been working to dismantle many of the claimed scientific certainties as they pertain to women. I have already alluded to the problem of understanding how the female body became naturalised in medical discourse, as exemplified by the work of Jordanova. Michèle le Doeuff,[57] like Jordanova, also examines Roussel's work but le Doeuff uses it as an example of a scientific metaphor about the female body which arises from what she terms the 'lettered imagination' of medical science. When this imagination presents its theoretical inventions, it simultaneously establishes a principle of competence because of its assumed authority to speak, in addition to its authority to think what it wishes. Both effects come from what she calls the 'terrain of doctorality' and result in an extraordinary sort of freedom to do what it will. For example, in the *Systeme physique et moral de la femme*, Roussel denies that a woman has any sexual attributes around her pubes but declares that everywhere else in her body is marked by the signs of her female sex, including her brain. He also concludes that menstruation is a sickness which can be eliminated with proper diet. When he argues in this manner, he exercises these joint principles of imagination and competence. He produces a version of the female body in line with his imagination which has, literally, doctoral authority so that even when medicine later comes along to disprove these 'wild imaginings', replacing them with another set of truths, the important thing is that medicine has learned to create the female body it requires. Just as with the work of Pomme, Roussel's notion is abandoned but the authority to pronounce is retained.

Science does not see its work as metaphorical but we, as women, must deal with the effects of their metaphors. Le Doeuff points to how a gendered anatomy comes into being, an argument that Londa Schiebinger takes up in relation to anatomical drawings of women in the eighteenth and early nineteenth centuries.[58] Although anatomists had been drawing human skeletons based on dissection and observation from the sixteenth century, it was during the eighteenth century that the first drawings of a distinctively female skeleton were published, in what Schiebinger relates as an intensifying search for sex differences in every part of the human physical make-up. Whatever about the individual idiosyncrasies of the anatomists, the general rule of law they put forward was that women's bodies were lacking when compared with the male body, the normal standard by which all else was measured. Women's smaller bones were equated with weakness, with having less muscle to support, less work to do, even with breathing less vigorously. This search for physical differences between men and women, Schiebinger argues, lent itself to the delimitation of women's role and position as modern bourgeois society took shape, not least because they could be used to account for social inequalities based on sex. These were transmuted into natural inequalities, based on natural differences. Women had less natural reason and therefore it followed that they required fewer rights in the social and political spheres than men.[59]

Roussel's interpretation of the anatomists' findings was an influential insertion into the debate about sex difference: he argued that the moral capacities of men and women could not be separated from their physical organisation, leaving women less capable of exercising morality because of their diminished physical capacities when compared with men. This claim was echoed in the work of Enlightenment philosophers like Rousseau and Voltaire and also found a fertile home in the nineteenth century in the work of the sociologist Auguste Comte, who argued that women's social role was determined by their biology. Schiebinger argues that because this developing thesis was generated from within science where there were almost no women as practitioners in any case, it had ample grounds as it gathered credibility to continue to produce both its gendered analyses and the reasons as to why women were naturally excluded from working in the discipline that was busy defining them.

So while the human sciences of anatomy and physiology held sway, their gendered accounts doubled back on women to further strengthen the initial assertions, with consequences for women in childbirth also. A good example can be drawn from the changes in birth positions. Women regularly used any number of diverse positions when giving birth prior to male midwifery, especially prior to its hospitalised variant. Jacques Gélis, in his archival work on modes of childbirth in pre-modern Europe,[60] has examined historical evidence on birth positions and concludes that women usually chose positions which could leave the body unconstrained for a job of work that actually requires great strength, despite scientific claims to the contrary. Indeed the uterus in labour is the strongest muscle in the body (male or female) and in order to speed its work, Gélis documents women's use straight across Europe of vertical positions in labour or positions where the body is on a vertical axis, such as standing, kneeling, all fours or squatting. These positions appeared to supply a freedom of movement and what Gélis terms 'maximum play' to the body to enable the baby to descend through the birth canal most efficiently.[61]

However, towards the end of the seventeenth century, the French man midwife, Mauriceau, advised that women be delivered in their beds in a supine position because it would enable them to conserve their strength to deal with the pain of labour.[62] It is true that initially not all men midwives approved of this shift. Henrik Deventer, the Dutch man midwife, writing at the beginning of the eighteenth century, not only recommended the birthing stool, which would permit women a vertical axis, but in instances where women were 'ill-shaped', 'round Shouldered', 'crooked' or 'asthmatick', he advised 'let them walk or stand, being held up by some Body, that the Infant is brought forward for Birth'.[63] But by the end of eighteenth century, men midwives, now reinforced in their views about women's physical weakness, found no place in their practices for this diversity; they directed women to assume a supine position, whether attending them at home or in a lying-in hospital.

And they found new and better reasons to support a change in practice. In Ireland, according to Fielding Ould, the Dublin man midwife who became second Master of the Rotunda Hospital, women still gave birth at home in the eighteenth century in various postures: 'on their Back, Side, Knees, standing, and sitting on a perforated Stool'. But Ould preferred to have women lie on their side for the actual moment of birth, not least because 'as the Operator and Standers by, are by this Means behind her Back, she is less subject to be disturbed by their Remarks and Whispers'.[64] This left lateral position became the favoured position for birth adopted in the Rotunda. One serious consequence of this change was that in instances of difficult presenting foetal positions, where women might have once made use of kneeling on all fours to aid labour, especially when there were instances of difficult foetal presentations, men midwives now dismissed this out of hand on the grounds of its being too animal-like and 'repellent to humanity'.[65] In place of a simple expedient like a change of posture or movement, a technique which the woman could accomplish for herself, men midwives offered obstetric expertise of exactly the sort that enraged Elisabeth Nihell, for it denied women their own physical capabilities and replaced them by alien and dangerous technologies.

Problematising Natural Childbirth

The 'terrain of doctorality', to use le Doeuff's phrase, has steadily changed how the pregnant female body is conceptualised, building on the concept of the natural gendered body which became such a vivid metaphor in the eighteenth century. If we are to think through the meanings of the female body, we must deal with the bundle of scientific accretions which have manufactured the body we recognise as female. This has already proved a difficult undertaking within the childbirth movement. The temptation to claim that there is a natural female body which is outside male culture, a body that can celebrate womanliness and the virtues of womanhood, that celebrates childbirth as the most essential attribute of being a woman, has provided a continuing focal point for many writers on childbirth.

Feminists who are committed to the notion of the natural female body have split on the issue of whether this body can be rescued from male patriarchy by privileging reproduction, especially the act of giving birth, or whether the reproducing body must be jettisoned, on the grounds that patriarchy can be defeated only when we are free of the biological burden of childbearing.[66] Women who believe in the former course of action have pursued what I have called the 'naturalist thesis' of childbirth. As the childbirth movement became organised and grew in numbers from the late 1950s, this naturalist thesis had great rhetorical power because it appeared to offer a genuine alternative to medicalised childbirth. The upward curve of protest about institutionalised childbirth which rejected such practices as the separation of mothers and babies after birth, rigid feeding schedules that limited the opportunity to breastfeed and excluding fathers from the birth itself, relied on an argument about the naturalness of birth.[67] It used an account of the female body as an instinctive entity which was somehow outside all cultural constraints and would therefore undergo a birth in an entirely 'unquestioning, unselfconscious, and uncomplicated' manner.[68] In this reading, women in traditional societies would know automatically how to give birth whereas women who had been subjected to medicalised birth needed to reclaim their instincts on birth which they had lost.

There was almost an element of make-believe in how traditional societies were used in this argument and yet the assertion that birth was a 'natural' process seemed the only sensible tactic to employ against an interventionist technology-driven obstetric practice. However, this argument actually created as many difficulties as it sought to resolve. One obvious problem was that women were drawing on the same natural body that medicine had invented and which was so often used to our detriment.[69] There was also the related and highly problematic notion of the female body being altogether outside culture. Lois McNay, amongst others, has asked how in logic we can try to argue that the female body is some pre-discursive pre-cultural pre-social essence, fixed for all time, and has urged us to consider if this form of essentialism should ever be invoked by feminism.[70] An unchanging female essence, after all, does not well equip us with the resilience we require individually and politically to deal with the constantly shifting mutations of our (patriarchal) social order. In the United States, for example, natural childbirth is in danger of becoming an expression of the extreme privatisation of health care, not confronting the social power of medicine nor attempting to change it for women in general. Moreover, the woman in this situation has often taken on a totally circumscribed feminine role within the domestic sphere, while her male partner has taken up the patriarchal role otherwise held by the male doctor, directing the labour and 'catching' the baby.[71]

The crudely idealised division between natural and medicalised childbirth does not hold up under scrutiny in any case, because there is a multitude of different meanings for different actors. 'Natural' can range from the birth at home – least subject to 'high-tech' machines and therefore most 'natural' in the eyes of its advocates – to the 'spontaneous' birth in hospital. The latter is recorded in hospital statistics as such even though the woman may have had her labour accelerated with hormonal infusions (and may well have requested an epidural anaesthesia to deal with her more acute labour pain) and may even have been given an episiotomy. So long as she did not give birth to her baby with the aid of forceps or ventouse and was not given a Caesarean section, and the actual moment of expulsion of the baby was unaided, from an obstetric perspective, the actual birth of the baby was 'normal'.[72]

These differences illustrate what Chris Shilling has described as 'the enormous utility of the body as a highly malleable ideological resource'.[73] And yet the naturalist thesis has made very little impact on women's considerations about how and where to give birth. The cumulative inputs of the childbirth movement, the home birth movement, the consumer movement and the feminist critiques of childbirth, which have all been influenced at some level by the notion of natural birth, have failed to dislodge the vast majority of women from going to hospital, the setting where the overall package of practices in labour and birth is still not in the hands of women. Political activism has whittled away at many aspects of institutionalised birth so that women may in certain circumstances be able to make some decisions, as with pain relief, birth position, or in Britain, birthing pools. But the balance of discretion still lies with the medical profession in the most liberal of hospital regimes, while in those institutes more rigidly encased in the medical model, choice in childbirth becomes a very relative term. Birth outside hospital is taken on by a very tiny minority. Of the 50,874 births in the Republic of Ireland in 1992, 215 or four-tenths of 1 per cent were born outside hospitals.[74] The figures for England and Wales, Denmark, Finland, France and Germany hover around 1 per cent. Only The Netherlands retains a significant number of midwife-assisted home births, 35 per cent of the childbearing population, although those births are contained within a system where a medical risk-scoring model determines eligibility for home birth.[75]

Neither of these settings, hospital or home, is free from legal constraints and quasi-legal constraints about who can be in attendance at the point of labour and birth. For example, in a labour ward which is extremely short-staffed, it is unthinkable for a staff midwife to ask a woman's partner or friend to step into the gap to help a woman if she suddenly begins to deliver; on paper at least, a woman must have a student midwife assigned to cover her in labour, the midwife herself being under supervision, regardless of whether the midwife can actually provide quality support to perhaps three women simultaneously. And as mentioned before, anyone without a trained medical or nursing background who attends a woman intentionally giving birth at home is liable for prosecution in Ireland and England, while in Canada and a number of states in the United States, midwives carrying out a home birth are engaged in an illegal act.[76]

However, I am not arguing that there is a repressive operation of power over the female body in labour, as we might commonly understand repression when we speak of a total denial of civil liberties, or policies of internment without trial. In relation to birth, whether women opt for home or hospital, doubts and anxieties about the potential for loss of life are an extremely powerful lever in how free or unfree, how 'natural', how open to choice the birth process can be permitted to become by all participants. Put simply, there is a problem of how we are influenced by the issues of risk and possible death.

There are other important dimensions also, including what Shorter terms 'the rise of the birth experience' which, he argues, has come about because obstetric science has rescued women from mortality in birth which, in turn, has allowed women to achieve greater intimacy and feeling in birth with their partners.[77] It is true that Western women are no longer dying in birth, and that both fertility rates and perinatal mortality rates have fallen drastically since the middle of this century. On close examination, we will see that obstetric science is unable to take the credit for these dramatic falls to the extent it has claimed. However, it is also true that many women have come to see the experience of childbirth as a critical moment where we can explicitly seek out an expression of ourselves as women and mothers and, in this way, it has become a significant arena for personal affirmation. This development can be seen to line up with what has been identified as an intensifying relationship with our selves, with 'self', arising from greater control over the body in sickness and greater possibilities of achieving and retaining bodily health.[78]

What I think we must acknowledge is that there are points of convergence and recognition between what obstetric medicine sees itself as doing and what we, as childbearing women, say we want. This is not a matter of collusion between women and obstetrics or of our unending gratitude to obstetrics. It is a problem of our relationship with scientific knowledge, in terms of how definitions of our bodies and physiologies and therefore our very selves, are achieved. There are in fact two fundamental issues: a problem with science and a problem with the self, with our subjectivity.

Pain relief during labour provides an instructive example. The use of epidural anaesthesia during labour is climbing steadily in Ireland. Patricia Kennedy, in her exploration of current maternity policies, records that the epidural rate for all women giving birth in the National Maternity Hospital rose to 36.4 per cent by 1993 (up from 4.4 per cent in 1986), while the 1993 figures for the Coombe Women's Hospital and the Rotunda stood at 43 per cent and 56 per cent respectively.[79] The technology itself has become quite effective, more effective than a narcotic analgesia in the first stage of labour, and that is its reputation amongst the general public, seemingly fuelling the demand by women to have this kind of pain relief. However, epidural use also has a tendency to prolong the first stage of labour and, as a result, for oxytocin to be used more frequently to deal with the effects of a longer first stage. If the epidural is maintained into the second stage of labour, which period some women at least experience as extremely painful, it may result in a longer second stage, predisposing to malrotation of the presenting part, and a substantially increased use of forceps to effect delivery. Thus use of the epidural in pain relief can cut across a fundamental norm in obstetrics, how long second-stage labour should be allowed to continue before failure to progress is diagnosed and an instrumental delivery is carried out. There is also recent data to suggest an increase in the number of Caesarean sections when epidural anaesthetic is used, once more because of what is seen as failure of the labour to progress. The middle- and long-term consequences, ranging from inadvertent dural puncture to significantly raised rates of morbidity from Caesarean section, can be substantive.[80] In other words, the reality of epidural anaesthesia is a mixed bag. Doctors argue that it is 'safe', meaning that they can control for these consequences through instrumental and operative deliveries (discounting the after-effects of these interventions for women); they also argue that they are responding to pressure from women to provide the epidural, implying that women cannot withstand the pain of labour.

Of course, the increasing demand for epidurals means that women are individually reconstituting meanings about pain in childbirth. But our decision-making cannot be separated from the medical context in which we give birth, where we are already subject to an organisation of our labours, into which the epidural slots perfectly. For just as women are demanding more epidurals in labour, the percentage of labours augmented by oxytocin is also increasing (increasing the demand for epidurals in an ever more circular movement); the percentage of women who are able to go through the whole of their labour in hospital, moving their bodies as they wish to help secure pain relief, is very small; so also is the number of women who go through second-stage labour and the moment of birth in a fully vertical position of their choice. These are not possibilities which appeal to obstetrics because they upset the tight organisation of the maternity hospital.[81] A key element in this organisation is keeping up the throughput of women and, whatever the rhetoric may be about individual choice, the bottom line is to ensure that the individual woman does not upset the system with her own demands or reactions to handling labour. The system is armoured against anyone whom it can define as a threat to its mode of organisation[82] and a liberal use of total pain relief must be seen in that context. Under such circumstances, it is immensely useful to the obstetric system to draw on variants of its own historically grounded argument about the natural unreliability of the female body in labour, which has been deftly extended to include the uncertainties of the female psyche, and which requires the additional assistance of pain relief. It is a fruitful ideology precisely because of its adaptability to new theories about possible sources of pathology and disruption.

While obstetrics always agreed on the natural female body, it was split over the naturalness of pain. In Mary Poovey's account of the controversy in the mid-nineteenth century about the use of chloroform to release women from suffering in birth, some medics sided with Simpson, who first promoted its use and who argued that childbirth entailed unendurable pain, which was 'unnatural' to permit if there was a medical alternative; others, like the obstetrician, Meigs, rejected this intervention, arguing that childbirth was a 'natural' process with 'no element of disease' and who therefore saw pain as a concomitant of this natural process, one which the woman was best qualified to judge. According to Meigs, 'to be in natural labour is the culminating point of the female somatic forces'.[83] It was still an essentialist naturalist argument but, in this instance, one which at least admitted some physical capacity on the part of women when giving birth. Meigs' reasoning can be said to have surfaced much later in the writings of Grantly Dick-Read in the 1940s on the naturalness of giving birth and the need to reinforce women's confidence, thereby reducing pain arising from the 'natural protective tensions of the body'.[84] However, Simpson's line of argument became dominant in the organisation of maternity hospitals. Thus when a woman makes a decision in contemporary settings to opt for an epidural in order to avoid pain in labour, no matter what the price, she reinforces that perspective of women that we cannot withstand pain.

One helpful way to view this conundrum is to look at the links between technologies of knowledge/power and technologies of self which Foucault has discussed. In his exploration of how we constitute self for ourselves, he argues that we can view the sciences as producing 'truth games', by which he means knowledges which seem self-evident, once they are created, knowledges like the 'natural body'. But these 'truth games' are in turn 'related to specific techniques which humans use to make sense of themselves'. These technologies of self do not function separately but entail individual training and modification 'not only in the obvious sense of acquiring certain skills but also in the sense of acquiring certain attitudes'.[85] In this way we can see that not only are our bodies inherently not the 'naturally' weak bodies of medical discourse but that we learn how to take on the attributes which enable medical organisation to think of us this way. We transform ourselves into those weaker bodies when we have to engage with medicalised childbirth which is concretely organised to produce these effects.

Elaine Scarry, in her sensitive appraisal of the politics of the body in pain, has written that the 'referential instability of the body ... allows it to confer its reality on whatever outcome occurred'.[86] This instability or malleability is especially marked in the medical knowledges that stream round the female body, in that new realities or truth claims about it are constantly being created. The female body in labour is not a natural entity (as medicine would have us believe) which has been inserted into medical schematisations but, like any body, is already profoundly embedded in a social and political system.[87] Therefore, in relation to childbirth, we do not need to learn what the body 'is' (because we cannot), so much as we need to discover how malleable our definitions and perceptions of the body are, in relation to how we interpret its actions (given the way power and knowledge operate, given the intent of obstetric technologies).

Current pain-relief methods pose a dilemma for obstetrics because they entail sequelae to which it must respond with further techniques that, in its terms, also up the odds of something going awry. An even greater dilemma about pain relief faces counter-formulations of the obstetric model. Opponents of medicalised childbirth argue that because there is 'no element of disease' in childbirth, pain can be interpreted as hard work for which a woman is perfectly able, as long as she has emotional support and encouragement in labour. Then she can retain control of her birth process. But, as it happens, the figures on epidural use in Dublin, which are quoted above, come from the National Maternity Hospital which has argued that they ensure an attendant to support each woman throughout her entire labour. Their system is failing for a cluster of reasons to which I will return, but the rising number of epidurals is presented, disingenuously, as women's choice, not as the system's failure. If there is also a rising incidence of instrumental and operative deliveries, this too becomes attributed to women's decision-making in favour of the epidural. Whatever about that claim, it is true that these epidural-driven experiences of pain-free but complicated deliveries, which often have immediate and long-term complicated consequences, become part of how women think of themselves.[88] If women are rejecting the construction of labour pain as hard work, then childbirth activists have as yet failed to communicate successfully how the demand for epidurals is part of a larger pattern of contradictory effects and outcomes. The latter point to a continuing reconstructing of the body within the hospital setting with its tremendous range of technical possibilities, where it suits the medical system to re-emphasise female fragility and unreliability, either physically or emotionally.

For me, pain relief is but one area which indicates that feminists and childbirth activists who challenge the agendas of obstetric medicine share a common necessity with women seeking epidural pain relief: to examine how obstetric knowledge and power work and why women accept what this system does to our bodies. It is difficult to see the obstetric system in its totality, but yet the system does have points where we can achieve effective resistance. Drawing together the full picture on pain relief illustrates what Scarry refers to as the

> ease with which power can be mixed with almost any other subject ... in strategies and theories that – whether compellingly legitimate or transparently absurd – increase the claim of power, its representation in the world.[89]

We can see how obstetrics invests in pain relief as part of its operations, while it seemingly attributes to women the decision about its unlimited use.

Nonetheless, despite the weight of obstetric power, which has produced some truly disturbing absurdities and which, in turn, women have accepted as truths, I am not arguing that its operations are for the dominating and against the dominated. Within their own system, they too are affected by a process of self-formation in line with their technologies: 'People know what they do; they frequently know why they do what they do; but what they don't know is what they do does.'[90]

An understanding of obstetric rationality should help indicate how this process works at concrete levels because there may be political potential here in shifting doctors and the midwives who work under their remit in the obstetric system; this can add to the potential being developed by birth educators, activists and research midwives already working to make sense of birth in a different way (I want to discuss this potential in the concluding chapter). However, a prime obstacle is the difficulty of contesting the scientific approach, for it is a deeply privileged one, deeply embedded in our culture. Therefore to stand outside that rational order may be a virtual impossibility. On the other hand, we must try to identify the sites where we can work to develop alternative definitions.

The Problem of Death

Lois McNay argues that we must understand how female bodies have been worked on historically and that what we should be developing is not a theory of the body, but a theory of discursive formations which catch and keep that body.[91] Reading obstetric discourse, we can read how the pregnant bodies of Irish women have been kept, bodies which are often weakened as a result of the diseases of poverty, and are then made weaker by the incursions of obstetric medicine; bodies which still recover strongly; women who go on to bear more children, clean wards, sell milk on the street corners or move away with their soldier husbands. Incidental details such as these occasionally enter into the clinical records kept by men midwives throughout the eighteenth and nineteenth centuries and even into the middle of the twentieth century (thereafter such comments are a rarity, perhaps because the focus is no longer exclusively on us because we very seldom die in childbirth and are seldom very seriously ill as a result of giving birth or perhaps because our ways of life appear predictable and more uniform).

Reading these texts, however, entails the much more daunting task of reading about their deaths. Because obstetrics is part of clinical medicine, it derives immense value from these deaths, of which it writes extensively in its first two centuries of institutionalised care. By the latter half of the eighteenth century, the rationales of clinical medicine and especially the work of dissection begin to convert death into a positive utility. Death becomes part of a trinity alongside life and disease but of those three, 'death is the great analyst that shows the connections by unfolding them and bursts open the wonders of genesis in the rigour of decomposition.'[92] This is Foucault in dramatic vein on the clinic, but the image captures both the excitement and the cool probity of the scientist (or so science would like to portray itself) whose domain of observation becomes limitless with pathological anatomy. Disease may not be curable (although that ambition is always there), but death can make it visible and therefore explicable. For the practitioner, disease becomes more graspable as clinical dissection becomes part of the teaching of medicine. In Ireland, early nineteenth-century practitioners like Robert Graves write about clinical dissection as the 'true way to study pathology'[93] so that pathology and medical progress go hand in hand.

But, as with the scientific project in general, the problem with death in childbirth is its radical and gendered split. Women become pregnant and give birth. If they die, men dissect their bodies to find out what death means. Thus with each pregnancy, women confront the boundaries of their existence while those who die in birth endlessly extend the boundaries of obstetric science, because their bodies yield the basis for the theory that is used to defeat the threat of death. Or so the science claims. How then are women making sense of death in birth?

In general, the way we think about death has been shifting across two centuries, as patterns of modernity have taken hold. The intensification of self that has been integral to the development of modern society, which now appears to affect our weighting of the experience of birth, has also posed new and special problems around death, itself characterised by its increasingly private and individual nature, amounting almost to a scandal about which one must remain silent.[94] This is another issue that many sociologists were slow to consider, outside the study of religion. Perhaps this reluctance is linked to what Chris Shilling sees as an inescapable reality which has become especially disturbing to modern people, because our self-identity is now so centred on the body.[95] Zygmunt Bauman, who has written extensively about modernity, self and death, argues that the elaborate, even obsessive, regimes of self-care, which have become so integral to our lives, function largely to defend the self against the ultimate limitation of death. Increasing our knowledge of our constituent parts and all that can malfunction is part of the way we avoid death itself, for if we know, then in theory, death can be prevented.[96]

However, once more there is a radical gendered split here for women as childbearers who occupy a paradoxical position, not least because the strategies to increase knowledge of our pregnant bodies that have legitimacy are not in our hands. Our individual regimes of self-care may reflect our belief that pregnancy and childbirth are not illnesses but are rather a common life experience with highly individual nuances, sensations and feelings, both physical and emotional. But our multiple variable concrete knowledges about ourselves and our modes of self-care are irrelevant to obstetrics and are dismissed out of hand. Our criteria about what is meaningful in pregnancy and birth are worlds apart from the performance-driven criteria of the obstetrician.[97] Hence the regimes of self-care we are asked to pursue during pregnancy relate principally to the self-care of the science rather than those of the woman, with whom it rarely chooses to discuss death openly. Inevitably, these regimes are premised on our inherent pathological potential.

The anxiety not to discuss death with us is not because death is not on their collective minds, far from it. There is a constant pressing need to present schedules of figures with ever-lower rates of mortality as proof of success of the various obstetric models of birth management. In this sense, the maternal and perinatal statistics which form the core of annual clinical reports from the maternity hospitals might be considered as a version of death-defiance or 'immortality strategies',[98] on the part of obstetrics. Bauman reminds us that such strategies have been used in all societies, commonly to maintain social stratification by underwriting the superior social standing of one group whose interests can be promoted even after death, like Egyptian kings. It is a kind of 'heroism' which protests against the inescapable human condition, but which also aims to secure further power or kudos for one specific group as a result of its immortality strategies. In the instance of obstetric science, its bid for immortality is linked to its own ambition and reputation, individually and collectively as a science which can face down death. In this sense, the death of a woman (a frequent enough occurrence until the 1930s) or her baby is a personal defeat, a blow to that ambition, rather than the terrible loss it is to a woman or her family.

As with the problem of pain and epidurals, there is work to be done here by feminists and birth activists. Indeed one can say that this is the problem which goes to the heart of the matter. When women and childbirth educators began to develop a platform of action in the late 1950s, we stopped speaking about death because we wanted to emphasise the normal everydayness of birth and the lack of risk, compared with the risk-laden account of childbirth obstetrics has historically presented. In contrast with their heroic strategies, we wanted to express that our immanence in relation to birth necessarily entails the ongoing experience of being a mother to a child, one which does not stop at the moment of a 'successful' birth (or even a child's death), as it does for obstetrics. Our criteria for success were quite different. We saw our emphasis on 'normal natural birth' as a way to contest the medical model and its 'shroud-waving' about our likely pathology, if we did not follow its regimes of care.

But we have not succeeded. Women continue to be pathologised. Our care is characterised by the medical injunctions of what we must and cannot do, about which injunctions we are not permitted to decide; we are unable to care for ourselves as we see best. Yet, when there are adverse outcomes, obstetrics continues to refuse to discuss death with us openly (most often denying its role also).[99] Obstetrics remains in a position to practise an immortality strategy quite separate to the needs and desires of pregnant women. Its strategy rests on the power it retains to pronounce on death and how it happens and this is the critical element in its historical relationship to childbirth. In securing its control over women's bodies, it used the knowledge gained in death to make a credible claim to be the experts who should manage childbirth. But it also killed a great many women in achieving its position, as we shall see in Chapter 3.

There are consequences stemming from the gendered relationship of a male science which has based itself on the female body in death. The first has to do with reinforcing passivity and victimhood when presenting death. In her study of male theories of femininity, Elaine Bronfen points out that as spectators, male doctors, anatomists and aesthetes (for these spectators cast themselves in the latter role as well) were able to project their own fantasies onto the dying because, while death was taking place, they could only see death externally and hence could make of it what they wished.[100] This level of projection permeates early obstetric writing about women, where, for example, the ongoing drama during the nineteenth century of puerperal fever in the lying-in hospitals produces almost stock descriptions in clinical reports of women 'sinking' to their deaths. This description belies the active physicality of deaths from puerperal fever which is never so kind as to permit women to gently take leave of life. But the image of 'sinking' fits in with the passive objectivity of women which the science is otherwise constructing. In its bid for immortality, the woman who has sunk to her death becomes the 'beautiful girl . . . lying on a slab under the male gaze',[101] a potent theme, while the scientist becomes the subject of the action.[102] Bronfen argues that: 'the feminine corpse inspires the surviving man to write, to deny or acknowledge death, while at the same time the corpse is the site at which he can articulate this knowledge.'[103]

In the production of this scientific knowledge, she remains (as corpse) objectified, the subject of his discourse. A second consequence is that women's passivity in death is then carried over into the views of women while pregnant and alive. Resonances about a woman's extreme victimhood work to make some 'facts' about her body appear far more visible than others as the lifeless sciences of anatomy and pathology draw conclusions from the beautiful lifeless body on the slab. These prove fertile for obstetrics in arguing against a woman's physical capabilities in birth: when an impoverished and malnourished woman, already suffering from pneumonia, comes into your lying-in hospital to give birth; when you put her to bed and keep her immobile for the entire first stage of labour; when she labours for six or more hours trying to push the baby out; when she is unable to expel the baby; when the head of the foetus has pressed for such a long time, unmoving, on the same spot, obstructing the discharge of urine, and leading to inflammation of the lower part of the bladder and the urethra; when finally the perforator must be used to release the trapped dead baby; and when the woman then dies as a consequence of the puerperal fever she has contracted from the infection begun where her tissues were starved of oxygen for so many hours because of the obstructed foetal head; when you finally come to dissect that body, you reach decisions about the cause of death and about how labours are best handled. These decisions are unlikely to include any version of labour management where, for example, you facilitate the woman's labour by moving her onto all fours, using the pelvis space to help deal with the dystocia which keeps the foetus from advancing any further. You will not see that possibility of movement and flexibility in the woman when she is dead and you carry back with you to living women that version of immobility. Cases like these are consistently recorded in the clinical records; in building obstetric theory, our bodies are caught and kept in ways which deny our capacities.

And, when women no longer die in such numbers, as obstetrics stumbles slowly towards what it has identified as solutions for maternal death in childbirth (the two developments are not linked in the way obstetrics has liked to argue, an issue I will discuss in Chapter 4), its practitioners feel able to shift their attention away from the mother, having secured sufficient ground for its version of how she works. With the downward sweep of maternal mortality figures from the 1930s onwards, obstetrics extends its boundaries to absorb the problem of the foetus and thus its immortality strategies begin to take in the forestalling of foetal death, managing handily to redistribute and redefine 'its procreative capacity'.[104]

There is a long timeline with this process, which begins in the eighteenth century when the hospital becomes a place of science where there is the chance to make and practise science because women come to its doors. Joseph Clarke, sixth Master of the Rotunda Hospital, from 1786–93, wrote of this space when introducing his clinical notes:

> All I have to urge in justification of myself, is that few have had greater opportunities of practice in so short a space of time; that I have always observed instruments to be most easily applied where least necessary; and that my experience of them was acquired in an Hospital, in a situation where I felt myself totally uninfluenced by any existing prejudices, and where the only object I had in view was to discharge my duty conscientiously between mother and child.[105]

Clarke's sentiments are interesting: he is conscientious, one of the most conscientious of the Irish men midwives and the obstetricians who follow after him down through the decades. The paradox for him is that in his conscientiousness, he is unable to see his knowledge-building as the ambitious bid it is, to acknowledge how he uses the femininity he thinks he perceives to confront the phenomenon of death. So it is with obstetric science in general. It is also worth noting that the concrete images of women's feebleness, details like emaciation and so on, vanish over time. There is an increasing sense of abstraction about women once clinical records are being kept in detail. Women become letters, numbers, symptoms, fragmented into body parts. What matters is the disease process that is thought to have killed them; that is what is named in vivid detail.

Using the Female Temperament to Claim Professional Competence

Ideologies about women's inherent incapacity to labour have provided the obstetric rationales for managing women in birth since the eighteenth century. Dating from that same period, men midwives also used their range of arguments about the nature of the female temperament to explain why women midwives were not competent to manage birth. At least one woman, Elizabeth Nihell, fought back on those same grounds as to why women were the only suitable attendants for birth. Although feminists in England and the United States have written about childbirth in this period in terms of the struggle between men and women midwives for professional control,[106] this conflict is not the direct focus of this book, not least because Ireland appears to have lacked trained professional midwives of the sort who worked in England, Germany, The Netherlands and France. And although Irish midwives and handywomen came in for more than their fair share of disapprobation by men midwives in their writing, there is no indication that they defended themselves in print, for example, and there were no pre-existing formal arrangements to be torn down.[107] Overt conflict was never as sharply defined here possibly because of the perceived lack of strong competition from women midwives. There was a specific aim in the Royal Charter granted to the Rotunda, on its formal establishment in 1756, to initiate schemes for training women midwives to work in the most remote areas of the country, where it was assumed that the services of a man midwife would not be available, there being no great professional inducement. However, these training schemes for women were a long time emerging, relative to training for men midwives and when they did, midwives were automatically subordinated within a medical hierarchy which was created from the top down, starting with the Master of the lying-in hospital whose appointment was for a seven-year term (the title appears to be exclusive to Irish obstetric establishments).[108]

Men midwives built a professional language to indicate their competence which also helped to differentiate them from women midwives. It was in that same professional language that they described why the female temperament prevented women from practising as midwives, as much as it prevented women from giving birth with ease. In the eighteenth century, the economic and political drive to stamp a new order on the social body by bringing order to the individual reproductive body, was a peculiarly invasive one, although it appeared as an essentially benign regime.[109] As we have seen, descriptions like Roussel's, linking a woman's 'soft parts' with her social role were commonplace distinctions within medicine by the end of the eighteenth century.

Men midwives were well placed to promote this ideology as a way of legitimating their practices because they wrote about their practices and published their texts in numbers which expanded even more rapidly than their institutional base of the lying-in hospital. What often began as a series of points for discussion or arguments evolved through a stage of persuasion and ended as incontestable facts presented to the world at large and which, as far as the non-medical person was concerned, could not be challenged except by bodies of knowledge which were already rejected as pre-scientific, like popular peasant knowledges.[110] Men midwives had a specific need to interpret events in such a way that their competence and probity were assured.[111] Thus, arguments about the pain and danger of childbirth were staple fare. The great challenge for the man midwife was to assist a woman who was stranded between those threats on the one hand and, on the other, her own natural weakness. This extract from Fielding Ould's 1742 treatise on midwifery illustrates how the argument worked:

> For in the most favourable Labours, poor Women endure as much Pain as Mortals are well able to undergo; and how wickedly cruel and hard hearted must he be, that would do any Thing except of Necessity, to increase their Misery?[112]

This can be seen as an application of what Joan Brown terms 'words that succeed'. Brown analyses how the professionals' use of metaphorical language often justifies their work without having to disclose how they have arrived at their own knowledge and so a powerful, simple metaphor rapidly organises the public view of the importance of that particular profession.[113] The 'Misery' of childbirth is one such metaphor which accounts for the importance of having a man midwife in attendance. The passage can also be understood in terms of what Ludie Jordanova identifies as a 'stiffening' of gendered polarities in the eighteenth century in which medicine produced relevant metaphors with which to anchor a definitive identification between women and the natural realm.[114] As Elisabeth Nihell herself noted, medicine successfully constructed metaphors around 'the phantom of incapacity in the women',[115] and this was linked to gendered words with feminine connotations, like soft and weak.

Other staple fare proffered by men midwives were: litanies of uncontrolled female emotion – 'some extraordinary Passion of the Mind, as Fright, Anger, excessive Joy, Grief &c.'; the wilful refusal of a woman to take care of herself – 'taking medicines improperly, or perhaps with that Design, some acute Disease, or perhaps a natural bad Habit of Body' which could disturb a pregnancy or labour 'whereby the Patient is in great Danger of being lost'.[116] These linkages had great utility in attributing a disastrous outcome to the woman's physiological processes and passionate reactions, which weakened her, or to her individual desire to be devious, or to refuse to care for herself and thus lose the pregnancy. The danger that her inherent tendencies courted was constantly brought to the fore. Deventer, the Dutch man midwife, for example, spoke of 'fearful, timorous women and passionate women' always being most likely to miscarry.[117] Yet another staple theme, one which indicates the necessary flexibility of these metaphors, was that women who were sexually active outside marriage were paradoxically stronger physically, and thus had better outcomes in childbirth and were less in need of assistance. Ould's version of this was:

> There are constant Instances of Women bringing forth both Child and Burthen without any other Assistance than that of Nature. This happens chiefly to those who have Bastards, Women at Sea, and in Camps.[118]

Brown argues that the secularisation of the word 'professional' has been coterminous with the building of modern society, and, for any newly organising group, has entailed the work of defining, organising and publicising their claims to expertise and authority, often by contrast with historical examples.[119] This strategy is evident in the texts of men midwives who presented themselves as makers of a new science, comparing themselves favourably with older non-scientific, non-rational practices of midwives.[120] Here too, they relied on a distinctive use of words, a professional language, to indicate the distance between them and women practitioners. Men midwives had a nobler duty, to preserve humankind, and a finer knowledge, as Ould argues in the introduction to his treatise:

> Nor is this Art, in any respect the meanest Province in the medicinal Common-wealth, but much on the contrary; as on it depends, not only the Preservation of the Species, but the various Methods of relieving distressed Women, from extraordinary Pain and Torture, innumerable Disorders and Death, the consequence of bad Practice.[121]

Across Europe, the process of institutionalising childbirth was marked by palpable hostility to women midwives, who were condemned for their 'bad practice', both those trained in institutions like the Hôtel-Dieu or as part of municipal corps of midwives and untrained women in local communities.[122] In England, Nihell pinpointed professional divisions between two broad groups: the surgeons, the apothecaries, the men midwives, many of whom got their start as barber surgeons, and a number of women and nurses who maintained that midwifery should be the concern of men formed one group who were in opposition to many of the old-style physicians who still believed that midwifery should remain the business of women.[123] Part of the hostility of the emerging professional group of men midwives had to do with the obvious need to create distance between the bearers of the old order and the new, even though both used the same or similar approaches to the problems of birth.

At the beginning of the eighteenth century, there were still writers who praised the skill of 'expert midwives' but this vanished by the end of the century; in a typical statement of the period, Joseph Clarke from the Rotunda condemns midwives in Dublin and also indicates that he speaks from a professional space legitimated by the state:

> Midwives in this city and its environs, are in general, ignorant, self-sufficient, and prone to drunkenness. I have no doubt they destroy many of those entrusted to their care; nor have we any law, either to prohibit or punish them.[124]

The deeply polarised account of gender which marked medical discourse operated to the disadvantage of women midwives, who saw their efforts dismissed as ignorant and non-scientific. Even when practices were the same, they were placed definitively outside the newly formed boundaries of professional male practice. If men midwives disagreed amongst themselves about whether to give a woman in labour 'strengthening broths' or 'heating cordials', it was an internal disagreement amongst scientific experts. If a man midwife favoured the former and a woman midwife used the latter, cordials were dismissed as a harmful practice carried out by superstitious midwives.[125] The nineteenth-century Irish physician, Sir William Wilde, tells us that untrained women midwives in Ireland used the *medoag*, a curved blade made from the point of an old reaping hook, in order to cut the perineum to enlarge the birth canal, a practice he and other male doctors condemned. Wilde also reported that Irish women midwives were known to force pieces of candle mould down women's throats to try and make them vomit, in instances where the placenta was not soon expelled after the baby's birth, in order to put pressure on the diaphragm and hence on the uterus.[126] However, variants of the very practices Wilde condemned were carried out by men midwives. Ould was the man midwife who was credited with introducing the episiotomy, the medical term for what the country women midwives were doing, that is cutting the perineum, into medical writing. It was also Ould who advocated putting fingers down the throat of a woman, a substitute for candle mould, to induce vomiting.[127]

Anomalies like these were absorbed into the science itself, leaving Wilde free to write that the importance of the establishment of the Rotunda was that it 'placed the obstetric art on a sure and scientific basis – and in so doing gave a blow to quackery in that department at least.'[128] Thus the legitimacy of a particular practice relied on who the practitioner was and how that related to a professional base, not on the practice itself.[129]

If professional competence is proven by employing an abstruse vocabulary, the next step in securing competence is to take this abstruse vocabulary and translate its meanings back into a common language while controlling how these terms are used.[130] Male midwifery worked to separate women from how they had related to their bodies through the use of a new professional language. This is illustrated by the evolution of the term placenta to describe the afterbirth. When the Dutch man midwife, Deventer, published his treatise towards the end of the seventeenth century, he used the term 'cake' to describe the placenta, that being a common everyday term.[131] As late as 1767, John Harvie, a London man midwife who wrote a treatise on the management of the placenta, used both the new medical term and the common word, seemingly without prejudice towards the latter.[132] But 'placenta' was more medical sounding than 'cake' and it became the dominant term by the end of the eighteenth century,[133] when male midwifery became institutionalised. Similar to other terms about female reproductive anatomy and physiology, the re-naming process of cake into placenta created a distance between women and their common language usage while strengthening professional medical control.

As I have noted above, a professional medical language was also crucial in strengthening the process of naturalising women's bodies. Nihell rounded on the efforts of men midwives to create a professional language which distanced and confused the laywoman. Yet she sought to deal with this problem by making the attributes of a gendered body the basis for a more knowledgeable and sensitive response to women in birth. 'I am myself a mother',[134] she wrote, and dismissing the accounts of men midwives about her number, she also wrote:

> All the knowledge, experience, dexterity, strength, prudence, tenderness, charity, and presence of mind, of which a woman is capable, are requisite to accomplish certain laborious deliveries.[135]

And here:

> Women, in those cases have more bowels for women: they feel for those of their own sex so much, that the feeling operates in them like an irresistible instinct, both in favour of the pregnant mother and of the child.[136]

This 'irresistible instinct' could support a woman through the pain of labour (which Nihell did not dismiss as insignificant), a quite different response to that of men midwives. Nihell argued that the latter used instruments under the 'temptation of a quick riddance to a violent state of pain'.[137] In difficult instances, she argued that men midwives always reached for their instruments while women midwives always used their hands. In breech births, for example, men midwives maintained a 'constant supposition' that it was impossible to deliver the head without the help of instruments; they argued likewise, when the foetal head became delayed in delivery 'having ingaged itself halfway' and 'the labour pains remit' that forceps were the only solution.[138]

In Nihell's judgement, all instruments, including the crotchet (a curved hook used to destroy the foetus in order to effect birth where there was an obstruction), were dangerous expedients for making short work of a labour, when what was really required was a different level of support altogether to bring it to a happy conclusion. In ironic vein, she wrote of 'those poor instruments of God's making, the woman's fingers'[139] and described the art of 'how to predispose the passages, and by gentle reductions to restore Nature to her right road',[140] arts not open to 'men dabblers in practical midwifery'.[141] She argued that 'Nature acting on ever surer principles than Art'[142] was far more to be trusted in securing a safe labour for women, with women themselves as the principal instruments:

> In women with all their supposed ignorance, you may observe a certain shrewd vivacity, a grace of ease, a handiness of performance, and especially a kind of unction of the heart, that all evidently demonstrate this talent in them to be a genuine gift of nature which more than compensates what she is supposed to have refused them in depth of study, though even of that they are not so unsusceptible, as some men detractingly think.[143]

And, if men midwives like Ould dismissed women midwives as 'ignorant women' or 'female adventurers',[144] Nihell tore out the heart of their term, man midwife, 'that hermaphrodite appellation':

> What is, at the best, a man-midwife? ... the common word for him in the English language is a contradiction in terms, a monstrous incongruity; a MAN-mid-WIFE.[145]

She turns their argument about their relationship with learning, science and rationality on its head and casts the man midwife in an entirely different light:

> In the men, with all their boasted erudition, you cannot but discern a certain clumsy untowardly stiffness, an unaffectionate perfunctory air, an ungainly management, that plainly prove it to be an acquisition of art, or rather the rickety production of interest begot upon art.[146]

Women midwives have talents accompanying their tender sensibilities and instinctive love to do 'both with the manual function in the delivery of women, and for all the concomitant requisites of their aid during the time of their lying-in', which talents are:

> superior to any possible attainment of the men in that art, though they should have sacrificed hecatombs of pregnant rabbits or have brooded over thousands of coveys of eggs in their search of excellence in it.[147]

So men midwives can at best use their inappropriate skills as anatomists to try to learn by imitation what is natural to a woman:

> A woman in labor requires a midwife to lay her, not an anatomist to dissect her, or read lectures over the corpse, he will be most likely to make of her, if he depends more on the refinements of anatomy, than on the dexterity of hand, and the suggestions of practical experience and common sense.[148]

And what of the consequences for women, when women midwives are attacked by these 'keen instrumentarians', these 'pudendists', when foreign to the dictates of nature men deliver women, what happens to midwifery?: 'Of good midwives there were never too many; but they are now much too few.'[149] Of course there have been too few, too few especially in Nihell's position, of being tough, skilled and articulate enough to challenge the male medical establishment.

It has been in the interests of male midwifery to write out, demean and downplay the substantive challenges to it. And, since Nihell's time, obstetrics has been aided in this not just because it has been able to build a power monolith of facts and knowledge but also because relations of power are differently formed once there are no longer dual systems of care in birth in direct competition with one another. By the time Nihell published her work in 1760, the discursive and institutional practices of male midwifery had already assumed the status of an official discourse which enabled it to either subordinate or see off all other systems of care, whether formal or informal, in which women had played the dominant role. Whatever about the potential to actually damage women physically, Nihell was acutely aware of the alienating possibilities of this new science and, in order to retain agency, she turned instead to using the femaleness which men midwives were intent on circumscribing. It was a strategy which failed, because the individual instinctive woman had no place of authority in the larger scheme of discursive practices being built around her. Nonetheless, this same strategy has periodically risen up, as women have struggled to work with a definition of self and subjectivity that will work in birth against the obstetric establishment. Many of Nihell's claims have such a contemporary ring because many childbirth activists are still working with those same possibilities. I am suggesting that we need to take on different strategies of self in order to deal effectively with obstetric power, strategies that will make sense to women whether they are uneasily aligned with obstetrics, as with women who request epidurals, or unwillingly, as with women who wish not to give birth in hospital at all.[150]

Understanding Obstetric Knowledge

Perhaps the principal problem of obstetrics has been that it has presented an ontological argument about the female body, in which certain concepts about the body become the basis for arguing that the body materially exists exactly as those concepts state, that there is one material unchanging female body. This is problematic because there is little about the female reproductive body that is unambiguous and unchanging (think for example of the shifting age downwards of menarche over the last two centuries). The multiple realities of the body are such that obstetric rationality, even though it claims a position of universality and authority, may be one of several or even many rational views of the body.[151] Our problem is to single out the elements of obstetric rationality and present them so that we can make some judgement about its version of the female body and, by extension, its claims to primacy.

One route into obstetric rationality is to locate its forms of argument, specifying how they emerge and how they shift over time. There are ongoing theoretical debates in obstetric science which gain new interpretations and new political possibilities, but these appear to be underpinned by themes which remain constant because they are a continuing preoccupation for its practitioners. However, the constancy of these preoccupations is not related to a great rational structure that is obstetrics, rational in the sense that science may want it to mean; they are curiously fragmented and inconsistent, as we shall see.

These preoccupations are often presented in pairs or dyads: as two objects bound together by the same outcome; as two alternatives; as cause and effect. This way of thinking is within the Western tradition of organising our concerns as dualities which can appear and reappear with new interpretations. Sometimes these preoccupations appear to be internal to the possibilities of the science, as with a point of physiology and how it is interpreted in different obstetric models of management at birth; sometimes preoccupations are external and intrude, as with public concerns about the rates of death amongst women in lying-in hospitals during the nineteenth century from puerperal fever; sometimes there are agendas which develop in separate but related spheres, where the immediate obstetric interests overlap with some other social dimension. This happens, for example, in the mid- to late nineteenth century with debates in ecclesiastical journals about destructive operations like craniotomy, where obstetrics accounts for its actions with terms of reference that displace religious interests.

The central pairing, the dyad on which obstetrics pins all its claims for existence, is that of mother and foetus. Complex agendas flow from and around this dyad but it is the essence of obstetrical argument that it is in the best position to preserve and protect the interests of both. This assertion about the preservation of life appears in the earliest obstetric texts and is an ongoing theme. Obstetric claims that it is the most essential medical science, because it is concerned with the survival of the human race through the mother and child, fit into several different arenas. While obstetrics is still working to prove itself to the rest of male medicine as a respectable sub-discipline, it is important for men midwives to argue that they have taken over a critical area of endeavour from women midwives who were never mindful enough of this onerous obligation to preserve maternal and infant life. One of the principal reasons obstetrics is poised for success in the eighteenth century and why it receives state backing for the lying-in hospital is that its argument about maternal life conveniently reinforces the control over the social and reproductive body, the 'biopolitics' which is so essential to modernity. In the Rotunda's charter, for example, the concern is primarily about the loss of maternal life without which the (economic) life of the nation will not be renewed, for, without bodies to turn the soil and produce the manufactures, there can be no thriving national economy.[152] There are vastly different political meanings and possibilities attached to the mother–foetus dyad between eighteenth-century mercantilism and twentieth-century discourses on maternal welfare policies but that dyad is always there as the essential organising principle for obstetric science.

The distinction between 'natural' and 'preternatural' is a second critical organising principle. Obstetric science consistently states that there are difficulties attached to the birth process, difficulties which they, as scientists, are far better equipped to identify and deal with than are women midwives, whether trained or untrained. However, what they must be able to do is to distinguish between what is natural and what is preternatural or abnormal; their science turns on that moment of identification. Consistency ends there, of course, in that moment. They are all agreed they must be able to identify this distinction but cannot agree about what defines that moment.

This ongoing and fundamental disagreement leads to a third pairing or set of distinctions in their theoretical debates, namely what is error and what is truth; contesting one another's theories and practices as truly meritorious or clearly erroneous quickly becomes an extensive practice in the eighteenth century. In Chapter 2, these organising principles or pairings are examined in detail, using eighteenth- and nineteenth-century debates, most often drawn from within Irish obstetric practice, to illustrate how they work. Getting to grips with these debates also enables the reader to become familiar with how male midwifery makes sense of its own categories.

In the third chapter, I am unravelling the problem of puerperal fever, also largely in an Irish context. As obstetric science and the lying-in hospitals grew in importance, it affected the lives of many thousands of women. But newly won legitimacy as a scientific specialism was also threatened by the widespread presence of 'childbed', or puerperal, fever in lying-in hospitals which often killed the women obstetrics had vowed to save. Dissection of dead bodies, which had become a knowledge-building strategy, entailed further death. Women were dying from puerperal fever and, in one form at least, this was the result of their contamination at the hands of male practitioners, who carried out dissections to find out how and why they died, thus infecting other women. The debates on puerperal fever were the most extensive and the most entrenched in the nineteenth century, as obstetrics struggled to deny the connections between its practices and women's deaths. The ideology of female frailty was crucial to its arguments about the fever.

The problem of defining what is natural and what is preternatural is gradually subsumed into the more contemporary problem of distinguishing the normal from the abnormal. This is bound up with the process of building modern society as well as with the development of obstetrics; that is, the concerns of the latter merge with the concern of modern society about establishing norms and normality as a mode of social organisation. Searching to establish normality has permitted an ever-expanding domain of the abnormal which is part of what we confront in obstetric medicine today. And for us, this is also critically bound up with the growth of the notion of risk and the problem of death. Marsden Wagner, speaking from within medical ranks, sees the increasing number of women who are labelled as being at risk as a direct consequence of obstetric power; women are captured by specialist obstetric regimes on the grounds that they have abnormalities in their pregnancies and during labour which will jeopardise the lives of their foetuses.[153]

I look at this transformation in the fourth and fifth chapters, examining first the growth of the risk model and the thesis that pregnancy and birth are only ever normal in retrospect and then examining how this thinking has contributed to what is termed the 'active management' of labour, including the third stage when the placenta is expelled. The 'active management of labour' played a critical role in Catherine Dunne's story of the National Maternity Hospital, referred to above, and has contributed substantially to the international reputation of Irish obstetrics in recent decades. The force of 'active management' as a concept cannot be separated from the obstetric attempt to measure risk and deal with death.

The history of our bodies in obstetrics is also the history of a science. I draw heavily on the work of Michel Foucault, Ludwig Fleck, Ian Hacking and Bruno Latour in dealing with the problem of science and power. But I am never far from our experiences as women and from how we have attempted to deal with obstetrics. The phrases 'old wives' tales' and 'horror stories' come to mind and I recall a popular paperback on pregnancy in the 1970s by an English obstetrician, Gordon Bourne, in which he upbraided women to reject these exchanges he presumed were happening between them:

> Probably more is done by wicked women with their malicious lying tongues to harm the confidence and happiness of pregnant women than by any other single factor . . . the final authority on any individual pregnancy is of course the doctor.[154]

I would submit that women's confidence and happiness have been profoundly affected by the way obstetrics has dealt with our bodies, and that how women speak to one another about childbirth is most crucially affected by obstetrics itself. Its reliance on 'horror stories' about what goes wrong during labour and birth in order to build up its understanding of how childbirth should be managed is integral to its history as a science. In the final chapter, I look at the notion of horror stories; obstetrics' stories about our malfunctioning bodies and our stories in reaction to theirs. I argue that agency in relation to reproduction and childbirth can best be established and sustained by establishing a position on their horror stories; this necessarily entails our taking a position on risk and death. Obstetric rationality is only one form of rationality in responding to an outcome which can never be guaranteed. In establishing the principle of our own agency in undertaking pregnancy and birth, I explore alternative possibilities which have been raised in the last twenty years, coming primarily (though not solely) from a midwifery movement, which has been revitalised and strengthened, one which would bring huzzahs of approval from Elizabeth Nihell. Carried by the challenge of building feminist theory, we are working actively to bring on those possibilities to a point where the exercise of obstetric power is displaced.

Davina Cooper and Janet Sawicki, amongst other feminist writers, have written that the way power operates suggests that those who seek to deploy power, as well as those who are subjected, can all undergo change because where power is exercised, there is always a way to modify and shift its effects: 'it suggests that in the deployment of power it is not only those subjected who are in a state of flux, but rather all forces involved, since all undergo change.'[155]

It seems to me that we need to recognise that obstetrics appears as a total success with a totalising account of the female body. Yet, in fact, it is an account which tends to fracture or to constantly require reinforcement, one which constantly regroups to face its critics. It has always been seen as a threat to women's well-being: also as a threat to women's modesty (Nihell); to their lives (public-health arguments over lying-in hospitals and the spread of puerperal fever); and now, to women's 'natural' status and role as mothers with the ever-unfolding possibilities of artificial reproduction, autogenesis and foetal experimentation. The challenges obstetrics provokes engage all areas of the political spectrum about the female body, areas where women themselves are in various stages of objectification and yet slowly coming to control aspects of these agendas. I hope this book can make a contribution to this regrouping of forces, for if feminist politics has any meaning in our lives, it is about taking control of and re-forming the knowledges of these, our bodies.

2

Obstetric Pairings and Knowledge Formation

Theory and Practice

Possibly the Dublin man midwife, Fielding Ould's, most famous contribution to the theories of management of childbirth is the operation which eventually became known as the episiotomy. This is how Ould describes the necessity for such an operation:

> It sometimes happens, though the Labour has succeeded so well, that the head of the Child has made its Way through the Bones of the Pelvis, that it cannot however come forward, by Reason of the extraordinary Constriction of the external Orifice of the Vagina; so that the Head after it has passed the Bones, thrusts the Flesh and Integuments before it, as if it were contained in a Purse; in which condition if it continues long, the Labour will become dangerous, by the Orifice of the womb contracting about the Child's Neck; wherefore it must be dilated if possible by the fingers, and forced over the Child's Head; if this cannot be accomplished, there must be an Incision made towards the Anus with a Pair of crooked Probe-Sizars . . . the Business is done at one Pinch, by which the whole Body will easily come Forth.[1]

This is the first time a description of the episiotomy appeared in an obstetric treatise and it presents a problem of evidence and how evidence is related to conceptions. The description of the head bulging against the perineum 'as if it were contained in a purse' is consistent with a woman giving birth in a supine position, where gravity is pulling downwards. But with the woman lying horizontally and pushing on that same plane, she is pushing against the perineal tissues and the result is that the force of her pushing is deflected from fully assisting the baby down the birth canal, often leading to tearing of the tissues.[2] Ould does not link his observation about the way the tissues bulge outwards to his preference for women giving birth lying down which permits him to retain most control over her labour. However, in order to resolve the problem he has created by insisting on this birth position, he comes up with the notion of pulling at the edge of the perineum, to 'force' it over the child's head. As a technique, this is a long way removed from the gentle movements Nihell advocates.[3] Ould's conceptual package: placing the woman in the horizontal position, positing the imagined dangers of the neck of the uterus closing round the baby's head, pulling forcibly at the edge of the perineal tissue and, if that is not successful in removing this impediment, cutting the tissue, forms a classic account of the way male midwifery seeks to overcome the female body, rather than to work with it. The question set by such arguments is how obstetric theory is built up in relation to how the body is read.

The production of theory is fundamental to all sciences. Inevitably, theory has played a major role in the development of obstetrics. The Dutch man midwife, Henrik Deventer, often called the 'father of modern midwifery' in obstetric histories,[4] wrote:

> Theory ought to go before Practice, as the Body before the Shadow. He that knows not what is to be done, knows not how to produce the Effect; much less does he know the Method of doing well.[5]

He adds that 'Those who only think it sufficient to grow wise by practice, without the previous Knowledge of Things, are often deceived' because 'our Members are not so ready in acting as our Minds are in perceiving.'[6] So, in his interpretation of how knowledge is built, Deventer insists that theory determines the direction of midwifery practice.[7]

Even in its infancy, obstetric science understood that its success would rely on the work of organising the 'Knowledge of Things'. In line with the aspirations of an emerging science, the treatises of men midwives began to take on a consistent structure of writing and presentation by the eighteenth century, one which became correspondingly weighty,[8] and in which they set out broadly similar arguments, citing a direct relationship between theory and practice. For example, Fielding Ould, who published his treatise in 1742, writes of the 'Theory and Practice of natural Deliveries'[9] and argues that his own contribution to the 'facts' about midwifery 'though they be but few and of little Moment, yet they have Truth and Demonstration on their Side, being confirmed by Practice'.[10] Frederick Jebb, who was to become the fourth Master of the Rotunda, argued in favour of the production of theory in a manner that strengthened the claims of male midwifery as a science:

> There is nobody so absurd as to advance that practice alone is sufficient to entitle an operator in the science to the claim of perfection. Practice in order to be solid must have precept for its foundation, indeed that precept or theory should be founded upon principles obtained from observation.[11]

Men midwives spoke of a science in which theory and observation establish a set of principles or axioms to underpin practice; this process informs further theory-building based on the observations of practice, and the theory-building itself is circulated and expanded by teaching and writing. The problem in this model is with the nature of facts, with their production. We have already seen that the way in which the facts about the female body are observed and transmitted can be shot through with ideology. The theory-building of obstetrics did not transcend these ideological constraints; indeed they were inherent to obstetric thinking. But how did the process of fact-making work? Ludwig Fleck, in his essay on scientific facts, says that within science, a fact should be capable of being distinguished from 'transient theses' because it is concrete, permanent, independently measured for its validity, and free from 'subjective interpretation'.[12] This is what science argues to the rest of us that it profoundly believes in, the discoverability and measurability of facts. Yet Fleck cautions that the history of scientific knowledge reveals something rather different taking place, where 'evidence conforms to conceptions just as often as conceptions conform to evidence'. Moreover, conceptions are not logical structures for, despite their creators' desires; 'they are stylised units which develop or atrophy'.[13]

Fleck's analysis suggests substantive problems in examining evolving theories in obstetric discourse. Firstly, we must allow for a content which is always ideologically laden, so that we have a female body which is constantly in the process of being reconstructed. Within that frame of reference, if obstetric conceptions, which should have a rigorous logical structure according to claims about the rules of science, are more commonly 'stylised units', how can we distinguish between these 'stylised units' and theories which reflect verifiable facts? What does a verifiable fact look like? Does it exist? In terms of the impact on practice, does it matter if these theories are composed of evidence which is made to conform to conceptions? What difference will the very articulation of a theory, and whether and how verification is sought, make to how it gets used on women in labour? The related issue is whether the development of obstetric concepts is linked to or guaranteed by the status they may come to assume. If one set of concepts becomes dominant, does this mean that evidence is used to support its further development in an uncritical manner and to the exclusion of other possible concepts?

From a related area of bio-social medicine, the pathological condition of hysteria provides an instructive example. Hysteria remains a vague and ill-defined concept within medicine; its root notion, a uterine disturbance that somehow unbalances the mind, contributed to its characterisation as a female 'illness' which came to prominence at the beginning of the nineteenth century, with a seeming epidemic of the illness amongst upper-class women. It would be difficult to ignore its ideological loading and application, as increasing numbers of women were diagnosed as hysterics. But whether women were responding to the constraints of an impossible social role by literally throwing fits, or whether they were diagnosed as such because it accounted for any behaviour of women not sanctioned by contemporary social mores, the notion itself appeared to have enormous salience which was taken up and transformed in respect of psychoanalysis. Its conversion into a touchstone for Freud's theories of the unconscious and away from a gynaecological disorder also suggests that, in the first instance, it had the status within gynaecology and general medical practice of an uncertain or less logical conception which evidence could be made to fit. However, this uncertain status did not prevent many thousands of women being submitted to bizarre forms of treatment and containment by medical doctors to effect a 'cure', before Freud's talking cure became established.[14] In other words, its salience impacted directly, whether or not its basis was proven. The problem women face with science, then and now, is the power-building capacity that is part of its fact-making. This is what Foucault refers to as power/knowledge: power as a set of relations which 'can materially penetrate the body in depth, without depending even on the mediation of the subject's own representations'.[15] Indeed, Foucault argues that the female body, in the guise of the 'idle woman' of the upper classes was the first to have its sexuality medicalised through the showcase of hysteria.[16]

How does the fact-making work internally? What actually happens? Within any given scientific discipline, there is a constant movement, with concepts being taken further or being let atrophy. Because there is always a social dimension to knowledge formation, some ideas are retained while others are neglected, forgotten, overridden, even derided. Fleck implies that scientific facts are more rarely based on proofs when he argues that 'the tenacity of self-contained systems of opinion' affects the 'operation of cognition'.[17] Another way of looking at the complex interplay between conceptions and evidence is to consider what happens in what Bruno Latour refers to as the 'simplest of all possible situations when someone utters a statement': either that statement becomes in time a 'fact', because others accept it, or an 'artefact' because they disbelieve or ignore it. Latour argues that a collective process of use moves the statement 'downstream' to become a fact or a collective process of abandonment moves the statement 'upstream' to become a 'fiction' or artefact.[18] We have already seen the example of Roussel's argument about menstruation being the result of faulty diet; we can say that the statement was pushed upstream to become an artefact (although the style of argument was kept intact). Reputations of individuals and of schools of thought are made or broken by the judgement, over time, of whether they have produced facts or artefacts. So, coming back to the treatises of men midwives, despite disclaimers like that of Ould's, about his theories being of 'little moment' or import, he and every other man midwife hoped that their individual discoveries would be of very great moment, moving 'downstream' to become a general theory.

In the stakes to build their reputations as men midwives, a rejection of the 'rules laid down by most practical Authors'[19] was often given as the principal reason for writing their treatises. It was commonplace for them to target their rivals in their treatises, like this swingeing condemnation by Ould: 'many of their Schemes are like those of some Navigators and Geographers, who never made use of a Compass, but in their Closet.'[20]

In her comments on this practice, Elizabeth Nihell captures perfectly the sense of competition and strife that marked the establishment of obstetrics:

> Have not some of our modern authors, especially the male-practitioners, who in these later times have treated of midwifery, added new and worse errors of their own to those bequeathed to us by the antients, whom they have insulted, as they themselves will probably one day be, but with more reason, by their successors, if the world should continue blind enough for them to have any in this profession? One would even imagine, that in the criticisms in which they indulge themselves of one another's sistems and instruments, they are inflicting part of the punishment due for their common offences against Nature, in the abuse of an Art, originally intended to assist her. At the same time, even from their own showing, nothing can be plainer, that their boasted inventions have, under the specious pretence of improvement, fallen from bad to worse, as is ever the case of superstructures on the crazy foundation of false principles.[21]

Nihell criticises male midwifery for not respecting the boundary between an art which can assist people and one which takes over the woman's body entirely. She also criticises the extent to which untested conceptions are let loose within obstetric thinking, as part of their search for individual reputations, and scorns the notion of theory determining practice as a 'crazy foundation'. Nihell's position, on the intuitive grasp women midwives have of the labouring process, and her total opposition to what she sees as a pretentious male science, leads her to make the case for a practice that stems from experience, one that is based on what she terms 'common sense'.

Nihell's arguments about midwifery as an art which assists, rather than takes over, and about the location of experience and common sense in determining workable theories, puts her at some remove from the men midwives, but all of them are struggling with the problem of how knowledge can be built. A close reading of the treatises of Deventer, Ould, Jebb and Nihell reveals these different positions but also reveals similar tensions in the ways they organise their thinking, tensions which are inherent in the relationship each posits between experience and theory. In turn, this relationship determines for them the nature of midwifery as a practice which either assists nature or displaces nature.

All four of these writers are concerned with the problem of 'crazy' or flawed foundations. All of them argue for a version of common sense insofar as they link common sense to what is knowable. Chris Weedon, writing about common-sense knowledge, argues that its principal features are a belief in the transparency of language, that is, that language unproblematically and always reports what already is; and an appeal to the value of experience which can act as a 'guarantee' of truth.[22] Furthermore, the 'common-sense' assumption, that language transparently contains pre-existing facts denies the role of language in shaping fact, thus changing our perceptions of it.

The development of obstetric knowledge for both versions of midwifery is complicated by an assumption that there are pre-existing facts which language can present transparently. Ould, Jebb and Deventer write about the common-sense work of developing linkages between observation, theory, and practice, the essence of scientific discovery. However, this enables 'Nature', in the form of the pregnant woman, to be treated as an unproblematic whole, there to be uncovered, discovered and conquered.[23] Nihell has a different line, one that emphasises the matter-of-factness, the naturalness of understanding birth, that is instinctively part of a woman midwife. In her construct, this instinctive aptitude is of a piece with women's location as being closest to nature, most instinctive and therefore most suitable. She does not reject the importance of theory for women midwives but she rejects a theory that does not allow room for a natural aptitude in the practice of midwifery for making sense of what presents itself during each labour and birth. And she connects this to the physical knowledge women midwives acquire on a case-by-case basis:

> Their skill in the manual function cannot but be improved by the addition of a sound and competent theory. But it should always be remembered, that the very basis or capital point of the art is the manual dexterity; and in that point the most learned of men must yield to the most ignorant of the women.[24]

This frame of reference implies that theory is built up from the experience of women midwives, especially their manual dexterity and the knowledge that arises from it. Arguing from her naturalist perspective, Nihell insists that the writing of men midwives is deeply unsatisfactory; it 'still leaves the mind unsatisfied' for 'too much is given to theory, and too little to the practical part, or manual function'. The 'causes of difficult labors are far from solidly or sufficiently explained'; 'they give us no tolerably sure method for preventing or remedying those difficulties'; 'the whole boasted improvement of the art is reduced, to a pernicious recourse to instruments, which cut at once the knot they cannot unty.'[25] This last, by the way, is a brilliantly apt image, of the too hasty and unknowing men midwives, this 'cloud of writers' whose theories are so unrelated to the 'sense' of the labouring body that they act to disrupt the labour process rather than sustain it.

In examining how the working concepts of obstetrics took shape and how particular versions of its thinking became legitimated as scientific, we will see that similar to other sciences,[26] practices were created through a process of often furious disputation, which advanced a number of theories abandoning other theories, while it stranded still other theories for long periods of time. As a result, the process has been contradictory and uneven for women; we have not had control over the many shifting currents of fact-making and yet we have had to deal with the ability of this fact-making to concretely impact on our pregnant bodies, in the form of obstetric schemes of management which we have been unable to withstand.

Natural–Preternatural

A basic problem which has been set for us is the relationship posed by obstetrics with the natural domain, as men midwives took on their fact-making work. Early scientific knowledge about labour and birth is organised around the distinction between 'natural' and 'preternatural', meaning outside the natural or ordinary course of events. This dichotomy represents a pivotal stage in the genesis of obstetric knowledge, in which all labours, no matter what their individual characteristics, must first be placed in one category or the other. The basis for arguing about the necessity for intervention in the labour process follows on from this division between 'natural' and 'preternatural', preternatural labours becoming most readily the focus of obstetric intervention. But not surprisingly, men midwives do not agree about where this division between the two actually comes, let alone about the best response to make.

In the twenty-third chapter of his treatise, Deventer writes of 'a natural or most easy birth' and lists fourteen conditions which must be met before a birth can be designated this way. The woman must be free of all infirmities and her womb must be sound and 'well placed'.[27] The baby must not be hindered in being born by a misshapen pelvis or any other defect of the birth canal or a disproportion between its size and the size of the mother. The baby has to be alive when birth commences (a baby which dies *in utero* is thought to make a difficult birth). The birth cannot be premature, before the full nine months, nor can the baby be 'monstrous', because any significant physical defect inevitably delays birth. The birth must be achieved by the force of the labour pains, which must be constant and which do not require assistance, and the baby must be born head-first, that is, in the vertex position. If there is a multiple birth, all must be born head first to be considered natural. The birth process can exhibit no untoward symptoms and the after-birth or placenta must follow 'without any remarkable hindrance'. If one or more of these 'requisites' is absent, it is 'a difficult birth':[28]

> Therefore by a natural Birth . . . we understand such a one, as is only performed by the Force of Nature, without Art or other Help.[29]

Deventer is keeping a 'Natural Birth here to stricter Limits, than other Authors do, because for that Reason it is the easier for me to describe a preter-natural or difficult Birth'.[30] In a natural birth, the midwife does her duty if

> she receives the Infant, cuts off the Navel-string, takes care of the Infant, by washing and nourishing it, or recommends that to be done by any of the gossips.[31]

Any birth that falls outside the criteria Deventer outlines for a natural birth requires 'Art and Assistence' and

> it is necessary for young Midwives to know how they may behave themselves upon any Occasion, that they may assist the Woman in Labour.[32]

Deventer tells his readers that his definition of 'preternatural labour' can help determine when assistance must be given to a woman and therefore it should become a part of the teaching for young midwives. But this division of easy and difficult labours was to have far-reaching consequences for obstetric science, well beyond the possibilities of instructing young women midwives who were still the main caretakers at the beginning of the eighteenth century. It gradually opened up the most amazing field in which the dense singularity of each individual birth process was made to conform progressively to averaged-out and normative criteria. It established that the scope for a birth attendant was non-interventionist only when such a range of contingent conditions could be met that almost nothing was excluded. Finally, it set in train the notion that only in retrospect could a birth be considered natural, for only at completion of the third stage of labour, once the placenta was delivered, could all these criteria be assessed. The consequence of this theorising was that a field of continuous surveillance and intervention, stretching to cover all births, was legitimated.[33]

Turning to Elizabeth Nihell's views on this issue of what constitutes natural and preternatural, the distinction which she puts forward appears at first glance to emphasise only the presentation of the foetus, that is, which part of the foetal body enters the pelvic inlet first, as it travels down towards the birth canal. Nihell defines a 'natural' birth as being 'that in which the foetus comes out in the most ordinary way, when it presents the head foremost' while a preternatural birth is 'when the foetus presents in the passage any other part than the head'.[34] However, Nihell does not argue that a preternatural birth, by definition, becomes a birth requiring intervention, for she establishes a crucial second distinction between easy and difficult births:

> The delivery is termed easy when the foetus comes out readily, and without the aid of art. It is termed difficult, when the labour of it is hard, and the foetus does not make its way out but with pain, and with the help and assistent industry of the midwife.[35]

She argues that both natural and preternatural births can be either easy or difficult. So a preternatural birth, where the foetal part presenting itself in the birth canal is not the head, as with a breech birth for example, can still be an easy birth in which the midwife's help is limited to 'receiving the foetus, tying the navel-string, giving the child to be kept warm, and then delivering the mother of the after-birth'.[36] For Nihell then, the scope for intervention is a more limited one:

> when the foetus presents itself promisingly, Nature is best left to her own action, and nothing should be precipitated in the manual function, unless some unexpected accident should intervene.[37]

It is the difficult births, regardless of the presenting part, which open up the field of assistance. This is at once a simpler and more complex division than that of Deventer. Nihell readily concedes that there are 'those cases of labor, which are much the less frequent, and require no extraordinary assistence' but assistance nonetheless. Her central argument is that in difficult labours, it is the skills of 'manual operations', rather than the instruments men midwives reach for too quickly, which will support 'the kindness of that Nature' and bring labour to a happy conclusion.[38] The ability to discriminate between an easy or difficult birth and therefore, whether or not a woman is in need of skilled assistance, is part of the midwife's knowledge and indicates the grasp she has of her art. In Deventer's scheme, no great judgement is required to establish when one assists a woman. Unless she is able to give birth with absolutely no help or support whatsoever, which cannot be completely determined until the birth is over, she must be aided.

Both Nihell and Deventer favour the practice of 'touching' or vaginal examination, seeing it as essential to gain knowledge of this fundamental distinction, and in this practice, not for the first time, Nihell aligns herself more closely with obstetric practice than with traditional midwifery practice.[39] Deventer describes the technique thus:

> The Touch is made with the two Fore-fingers of the Right or Left Hand, as the Posture of the Person, or the Womb will admit . . . two Fingers are applied to the Touch, that every thing may be better distinguished by the Sense; for with two Fingers we may encompass and measure any Thing, which we can scarce do with one.[40]

Nihell agrees that 'thence are derived the surest prognostics for preparation'.[41] Only by touching can the midwife be certain of whether the os uteri has begun to dilate, what foetal part is presenting, whether the membranes have ruptured. She even quotes, with favour for once, her arch-rival, the London man midwife William Smellie, on the importance of touching.[42] Deventer argues that the midwife will know she is dealing with an easy birth when she 'can easily touch it [the foetal head] in the Borders of the Vagina and hath no occasion to press her Fingers further into her Body.'[43] Conversely,

> when the Midwife tries the Woman by the Touch, and finds the Mouth of the Womb higher, but a little, or not at all open, sharp, thick and hard, or the Humours [membranes] pressed up lengthwise, then there is occasion for the greatest Caution.[44]

Of course, once touching is put forward as a way of monitoring a labour, the grounds for intervention open up anyhow because the basis on which there can be a 'natural', that is, unaided birth, is discarded. Birth is already subject to the authority of examination and an authoritative voice other than the woman.[45]

Deventer's thinking on the value of midwifery and on issues like skilled women midwives handling birth as a matter of course, or the avoidance of instrumental deliveries, are close to Nihell's position some eighty years later. This is not surprising, given that he is writing when women midwives still command the field of childbirth care. However, despite his acknowledgement of women as primary caretakers on birth, his expanded concept of preternatural birth, along with what he sees as the appropriate forms of assistance to deal with circumstances which can be designated as preternatural, constitute a new and convincing model for the emerging science.

As the eighteenth century wears on, the disquiet about preternatural births lines up with the notion of inherent incompetence of both labouring women and women birth attendants. Fielding Ould's writing exemplifies this process. In his book, *A Treatise of Midwifry in Three Parts*, Ould argues that although 'the concurring Circumstances which contribute to Parturition are surprizingly beautiful . . . these are frequently impeded, from various Causes both internal and external'.[46]

Doubt about the reliability of the female body is balanced by certainty of observations and techniques, 'which have Truth and Demonstration on their Side, being confirmed by Practice'[47] that can come to the assistance of that unreliable body.

In a manner that appears similar to Nihell's categories, Ould distinguishes a natural from a preternatural labour on the basis of foetal presentation alone, a natural labour being the head presenting first. But his is a tripartite division, in which he presents instructions on natural labours, preternatural labours, and preternatural labours where 'Hands alone are not capable of affording Relief'.[48] Importantly, however, he also states that intervention is required for all labours. These include 'labours which are difficult and against Nature, though the Child be in a natural Direction' and those where 'the greatest Danger arises from the indirect or preternatural Situation of the Child in the Womb'.[49] But, when Ould argues that 'accidents' can 'render the most natural Labour, preternatural',[50] he shifts the meaning of preternatural to include anything which can go wrong and from there argues that this is why all labours require intervention and tight control:

> We are to consider the natural Situation of the Child in Time of Labour, with a little more Circumspection than has hitherto been observed . . . for want of a strict Regard to this Circumstance, many natural Labours have become in the End, very tedious and dangerous; nay, in all probability often mortal to both.[51]

By 'tedious' Ould means a labour that is progressing too slowly. With the category of natural labour now subdivided into 'natural tedious labour', the problem of time enters into the picture for male midwifery. And whether a labour should be allow to go slowly or be hastened along is destined to become an important criterion in determining whether a woman is exposed to danger in birth.[52] Here, with Ould's assertion, we can also note that if all labours have the potential to become dangerous, the designation 'natural' loses its meaning of birth being able to be accomplished without external aid. A 'natural' presentation is no guarantee in itself against disaster and the 'Operator', as Ould aptly designates the man midwife, must always be ready to intervene:

> The assistance of a surgeon particularly instructed in the art of deliveries is generally necessary in the most natural labours; first as they have it in their power from their skill of the art, founded on their knowledge of the animal oeconomy in general and the surgical operations in particular to prevent at least one third of the pain [which] without their assistance must happen. And secondly by their preventing labours originally natural from becoming the contrary which is too often the case under the misconduct of female midwives of which we have frequent opportunities of being convinced as the existing Treatise will sufficiently prove.[53]

Note also his declaration that women are too feeble to survive labour unaided and that midwifery is not safe in the hands of women midwives.

Ould's conviction that speed in delivering a baby was essential lest the birth begin to move towards calamity was reinforced by his belief that women were unable to sustain the pain of labour and led to his developing a slate of interventionist tactics, applying them to both classes of labour, natural and preternatural.

For natural labours, Ould taught that the amniotic sac or membranes should be ruptured, if they have not already ruptured of their own accord, by piercing them with a fingernail or a pointed instrument; he recommended sweeping round the edge of the cervix with the fingers to force dilatation; he also favoured thrusting the thumb into the anus and pulling back the coccyx and so 'assisting a weak Patient in her last Labour-Pains'.[54] The purpose of this latter manoeuvre was to 'fix it under the Child's Jawbone' to pull 'the Child forward with the Finger bent under the Jaw'.[55] This method had 'never before been taken notice of by any Author . . . which I wonder at, for the good Effects of it, are obvious to the meanest Capacity'.[56] Ould is pulling up the baby's chin and extending the head, making the diameter which must clear through the pelvis and birth canal wider, rather than flexing it to make the diameter smaller; his manoeuvre actually makes it harder to give birth to the head. The description and Ould's justification are an excellent example of fact-making where evidence is made to conform to Ould's conceptions of the body.[57] Ould is still dealing here with a natural labour, according to his definition, but he has already concluded that the woman is too 'weak' to push out the baby unaided.

Remembering as well the rationales he produces for the episiotomy, it can be said that Ould is strongly representative of the first of two strands in male midwifery, which was committed to intervening and overruling the body in labour rather than supporting it. The second strand, where men midwives wrote about not acting hastily, was not destined to become the dominant paradigm. Gélis argues that the first strand, an interventionist one, was at least as evident in the work of women midwives as of men midwives, based on historical accounts of many local and regional practices in France; he further argues that the time of labour was perceived differently by obstetricians and women midwives, the former because they had an understanding of the mechanism of labour based on allowing Nature to do its work unaided; the latter working with a metaphor about nature based on changing seasons.[58] We shall see below that even this reading of Nature by men midwives was strongly disadvantageous for women and that it still presented a deeply gendered and thus a flawed account of the physiology of labour and birth. If women midwives in the rural areas of France urged that the fruit of pregnancy, the baby, like the harvest, must be gathered up quickly, such views on speed, if not the precise metaphors and techniques, were to re-emerge and become deeply entrenched in the practices of men midwives.

Ould's interventions are the more curious when viewed from the perspective that theory is based on observable facts; indeed it was one of his claims that he made the 'strictest examination' of every woman he delivered or saw delivered. Yet in his 'Direction for the Management of Women in natural Labours', he instructs the 'Operator' to 'stay nigh' the patient 'for the Hand is of Service in the most easy Labours'. He argues that because

> the same Efforts that break the Membranes, thrust the Head into the Orifice, which is not yet large enough to give it Passage without Violence; wherefore the Assistance of the Hand must be administered in this Manner: It must be introduced as the Pain begins, and as the Head is forced down, endeavour to thrust the Edge of the Orifice up; and do all that is possible without committing Violence, to make the Orifice quite pass over the Head; by this Means, the Labour is not only hastened, but the present Pain much lessened.[59]

The force of the descent of the foetal head is what enables it to move unaided out from under the symphysis pubis, which Ould describes as the 'Edge of the Orifice'. But his insistence on hastening labour gives rise to an analysis of the labour process which distorts this observable reality and this from the man who was the first writer to commit to print the description of the internal rotation of the head during labour. His comments are an instance of a practice erected on what Nihell termed 'the crazy foundation of false principle';[60] in Fleck's terms it might also be described as an example of a 'self-contained system of opinion', which is so difficult to contest from outside the science.[61]

I have suggested that not all practitioners were agreed on such an interventionist regime as Ould's, being inclined to let 'Nature' do the work of labour. William Dease, who was surgeon to the hospitals of St Nicholas and St Catherine in Dublin towards the end of the eighteenth century, was one such who wrote a treatise, *Observations in Midwifery Particularly on the Different Methods of Assisting Women in tedious and difficult Labours*, in 1783. Dease preserves the basic distinction of natural and preternatural labour, based on the presenting part, but he argues that 'natural labours are best terminated when the surgeon intermeddles least'.[62] Dease is opposed to techniques like manual dilatation, forcing back the coccyx, and to artificially rupturing the membranes, and he advises shielding the perineum as the foetal head crowns in labour, rather than resorting to pulling at the perineal tissues or to the episiotomy. He argues that there are 'tedious natural labours' which frequently occur with women in labour for the first time where the 'only line of conduct the surgeon should pursue, is to wait patiently the efforts of nature, and to avoid teizing the woman by fruitless endeavours in dilating the os uteri'.[63]

But there are also 'difficult' natural labours, where 'neither the efforts of the woman, nor the hand of the surgeon can effect delivery', without resorting to instruments. The head presents in a vertex position but there are problems of pelvic disproportion, maternal haemorrhage, convulsions or frequent fainting, where the woman has become too weak 'to assist herself', or where the 'head of the child is morbidly enlarged'.[64] Finally, there are preternatural labours which are a 'wrong presentation of the child'. The 'axiom' found in the various discourses is to 'immediately proceed to delivery by the feet' which 'operation' the surgeon carries out manually, introducing his hand into the uterus when he finds the os uteri 'soft and dilated and that the membranes have burst, or are just ready to burst'.[65]

In Dease's work, we can see the complete system of categorising birth which soon becomes standard in hospital practices: it moves from easy natural births to tedious and difficult natural births to preternatural births. Deventer's definition has thus remained substantially unchanged; what has been added are discrete subcategories, like tedious labour. Nihell's account of easy preternatural labours, where a breech birth can take place without any great assistance, has been excluded entirely. And, despite his statements about not intervening, Dease's treatise serves as an indication that obstetric thinking is also becoming characterised by the problem of frequency – how frequently the less than easy natural birth occurs. Notwithstanding 'the great variety that exists' amongst births, practitioners are bedevilled by how many things go wrong:

> Although women, in general, are enabled by the efforts of nature, with very little assistance, to bring forth their children; yet many cases frequently occur in practice, which require the utmost exertion of the surgeon's abilities.[66]

The political problem which the category of frequency poses for women is that modes of management, based on the premiss of what has gone wrong, are soon extended to cover what *might* go wrong.

One of the odder aspects of this argument on frequency is that 'malpresentations' are observed to be class-related, yet the idea of frequent occurrence is applied to labours in general and theory develops on the latter assumption. For example, Ould observes that 'the poor who are by much the greater number [are] most subject to misfortunes in childbearing.'[67] The man midwife who attends women from the poorest sections of the community encounters women who may well be in a physically vitiated state, suffering in far more frequent numbers from malnutrition, anaemia, and rickets, all of which complicate their well-being in childbirth; rickets, for example, will predispose them to problems of malpresentation in labour as a result of their deformed pelves. But the connection between poverty and maternal ill-health is made and just as soon abandoned. Dealing with the social conditions which might contribute to maternal ill-health was never going to be the bailiwick of obstetrics.

Retrospectively, we can locate two broad reasons for these 'accidents' of labour, the first being the problem of a woman who has been pregnant too many times. The muscles of her abdomen become stretched and flaccid, giving rise to problems during labour, like increased instances of a transverse lie, where the foetus lies across her abdomen and never engages; or because the uterus is less able to contract, she experiences post-partum haemorrhage after the baby's birth. The second broad set of reasons is related to the general ill-health and poor nutritional status that inevitably afflicts women living in poverty. The overall political problem is how frequently these events impact on birth outcomes and how this might be responded to in schemes of birth management. Going back to the issue of rachitic pelves, for example, Louden estimates that the incidence of rachitic or contracted pelves in European lying-in hospitals in the eighteenth and nineteenth centuries ranged from under 1 per 1,000 cases to 12.8 per 1,000 cases, with corresponding problems during labour.[68] Shorter estimates that there was a possible 25 per cent total risk for women from all complications arising from pregnancy over the fertile years, or a one-in-four lifetime chance of experiencing a serious difficulty,[69] but these odds always increased in relation to poverty. The obstetric concern with frequency of preternatural labours was ultimately related to the consequences of possible maternal death for its reputation. Allied to the business of building schools of thought and reputations, statistics to illustrate the problems of labour and the beneficial outcomes for women under particular schemes of childbirth management became commonplace in obstetric writing, albeit without the political dimension of women's broader welfare.

In what is effectively the first clinical report of the Rotunda Hospital, Joseph Clarke, its sixth Master, offers statistics on 10,387 births. These are divided first by the categories of natural and preternatural labours. The natural labours are then subdivided into 'ordinary', 'tedious' and 'laborious' births while the preternatural births are further subdivided by presenting part, whether 'footling', 'breech' or 'cross'. Their use indicates that not only are these distinctions moving 'downstream' in obstetric thinking and writing, they are also accompanied by an increasing density of description and numbers to underscore their relevance, marking another stage in the evolution of scientific language about labour. Clarke writes of the conduct of 'ordinary Natural Labours' with an approach similar to Dease on non-intervention:

> It contributes greatly to the safety of the mother and the child, to allow the uterus gradually to empty itself during delivery, first by expelling the head of the foetus and afterwards the shoulders and body, by subsequent pains, with little or no aid.[70]

Clarke is concerned about a natural labour which is rendered 'tedious either by causes weakening the expelling powers of the mother, or increasing resistance to the passage of the foetus' and suggests a regime of mild nourishment and medicines, including opiates, in the belief that although such labours are 'not without danger both to mother and child', 'the powers of the constitution' seldom fail in bringing labour to a safe conclusion.[71] On the other hand, 'nothing but mischief' can be expected from using the forceps in these cases. Although he concedes their use in fourteen cases, sometimes swayed, he writes, by 'the sanguine expectations of my assistants', he concludes that forceps are 'rational and justifiable' only when 'the expelling powers are impaired by debilitating diseases'.[72] Clarke relates that forceps have been used during his Mastership in the ratio of one in every 728 deliveries, in a total of 10,387 births. He also states that it has been so long since he even thought of using them in his private practice that 'I am persuaded a fair opportunity of applying forceps with good effect will not occur to a rational practitioner in one of a thousand cases.'[73]

Here once more is this notion of class difference, suggesting that women in the upper classes experience fewer instances of some forms of hardship in birth.[74] Clarke has a number of observations on class-based differences in birth outcomes. For example, he writes that poorer women suffer more frequently from 'cross presentations', that is when the foetus presents in a transverse lie across the mother's uterus rather than on a vertical axis; and because impoverished women call in midwives who proceed to try and perform version and turn the child in the uterus, their outcome is poorer:

> Our practice in the hospital must appear unsuccessful, but much of this is to be attributed to injudicious attempts to turn, and sometimes to pull away, the foetus by the presenting arm before the admission of the patient ... among the lower orders of women in this city many of such mismanaged cases occur.[75]

Cross presentations are probably most directly related to parity; the more children a woman bears, the greater is the laxity of her abdominal muscles. They can often result in an obstructed labour with either an arm or shoulder presenting itself first. In his history of reproductive care, Shorter has argued on available figures, that a woman who gave birth five times ran a one-in-ten lifetime chance of a transverse lie, thus requiring internal version.[76]

Clarke is anxious to defend his hospital from the charge of mismanagement, once they have taken in these difficult cases. If internal version or pulling on the arm or feet have already been tried and have failed, it is extremely hard to do anything else to mitigate the conditions of labour and he advises performing a destructive operation, to afford a 'better chance to patients so situated'.[77] Forty-eight cases of cross presentation occur while he is Master; six end in the woman's death; in only thirteen does the child survive birth.

'Laborious parturitions' are largely the result of the problem of misshapen pelves, again occurring more frequently amongst the poorest women. The practitioner faces this with dread, for where the available space for the foetal head is reduced to three-and-a-half inches or less, compared with four-and-a-half or more in an 'ordinary natural labour', 'a violent struggle ensues during labour'.[78] With the foetal head compressed for many hours, great damage is done to the woman's bladder and the urethra with the result that 'mortification' sets in, or as it would now be described, when these tissues are crushed for a long time and thus deprived of oxygen, they provide a breeding ground for anaerobic bacteria. This is frequently followed by a woman's death. If women remain undelivered, due to obstruction, they will die in any case. They may also die as a result of the effects of the operation with perforator and crotchet to release the foetal body. There are forty-nine 'bad pelvises' in his years as Master amongst his 10,000 plus cases, on which number he comments 'I cannot help remarking the goodness of Providence to the female sex . . . [this] is surely a very small proportion.'[79] But Clarke is essentially conservative and the small number does not persuade him to pursue an operative midwifery on a greater number, just in case anything might be awry. Nevertheless, he seeks observable facts to support his conclusion for his work is part of a science. Only after dissecting 'the bodies of many women, who died following tedious and laborious labours', does Clarke conclude that three-and-a-quarter inches is the very smallest diameter he has seen through which a full-grown foetal head has passed 'entire', although the foetus had died sometime before in the uterus, making the head more pliable than that of a live child.[80] Clarke writes:

> Under the best management, and where an accoucheur does his duty conscientiously towards the foetus, a laborious parturition is attended with great danger to the mother. Our hospital abstract shews that one in three died; but as I had occasion to remark of tedious cases we frequently received our patients after having suffered greatly by mismanagement.[81]

He refers here to a tension between what it is possible to do for the foetus and what one has to do in the interests of the mother, a subject to which we will return below. Not all practitioners are in agreement with him for, as he tells us, his own assistants are prepared to use the forceps in slow labours. But he is in no way convinced by their results that it is a safer practice for the woman with a slow labour.

An especially notable feature of Clarke's registry is his punctilious attention to recording detail, in comparison with earlier treatises. He sets out the problem of managing difficult natural labours in a recognisably scientific frame of reference. There are statistics, intervals of occurrence, a specialised language which draws on the lessons gained from dissection, and references to modes of practice for particular circumstances advanced by other men midwives. His subdivisions of slow (tedious) and obstructed (laborious) labour are convincing scientific definitions, above all because they are delimited by conditions thought to be measurable. The former is distinguished by a limit on the length of time beyond which a labour is thus classified, twenty-four hours, and by the caveat that there must be no pelvic disproportion involved. In other words, this labour can be brought to a conclusion without using destructive instruments. A laborious labour will be 'protracted beyond 24 hours' and additionally, because of severe disproportion 'between the head of the foetus and the pelvis' will require the use of instruments 'to diminish the bulk of the former to save the life of the latter'.[82] Each individual labour must begin to conform to specific criteria for purposes of classification, but the scheme of classification itself is delimited in part by the recommended treatment. Finally, it should be noted that by far the greater bulk of this medical report is taken up with the problematic and irregular instances of labour, the complications of which, though numerically tiny – there are 9,748 cases of ordinary labour amongst his 10,387 women – are the basis for obstetric medicine.

Classification and Treatment: Constructing Black Boxes

The natural-preternatural dyad is firmly in place as a fundamental element in obstetric knowledge production by the 1780s, operating rather like a 'black box'. We have come to understand a 'black box' as a complex set of constructs about which one need have only the most basic information in order to use it.[83] Belief in a 'black box' as a fact is actually strengthened through usage. So for instance, men midwives accept that the complexity of labour can be adequately expressed by reference to this division between natural and preternatural labour (rather than speaking of labour as a time when like the ripe fruit dropping from the tree, the baby is born). There is broad agreement that the criteria generated by this basic dyad can be objective, measurable and transferable from case to case while debate and controversy apply not to the dyad itself but to definitions and modes of treatment within its subdivisions.

Comparing the work of Clarke, Ould, and Nihell is instructive on how arguments emerge about these subdivisions. Clarke's analysis of tedious natural labours, for example, is grounded in the concept or precept that within certain limits, a woman's own constitution can be relied upon to revive sufficiently to bring labour to a close. Therefore, he justifies a conservative management which rules out the use of instruments and also techniques like Ould's, of pulling back the coccyx, or pulling back the upper edge of the vaginal outlet. Clarke advises 'mild' rather than 'stimulating' nourishment and medicines and a continuation of what he says is the established hospital regime, of keeping women in a 'cool atmosphere' and 'prevent[ing] them making voluntary exertions during the dilatation of the os tincae'.[84]

And, despite Clarke's opposition to women midwives, he is not too far removed from Nihell's stance on 'difficult' natural births, wherein she demands a non-instrumental approach. Yet differences have emerged by the time Clarke is practising which have a concrete impact on labour. Clarke's comment on restraining women is more than just evidence that women are not able to exercise their own preferences during labour in a hospital setting. It also betrays elements of the male midwifery discourse about the female body as a fragile entity.[85] In cases of protracted 'natural' labour, Nihell takes a more active role, seeking to support a woman's physiology rather than accepting her body as a passive inert object on which 'Nature' works:

> When the membranes are not too soon pierced and the waters let out, when the pains are not provoked, when time is given to Nature to form to herself a passage . . . when due care is taken to procure all possible ease of body and mind to the patient; who may vary her posture, sometimes lying along, sometimes sitting up, or well supported when she walks: little by little the head will frank itself a passage with the weight of the body acting by an innate energy, and with a little due assistance of the midwife's art: and with this practical advertence, that in these arduous cases, much may be safely left to Nature, but not every thing.[86]

The angle at which women are sitting, lying or standing is, as Nihell indicates, not just a matter of custom but germane to actively assisting the labour in progress, with the woman herself making the decisions about what is best for her. By contrast, Ould's preference for having women lying on the left lateral side during labour became the norm in the Rotunda, gaining for the men midwives who followed on after him the advantage in being able to see the birth outlet, but losing the clear physiological advantage that Nihell had observed in her practice. Ould's interventionism arises because he has theorised the body as enfeebled female material that requires total management to rescue women from the pain and death which he otherwise predicts as the too frequent outcome of labour. Clarke is curiously ambivalent, theorising the body as having natural powers to recover, if the man midwife waits, but also seeing the body as fragile and irritable and therefore not to be manipulated if at all possible. Nihell is unafraid to use her midwife's skill to actively support the body, which skill will bring about a safe labour.

These differences enable us to see that observation does lead to discovery, to theory, and feeds back to practice, but theory is as variable as the observations on which it is based and the practices to which it leads can range from the uncomfortable, like being confined to bed while in early labour, to the disastrous, as with the use of forceps. Thus a self-contained system of opinion impacts on the process of observation, on what individual practitioners see as happening and what they subsequently interpret on the basis of their observation. What also becomes more visible is the one obvious aspect that drops out of the texts, the skills to support the woman's body in labour, especially with the hands. In the wake of this loss, it can be argued that male midwifery becomes influenced almost exclusively by instruments and whether practitioners are for or against their use being expanded.

The process of building the natural-preternatural dyad in the eighteenth century also enables us to see what an essential role is played by the circulation of emerging theories. Dease, Clarke, Nihell and Ould all refer in their texts to the work of others. Nihell references her work most extensively, citing no fewer than twenty-four men midwives, many of them French, but also English, Dutch, German, and Danish practitioners. She is especially thorough in reviewing the arguments of various men midwives for using instruments and the types of instruments they are advocating. Ould concentrates on opposing the theories of Deventer and Mauriceau, while Dease reviews the theory and practice of the seventeenth and eighteenth centuries, including Ould's work. Clarke refers to many of his contemporaries, the men midwives already working within a lying-in ward or hospital, like Charles White in Manchester. Clarke is also writing during a period when theories are first being floated in essays in the medical journals which have begun to mushroom, some of which Clarke quotes. These represent the beginnings of what Fleck terms 'journal science', that is science for experts, where the notions are often still provisional and personal but are nonetheless gaining broad exposure.[87]

By the end of the eighteenth century, the sheer volume of obstetric writing is itself decisive in advancing this newly legitimated field. The circulation of journal articles and treatises alike indicates the collective nature of the process of fact-making.[88] Despite the thoroughness of her work, Nihell's writing does not become scientifically legitimated in this expanding literature, but gets pushed 'upstream' as artefact or fiction. She survives into the twentieth century in orthodox obstetric histories as the midwife who attacked William Smellie with 'venom' and is otherwise associated with 'rubbish' and 'superstition'.[89] Once the perspective that she represents was lost, on using hands as an essential part of training for midwifery, it is arguable that obstetric controversies became over-determined by the existence of instruments. Certainly, within obstetrics itself, the precept of 'watchful waiting' which was seen as the obverse of 'meddlesome midwifery' arose partly in response to the terrible damage that was observed from wholesale intervention, whether the source was untrained women midwives, manipulating uteri and pulling at the placenta, or men midwives, eager to 'hasten' labour through forceps, amongst other instruments.

Such experiences clearly influenced Clarke, for instance, who rejected on the one hand, 'ignorant' female midwives and on the other, men midwives who favoured overt intervention. But what Clarke dismissed as inadequate and even unsafe practice, other practitioners, with equal conviction, argued was correct, a disagreement which turned on the interpretation of one of the subdivisions within the natural-preternatural dyad. We will examine this debate in the next section where we see an example of how obstetrics attempts to come to terms with the problem of its own errors.

Error/Truth: the Hamilton–Collins Dispute on Time and 'Meddlesome Midwifery'

Writing of science in the making, Latour points out the benefits of examining the process of fact construction before constructions achieve the status of a black box. There is often fierce controversy in which the disputants push one another's arguments 'back into their conditions of production' and from that vantage point, we can see more readily how they actually come to accept their black boxes.[90] So, in order to trace the lines of any given controversy, we must not only open the black box but reopen the controversy which precedes it.

Although the natural-preternatural dyad was achieved with relative ease (and perhaps because perspectives like those of Nihell could be so conveniently ignored), an interesting controversy then arose on the subdivisions of natural births. Clarke had already expanded these to include criteria on time, on how long a labour could continue and still be in one rather than another category. In 1837, an article by Robert Collins, twelfth Master of the Rotunda, appeared in the pages of the *Dublin Journal of Medical Science* on the subject of artificial dilatation of the cervix during labour. Collins was responding to a two-volume obstetrics text, *Observations on Midwifery*, written by Professor James Hamilton of Edinburgh, in which the latter had disputed both the statistics and the approach to labour management described in Collins' own *Practical Treatise on Midwifery*, published in 1836, a volume which covered over 16,000 deliveries in his seven years as Master. The issue Hamilton had raised was whether a woman's safety in childbirth could be maintained, if the length of time the first stage of labour, when the cervix was dilating, was allowed to continue beyond a specified period. Hamilton devoted a huge portion of his work to setting up his argument that the first stage of labour must be completed no later than fourteen hours after labour commenced, for, after that time, the 'natural efforts' of the body could not be relied upon to carry labour to a safe conclusion. Hamilton had been directing midwifery practice in the main Edinburgh hospital since 1800 and had always instructed his pupils to terminate the first stage of labour after fourteen hours by artificial dilatation, followed by a forceps to effect delivery, bringing the labour to a close quickly and thus, he argued, preserving the mother's life.

Collins, who was Joseph Clarke's son-in-law, had been deeply influenced by the latter's teaching on non-interference with tedious labours, the 'watchful waiting' of conservative midwifery. In his treatise, Clarke argued that as long as the pulse was good, the bladder and bowels were regulated to function well, the 'soft parts' remained free of pressure, and uterine action continued, labour could proceed with no harm to the mother and, indeed, stated he could guarantee her safety under such conditions.[91] Collins worked in a similar manner and in 15,850 of his 16,414 cases in the Rotunda, where the length of labour had been noted from its commencement, '15,084 were delivered within twelve hours, 15,586 within twenty-four; leaving only 130 above that period.'[92] Collins expressed dismay that what he saw as the successful course first pursued by Clarke, was not universally adhered to for the greater safety and well-being of women who had tedious labours. He resolutely opposed 'mischievous interference to promote hasty delivery'[93] and was dismissive of Hamilton's prognoses: 'Surely no experienced practitioner would be guided as to the safety or otherwise of his patient when in labour, by the number of hours but by the present symptoms and previous history.'[94] Collins later argued that these 'unsound doctrines' could be rebutted by 'the unquestionable truths' that were recorded in the statistical profiles of the Rotunda.[95]

When a scientist speaks of 'unsound doctrines' and 'unquestionable truths', what can be his basis for making such assertions? When men midwives considered the problem of 'truths', they were drawing on a discourse about the certainty of hard facts that has a lengthy history in Western culture. Descartes, for example, in his *Discourse on Method*, reasoned that it was both possible and necessary to construct a method whereby error was avoided in order to arrive at truth which was discoverable. He argued that he could 'discover the falsehood or incertitude of the propositions I examined, not by feeble conjectures, but by clear and certain reasonings'.[96] Collins' comment perhaps looks back to this tradition but significantly looks forward to the potential that statistical measurements will hold for science to make its facts still harder. Whatever the growth and subsequent splits in different methods of scientific enquiry, this discourse about creating true, hard facts has continuing resonance for its internal disputations (because the more of your fellow scientists you can convince of your arguments, the more these are rendered into hard facts). But the discourse of hard facts is also viable in a different way when science presents its work to non-scientists, for certainty is the face science puts forward to the outside world to justify its endeavours. Latour refers to this as one side of the Janus-face of science. Latour also comments that harder facts are the exception in science rather than the rule and are necessary in only a few cases in order to 'displace others on a large scale out of their usual ways'.[97] The usefulness of the rhetoric about hard facts, is, I think, undeniable for obstetric science in the making, which was trying to account for its newly occupied territory.

Deventer gives us a good early example of adherence to the notion that truth can be separated from error on the basis of observation when he writes: 'I do not spend my Time in trying this or that Method, but proceed in that which is the shortest and most certain.'[98] Similarly, Nihell is completely convinced that it is 'not by authority but by reason that truth claims acceptance from reasonable beings'.[99] Nihell inadvertently summarises the debate that is to follow when she writes of tedious labours, 'where nature is slow, as she sometimes is in her operation . . . a quicker expulsion would only destroy [the patient]' and she then attacks the men who 'from their natural impatience' rely on their 'infernal iron and steel instruments' to terminate labour.[100]

The problem in the Hamilton–Collins debate is that each exactly applied, so far as he was concerned, a rule of method to interpreting the available evidence and emerged with radically different conclusions. Collins declared of his position:

> These truths are all clearly shewn in the tables published by me, and markedly exhibit the great utility of registering simple facts, which, if accumulated sufficiently overpower all theory or argument opposed, and alone can form the basis of sound reasoning.[101]

Hamilton replied to Collins, first in the *London Medical Gazette* in 1837, and then in the *Dublin Journal of Medical Science* in 1838, reinterpreting Collins' regime on protracted labour and his reported cases and seizing on Collins' mortality figures to argue that the Rotunda method of treatment of tedious labour had not only resulted in higher mortality figures than were necessary, but also in a greater number of destructive operations, using the crotchet when compared with similar institutions elsewhere.

The Hamilton–Collins debate was carried out in the context of birth becoming a dangerous event, in certain circumstances, with a question mark over the issue of how long a woman could continue in labour without danger to herself. According to Shorter, before 1900, labours lasting longer than twenty hours were a common enough event. The complications which a woman facing a prolonged labour may encounter, excluding obstructed labour, are increased incidences of infection, physical trauma and shock, all of which can lead to maternal death.[102] But there is no easy prediction of these complications and there is also the problem of how to define 'prolonged'. Reluctance to intervene at all came into this equation. We have already seen how resolutely opposed Clarke was to any form of intervention, but time itself now became an issue. Hamilton said of Collins that he refused to be guided in his treatment by a scale of time. He reiterated his position from his own treatise, that labour would be beneficially hastened, and the safety of the mother secured, by adopting the method of artificial dilatation first advanced by his colleague, Professor Burns of Glasgow, namely 'dilating gently with a finger if the os uteri be flat and if it be projecting by introducing two fingers, and extending them laterally with gentleness during a pain.'[103] The forceps could then be introduced rapidly, once dilatation had been achieved. Collins had already argued that when there were weak contractions for whatever reason, if the fingers acted in place of the uterus, they forced the head against the pelvis which brought its own hazards. He suggested that because the newly introduced stethoscope could be used to monitor the woman and determine whether the foetus was still alive, it made it easier to permit a labour to continue, rather than to end it abruptly with forceps which so often had disastrous consequences for both mother and baby. If foetal death *in utero* did occur, Collins had to intervene operatively, but taking this risk was preferable to early interference.[104] Hamilton rebutted this argument by publishing comparative statistics on the use of forceps, while the foetus was still alive, and the crotchet to release the dead foetal body. The following is a table of the composite statistics he presented:

Table 2.1: Statistics on Operative Midwifery

City	Ratio of Forceps to Normal Births	Ratio of Crotchet to Normal Births
Paris, Hospital de la Maternité	1 in 344⅔	1 in 1417
Edinburgh	1 in 109	1 in 481
Dublin, Rotunda	1 in 608	1 in 210

Source: J. Hamilton (1838). A letter from Professor Hamilton of Edinburgh in reply to the Objections made to his Practical Precepts in Midwifery by Dr Collins. In *Dublin Quarterly Journal of Medical Science*, vol. xiii, p. 219.

The essence of Hamilton's argument was that the Rotunda's insistence on 'watchful waiting' ultimately led to a far higher number of destructive operations because the hospital relied overly on the crotchet to deal belatedly with a situation which, by then, could be saved in no other way. Hamilton culled through Collins' case notes, re-presenting some of Collins' data to back his own interpretations. 'No. 665' was a classic instance, Hamilton charged, of this mismanagement. Quoting Collins, Hamilton retold how the woman was:

> 'thirty-five hours in labour of her first child, for the last 24 of which, the head had not made the least progress. Her strength being exhausted and the child being some hours dead as ascertained by the stethoscope, delivery was affected by lessening the head (the crotchet). She continued to recover favourably until the fourth day after delivery when she was suddenly attacked with the most acute pain in the abdomen which resisted the most active treatment and she died in 48 hours. On dissection a large quantity of deep, straw-coloured fluid was found in the abdominal cavity ... the vagina was in a sloughing state.'[105]

Hamilton contended that manual dilatation of the cervix, followed by forceps, would have saved the woman's life, rather than using the crotchet so late on that she lost her life, after the infant had also perished. As it happens, what the dissection notes reveal was that 'No. 665' contracted peritonitis, probably by either the crotchet being introduced into the uterus or an infection setting in where the tissues had been starved of oxygen in the birth canal, and the woman died as a result of the peritonitis.

Of course, the introduction of Hamilton's fingers to force dilatation, and the use of forceps to effect delivery, could easily have ended in the same loss of life, infection and peritonitis setting in as a result of his interventions. However, this debate between him and Collins did not focus on the causes of puerperal fever, if only because of the tendency to think of the labour process in fragments, which isolated puerperal fever as another accident of labour rather than a consequence of practice.

Nevertheless, Hamilton's argument, which linked the Rotunda regime, as it was known in the journals, with the over-use of the crotchet, was damaging to the hospital because individual hospitals were always sensitive to charges of treating maternal and infant life carelessly. So, it was no surprise that there was a further lengthy contribution in 1839, this time by E.W. Murphy, a Dublin obstetrician, in which he attacked Hamilton for looking at only one part of the whole of Collins' work. Tedious labour, Murphy argued, constituted 'perhaps the most difficult description of cases that is met with', for the 'very weakness of the constitution may retard the labour'. The cause of the delay was 'mental influence' and the practitioner had to respond to this 'constitutional disturbance', as best he could, lest any untoward action hurry on to catastrophe.[106] Because energy was so often lacking, and contractions ineffectual, the Rotunda regime of keeping the patient cool and quiet and administering opiates to suspend uterine action altogether, until the patient recovered her strength, was a sound procedure; because danger was ever present it was always necessary to impress on students that labour 'is a complex function performed by living tissues whose properties and energies are regulated by the peculiar temperament of individuals'.[107]

Murphy argued that the danger of Professor Hamilton's regime was that the inexperienced junior practitioner, who was anxious about a tedious labour, would adopt this 'meddlesome midwifery', finding it difficult to maintain his 'self-possession', especially when the friends of the patient might interpret his 'passive watchfulness' as a sign of ignorance.[108] Professor Hamilton's arguments were proof that

> if there be any error more prevalent in medical writings or more calculated to deprive medicine itself of any claim to the name of science, it is the habit of founding general principles on a few loosely collected facts in which everything, which might be made to support some pre-conceived theory, is put prominently forward and anything of a contrary tendency with equal care concealed.[109]

These are serious charges that Murphy makes, about what he judges to be a flawed application of the scientific method, especially when Hamilton's figures from his Edinburgh practice (which, by the way, are an early use of ratios) are put alongside Collins' summary figures. After all, Collins saw 16,414 women delivered in his seven years; 164 maternal deaths; 1,329 infants either dead when delivered or dead before the mother is discharged from hospital. Death is there, of course, but perhaps it is not the damaging all-inclusive threat that Hamilton's ratios might suggest and, besides, there is incomplete information from Hamilton on his rates of maternal and infant death. Collins' approach appears the more thorough, using 'present symptoms and previous history' of the individual woman, rather than relying on a rule about the length of labour applied across the board, like Hamilton's fourteen-hour rule. Collins' method seems the closer to getting at truth and discarding error. Interestingly, he is prepared to see labour as a highly individual process. Yet in using Clarke's work as his basis, Collins has continued on with a conservative management of women which still emphasises women's frailty: the woman is restrained in a supine position throughout labour, for example. His management also has physical consequences, contributing to longer labours for women which, despite the safeguards of his criteria for monitoring those labours, may inadvertently help contribute to their deaths.

Both the Clarke–Collins regime and Murphy's extension are an excellent example of Fleck's thesis that

> whether an individual construes it as truth or error, understands it correctly or not, a set of findings meanders through the community, becoming polished, transformed, reinforced or attenuated, while influencing other findings, concept formation, opinions.[110]

Over time, an interesting range of concepts in this specific debate spread into the general obstetric community: the critical part of Hamilton's argument, one that was to continue to be a determining influence on theories of obstetric management into the late twentieth century, was that the absolute length of labour, beyond which it becomes dangerous, can be determined by a set rule, and that it is then in the power of the practitioner to judge how to achieve delivery to meet that set rule. The logic of Hamilton's argument, which opens up the female body to multiple interventions, strikes a deep chord in Western medicine, a hospital-based medicine, where, as Ronald Frankenberg observes, time is the most important basis of medical power and control.[111]

The timing and staging of the body becomes a central concern in childbirth, as elsewhere in modernity, in an application of industrial time.[112] What one might say is that the stages of labour, an obstetric concept, subsume the action of labour which is an individual action. The individual woman's rhythm, and the work she accomplishes, is taken over by the averaged times which obstetrics allots to each phase of labour. This take-over of industrialised timing occurs simultaneously to women being subjected to techniques and procedures within the obstetric system of management which, in any case, tend to impair their capacity to labour within this pre-set time-frame. Given the self-containedness of obstetric thinking, which is so adverse to absorbing theories which do not come from within its own boundaries, partial notions like those of Murphy's explanation of tedious labour as psychological in origin, merge neatly with arguments about the need to control the length of labour, while Nihell's model, where the woman determines her own movement, as a possible strategy for dealing with labour is out of the running altogether.

The Mother–Foetus Dyad: The Challenge of Operative Midwifery

The Rotunda's original purpose, its charter stated, was to assist the 'many poor and distressed women, great with child, who by the sickness, death, absence, neglect or extreme poverty . . . are in lying-in frequently themselves and infants lost'.[113] Its purpose as a philanthropy was convenient to the intentions of the bio-politics associated with mercantilism and the reason why it received state funding from its foundation; the lying-in hospital was designed to support the economic function of childbirth because a population increase was held to be a necessary step to secure greater national wealth,

> for the increase in inhabitants most to be desired is amongst the lowest ranks ... to supply hands for tillage ... for the carrying on of manufactures, for doping the laborious part and drudgery of mechanics, for maintaining the safety and glory of the nation in the warlike forces of both elements, sometimes at present filled up not without difficulty.[114]

This was a typically grand ambition of the period, but in one sense the men midwives tended to even grander claims about their science, quite apart from their remit to rescue the women and children of the working classes. In their scheme of things, the dyad of the mother–foetus and their understanding of it was spoken about not just as the focus of their work but as their contribution to the basis of human civilisation. Ould, for example, wrote:

> It is the Duty of every one conversant in this Branch of the Art of Healing, to study, not only the Welfare of those particularly under his Care, but that of the whole Species ... for if his Design be honest, and visibly for the general Good of Mankind, I think there is no doubt but the more valuable Part of the World will esteem him for it.[115]

Measured against either goal, charity or the science of midwifery, their success was more limited than their claims. Between 1757 and 1828, the Rotunda recorded the following cumulative totals:

Table 2.2: Rotunda Statistics, 1757–1828

Category	Totals
Number of patients admitted	123,796
Went out not delivered	5,806
Delivered in the hospital	118,187
Boys born	62,647
Girls born	57,421
Total children born	120,068
Women having twins or more	1,903
Children died	5,408
Children stillborn	7,091
Women dead	1,420
Proportion of children dying in hospital to those living	1–21
Proportion of children stillborn to those born live	1–17
Proportion of women dying in childbed to those who survived	1–89

Source: *Reports of the Commissioners on Certain Charitable Institutions in Dublin, 1830, Appendix No. 6*, London: Irish Office, 1830.

Leaving out the curious item of the 5,000 women who left the hospital before they gave birth, about whom in the official histories, there is otherwise complete silence, just over 10 per cent of the women giving birth went home without a live baby.[116] Of the women who died, the overall average ratio of 1 to 89 ranges from 1 in 229 in 1795 to 1 in 30 in 1826, the first year of Collins' mastership. By the standards of many European lying-in hospitals, these were reasonable rates and their survival rates were key to the hospital's rationale about its ability to preserve maternal life. This was perhaps more easily asserted than that of preserving infant life, as long as the threat of epidemic puerperal fever did not materialise.

Edward Shorter argues that before the 1930s doctors had little interest in the foetus and that their concern over labour management had to do almost exclusively with the mother's life[117] or, as Clarke put it, with the '*safety* and *speedy recovery* of a puerperal woman'.[118] On the other hand, Shorter is not altogether accurate. There was less they could confidently argue that they could do on behalf of the foetus. But they did not avoid the issue altogether. The debate about forceps in the eighteenth century turned precisely on the claim to preserve infant life. Interventionists like Hamilton continued to make the case that such an approach to childbirth management increased the survival chances of both mother and foetus. And, on the other side of that divide, in the school of 'watchful waiting', Clarke wrote this about '*ordinary* Natural Labours':

> It contributes greatly to the safety of the mother and child, to allow the uterus gradually to empty itself during delivery . . . it is of some importance also to the infant, and especially to infants born in a feeble state, to allow the circulation in the umbilical chord to cease spontaneously before a ligature be applied.[119]

Clarke touches here on the issue of the third stage of labour, when the placenta is expelled, and the allied problem of post-partum haemorrhage. He argued that there was a measurable benefit to the baby in gaining the full quota of the placental blood supply available by not cutting the cord until it had ceased pulsating; in other words, he argued for the protective effect this would have for the newborn infant, especially if it were struggling to survive.

Nonetheless, there were tensions between the claims to preserve both maternal and foetal life and what could actually be done. The balance of arguments which favoured the mother, from the seventeenth through to the end of the nineteenth centuries, was largely determined by the inescapable reality of her death if she remained undelivered which was, of course, the originating point for the work of barber-surgeons.

It was not just male midwives who recognised that there was a problem in maintaining a balance of interests between mother and child. Nihell argued that the skills and management of women midwives 'prove more efficacious towards favouring both mother and child; always with due preference however to the mother'.[120] She expanded on what she saw as the mother's claims and, following on from these, why the physician, as distinct from the man midwife, was needed when the woman who was giving birth actually became ill:

> It is precisely in those disorders . . . that the greatest skill and knowledge of physic are required. Then it is, not only the preservation of the mother claims regard, and certainly the preferable one, but even that of the child is no indifferent point. And to save both, the state of the mother's constitution must be carefully considered.[121]

In instances where the woman does die, whether from a post-partum haemorrhage, obstructed labour (in instances where it is judged that the forceps can be applied, rather than the crotchet) or puerperal fever, the fate of her baby, if it has survived birth, is covered by the use of the sparse phrase of 'the infant lived' or 'died'. In clinical reports from the Rotunda compiled by George Johnston much later in the nineteenth century, there are occasional details on the baby itself. When an outbreak of 'scarlatina' occurred (the streptococcal infection often appearing in lying-in wards), four women 'with their children, were discharged convalescent';[122] during an outbreak of smallpox, an unmarried woman gave birth to a boy 'healthy, in good condition' but who on the ninth day developed a purple rash on his forehead – he 'became low and weak, was given wine-whey' and died '46 hours after the first appearance of the rash'.[123] Johnston, who was exceptionally keen on the use of forceps, also recorded details of a birth where the head never entered the pelvic brim, that is, the baby was still above the bony edge of the pelvis, forming the entrance to the birth canal:

> He applied the forceps, and after three-quarters of an hour's exertion, he was enabled to extract the child. It was alive. And on the left parietal bone there was a depression of three and a half inches by one and a half inches. He never thought it would recover but the mother and child went out quite well.[124]

There is no comment on how the woman recovered, physically and otherwise, from this traumatic birth and of course there can be no indication as to the condition of the infant and how it survived such a damaging birth. But this account illustrates the difficulties of operative midwifery. The forceps could be used successfully to bring the foetus through the birth outlet but the obstetrician often did so, not convinced that the child could survive the operation.

Of the possible range of techniques that comprised operative midwifery (excluding the episiotomy), six offered any real possibility of salvaging the life of the foetus, as distinct from the mother. The Dublin man midwife, Fleetwood Churchill, lists both categories in his book on operative midwifery published mid-century:[125]

> artificial induction
> version/turning[126]
> perforator and crotchet
> vectis/lever[127]
> forceps[128]
> Caesarean section
> symphysiotomy

In theory, only the first two operations were open to women midwives to perform, the others being the exclusive preserve of obstetrics; certainly, the individual reputations of men midwives in the seventeenth and eighteenth century were founded on the various designs and refinements that each employed to deal with impacted labour. Dease argues that because midwifery was largely restricted to women practitioners until the eighteenth century, when barber-surgeons were called in:

> they were at a loss in what manner they should assist women in preternatural or difficult cases, which led them to imagine and adopt not only many absurd, but too often destructive methods to accomplish delivery.[129]

Internal version, for instance, which might be attempted where the presenting part was not even able to effectively enter the birth canal, was far more than just painful. According to Dease, if it were attempted before the amniotic membranes had ruptured, when the neck of the uterus was still 'rigid and not prepared to yield', 'the os uteri will not admit without great violence the operator's hand' and the same applied if 'the waters' had 'run off' and the uterus was in a 'spasmodic state of contraction'.[130] He preferred administering an opiate drug to relax the uterus, before proceeding, in order to avoid 'the most fatal consequences'.

If internal version failed, either the fillet or the crotchet was needed to deliver the foetus in pieces. The fillet was a wire thread or string used to decapitate the baby, thus unblocking the birth passage. Alternatively, the foetal head could be 'opened' with a knife or tire-tête (this latter was designed by Mauriceau, the seventeenth-century French man midwife) and then extracted from the uterus by the crotchet. Of such operations, Dease wrote:

> Those expedients frequently proved shocking to humanity, as children were brought alive, torn in the most miserable manner: Besides, from the crotchets, or rather the sharp hooks then in use, often slipping, the unhappy mother was torn in such a manner, that it were better a period had been at once put to her existence.[131]

Even the flamboyant Ould was wary of instrumental use, declaring that:

> where the Mother's Life is not to be saved, but by bringing away the Child, either whole or separately by the Help of Instruments . . . it is absolute Danger, not to say Death to the Child, and the Mother is never wanting in her Share of the Risque.[132]

In his instructions to men midwives about dismembering the foetus, he wrote that there must be a certainty of the 'Infant being dead' and the operator must also be sure that there was no possibility of bringing the foetus forth with the hands before instruments could be used. This instruction was only feasible in the wake of the introduction of auscultation in the 1820s which enabled practitioners to hear the foetal heart; certainty about foetal death before operating had not been possible up to this time (but as with so much of the territory new obstetric interventions opened up, auscultation too was to become a double-edged weapon, for it could be and was used to invade and disallow the woman's voice as much as to support the foetus).

The invention of the lever (by Roonhausen in Holland) and the forceps (by the Chamberlen family in England) made it possible, in theory, to deliver alive, foetuses in instances which had hitherto proved undeliverable. In practice, both were difficult to use without doing injury to the woman. Dease wrote that his experience of the forceps had been more extensive than he wished because he was 'fixed in business' in the most populous and poorest part of Dublin where 'difficult cases' often occurred. He was under pressure to save the woman but found it 'impossible to introduce them [forceps] without alarming the patient and assistants'. Eager to get the worst over with, he often miscalculated the position of the head: 'from imagining the head to be lower in the pelvis than it really was, after (with difficulty) fixing the forceps, and proceeding to the extraction, they slipped.'[133] Dease's conclusion was that although men midwives said they could deliver a head when it was 'high up', the reality was that they would not be able to grasp the head with the forceps and, on the basis of his experience, he sought to improve the lever, eliminating the forceps. In effect, he also eliminated the possibility of delivering the foetus alive.

Forty years before Dease reached his conclusions, Ould introduced a refinement to Mauriceau's tire-tête to deal more effectively, as he reasoned it, with the destructive operation. His account is one of the many instances when women's fragility was used to tighten the association between birth and acute suffering despite the fact that it was women who had to face the ordeal of their possible death, whether they were fragile or not. The assumption of fragility was set against images laden with violent sexual penetration, as with the following passage, where Ould argues that his own invention was an advance on the tire-tête:

What Danger must the Mother be in of being wounded, at the introduction of this two-edged Weapon? And how impossible must it be for her to escape, when by any of the above-mentioned Evils, the Head is at a greater Distance from the external Orifice of the Vagina, or inclosed by the above Swelling? This will appear plainer when we consider that the texture of the Vagina is such, that though it will give Passage to a large Body, yet if we introduce a Body into it no bigger than a Goose-Quill, it will be contiguous to the Vagina on all Sides . . . add to this the Patient's constant Motion of her Posteriors from her Pain, Weakness and terrible Apprehensions, and what must be the Consequence of the least Motion of those Parts, when this Knife is naked in the Vagina? I hope the humane Reader will paint in his own Imagination, the dreadful Danger of a distressed Patient in these Circumstances, in much livelier Colours than is in my Power to express, whereby he may be inclined to favour any Attempt . . . to prevent this Grievance.[134]

The pain-ridden, fearful, weakened woman of Ould's imaginings, turning and turning on her bed in desperation, which this passage reveals, also presents the female body as a highly sexualised object and a passive one, open to penetration at the physical and ideological levels in ways that suggest nothing less than an eroticised violence on the part of the man midwife. With this verbal portrait, the 'humane Reader', designated 'he', requires no other image. Jordanova argues about the English man midwife, William Hunter, that his so-called 'realistic' drawings of the pregnant female body exemplify a 'representational' violence that is preoccupied with gender, passivity and pathology. She discusses a line drawing of a pregnant uterus in which a clitoris is shown cut in sections, a completely unnecessary detail to what Hunter claims to be portraying, but vital to the ideological work that obstetrics is accomplishing during this formative period of the science. As Jordanova observes, this linkage results in what she terms a 'double female body image' idealising and violating women simultaneously.[135] Ould does this largely linguistically, although he does include line drawings of the principal operative instruments, including his own device, which he called a *terebra occulta*.

He tells us he designed the *terebra occulta* after an incident of impacted labour which he recounts, in his usual vivid detail, to illustrate the dangers on which he has already discoursed so eloquently:

In June 1738, I was sent for to the Assistance of a Woman on the upper Comb, who had been in Labour two Days and as many Nights; the Midwife who attended her told me, that notwithstanding her Pains were very strong during the whole Time, yet she could not determine what Part of the Child presented, which upon Inquiry, I did not much wonder at; for the Space between the Os Sacrum and Pubis was surprisingly narrow, insomuch that the small Portion of the Head which was forced between them, by the long Continuance of her excessive Pains, was not above two Inches thick.

Though there was no Doubt of the Child being dead, and though there was no method of bringing it forth but by evacuating the Brain; yet to avoid Censure, I told her Friends the State of her Condition, and at the same Time desired a Consultation, which they seemed much surprized at, however they granted it; we immediately agreed to lessen the Size of the Head.[136]

He then describes that because 'the Part whereon I was to operate was at a great Distance from me, which still increased my Antipathy to cutting Instruments, I thought a Pair of Sizars might be at least introduced through the Vagina with less Danger than a Knife'. He accomplished the operation with these even though it required 'all the Strength of my Right Hand'. Typically, he does not tell us how the woman sustained this trauma or even whether she recovered. But he does describe the instrument he then went off to design, its principal feature being that it shielded the blade needed to pierce the foetal skull, the *occulta* of its title.

This last passage is striking for the brief glimpse it permits of the social relations that men midwives had still to negotiate before the sanctuary of the lying-in hospital and a professional hierarchy dealt with the problem of the individual man midwife trying to 'avoid Censure' for a particular line of treatment. The passage also indicates that even when the woman was clearly in great difficulty with the labour, with a craniotomy as the only proffered solution, there remained an area of negotiation around whether the foetus was alive or dead.

Accounts of heroic rescues are rife in the works of men midwives and it is little wonder that Nihell waxed so furious on the subject of 'keen instrumentarians' whose work rarely failed 'of destroying the child, or at least cruelly wounding it, and never but injure the mother'.[137] If the unavoidable instances of operative midwifery were not as many as were claimed by the 'instrumentarians' (and, if one accepts Nihell's argument, could have been fewer still with different practices),[138] the impact of the consequences for women nevertheless affected practitioners committed to 'watchful waiting', leading to the circumstances which produced the Hamilton–Collins debate. The other side of that problem was that the rationale on how to deal with a clearly dangerous set of circumstances, like a severely contracted pelvis as the result of rickets, was extended to cover other instances where a change in practice alone, like mobility in labour to encourage descent of the head, might well have produced a better outcome for women. But they had already been ruled incapable of sustaining any other approach, save an instrumental one, which also put their lives at risk.

Even the conservative men midwives had to carry out destructive operations. In the instance of severe pelvic disproportion, Clarke advocated perforating the head of the foetus early in labour, then leaving it to 'be forced into the pelvis by pains' and only then to attempt to extract it with the crotchet. In a transverse lie, if the foetus was already dead, and 'spontaneous expulsion' was not going to occur, to afford a 'better chance' to the women, he suggested 'perforating the thorax or abdomen so as to lessen their bulk' before proceeding with a crotchet.[139] He admitted to his own unhappy reactions sometimes intruding in such cases, as in this account of a 'tedious natural labour':

> E.F. Admitted on the 6th of November, 1788, had strong labour pains till three o' clock. This was her second child. – As the head of the foetus was out of the reach of the forceps, it was turned and brought footling with some difficulty through the pelvis. The head could not be got away without perforation, and in doing this, Doctor Evory . . . was very apprehensive of injuring the intestines which he thought he felt in the vagina. After suffering a great deal from diarrhoea, pains in and round the pelvis, hectic flushings, &c. she was dismissed valetudinary [infirm] at the end of a month, and was seen twelve months after selling milk about the streets. On the day of this patient's illness I had suffered so much from fatigue and anxiety of mind, that I was unable to interfere further than by requesting she might be speedily delivered, as her life appeared to me in imminent danger.[140]

Clarke's insistence on acting 'conscientiously' on 'E.F.'s' behalf and his admission of his own overwhelming anxiety are in striking contrast to the pose of intrepidity that Ould favours. The description of E.F's vagina during the attempts to resolve this impacted labour is not meant to be lurid sensationalism as such. If Clarke writes in a tradition of benevolent patriarchy, disempowering women and denying them agency, he does not write as a conquering hero. Nonetheless, the practice is violent, a literal violence in Jordanova's terms, and in this instance inescapable for 'E.F.' who, from this description, contracted a puerperal infection in the wake of her operative delivery. The problem with the actual violence entailed in operative midwifery is the way it was redeployed within the area of 'representational' violence. When these two become intertwined, the latter is used to legitimate the former and even encourages actual violence, becoming ever more tangled on the issue of female vulnerability and the need to rescue women from their own bodies.[141] But it was 'E.F.' (and many more unnamed women) who had to work beyond her posited frailty, to recover her strength and return to the streets to sell milk. And, had she not recovered, she, and not the men midwives, would have had to deal with facing her death.

The options in responding to the problem of women who could not be delivered in any other way but instrumentally were only slowly expanded to include alternatives which were potentially safer for mother and foetus (this movement was complicated by the problem of sepsis). The style of argument that was used to support operative midwifery continued to focus on the preservation of maternal life while keeping the balance between maternal and foetal life where possible. In order to support any expansion, however, it was always urgent and, in a sense, apparently simple to come back to the dead corpse on a table and see the possibilities of resolution of an impacted labour from the anatomy and physiology which was based on that dead corpse. A practice of invasiveness was established in order to save life, they told themselves and us, but other directions were seldom explored and the invasiveness itself was to create further problems of practice and rhetoric which we are still confronting and attempting to disentangle. This is not least because incidents of the extraordinary and the pathological were permitted to determine the frame of reference for the ordinary but, always, without reference to the woman herself in making a decision about her body and her future.

In this context, it is worth recalling that Clarke himself had noted how small the incidence of contracted pelves was, relative to the numbers of women giving birth. Nihell's argument was that the number of operative interventions could be reduced or replaced by the skill of the midwife who 'uses all patience consistent with the safety of life to the mother especially'.[142] The skills she advocated for women midwives were grounded in a physiological model, using such techniques as supporting the woman to walk so that 'little by little the head will frank itself a passage with the weight of the body acting by an innate energy'[143] or manual skill in easing the presenting part out from under the symphysis pubis. Her model of female physiology was different to that of the men midwives and, not surprisingly, it lacked the dimension of violence that appears in their work. It is also arguable that the boundary of her work, that is, what could be done consistent with the safety of the woman, was a boundary that was more readily crossed by obstetric science, given their radically different reading of the female body; at once a more rigid, fragile body and more easily taken over. In the work of accomplishing that invasion, it also became possible for obstetrics eventually to reconfigure the mother–foetus dyad, facing us with our contemporary dilemmas to do with the status of the foetus as equal to the mother.

The Caesarean operation was key in securing this equal status, although initially it had an extremely high maternal death rate, attributable to the lack of an aseptic regime in operating and to not sewing up the uterine incision. In the seventeenth and eighteenth centuries, the Caesarean was not enthusiastically endorsed by men midwives, except in France.[144] Ould objected strenuously to the Caesarean which he termed 'repugnant, not only to all rules of Theory or Practice, but even of Humanity'.[145] He thought that its use might have arisen 'from an article in the Roman Catholic faith whereby they don't allow salvation to unbaptised infants'.[146] The problem, he argued, was whether rules to bind men midwives could be laid down, as the Sorbonne doctors of divinity had done in 1733, 'when and in what Cases, you are to prefer the Life either of the Mother or Child'.[147] He judged that the operation was best seen as an artefact of a period 'before the Art of Midwifry arrived to any Degree of Perfection'.[148] Surgeons employed the operation in preternatural labours where it was easy to imagine the lack of skilled assistance, attributable to 'the Ignorance of the present Female Operators', and

> by this Means became acquainted with the situation of the Child in the Womb, and the particular Anatomy of those Parts. And this consequently put them upon endeavouring to bring the Child, though in a preternatural Situation, into the World, without destroying the Mother.[149]

Despite arguments advanced in its favour, the operation was almost certainly fatal for the mother and thus 'barbaric'.[150] Dease was similarly convinced of the 'barbarously destructive' nature of both the Caesarean and the 'section of the symphysis of the pubis' or symphysiotomy, where the symphysis was sawn apart to deal with an obstructed labour. He wrote that 'the consequences of those operations have generally proved fatal to the mother, and seldom successful as to saving the child.'[151] Although the Caesarean was not used by men midwives in Ireland until the end of the nineteenth century, there is one instance of its being performed successfully outside the hospital system. In a 1742 pamphlet published by Thomas Southwell, a Kildare man midwife, who was intent on attacking Ould's work, he recounted the work of a local woman midwife, not to extol her skill of course, but to refute Ould on the worthlessness of the Caesarean:

> One Alice O'Neal aged about 33 years, wife to a poor farmer near Charlement and mother of several children, in January 1738–9 took labour but could not be delivered though several women attempted it. She remained in this condition twelve days, till Mary Donally, an illiterate woman performed the Caesarean operation with a razzor: at the aperture she took out the infant and the secondaries, and held the lips of the wound together till one went a mile for silk and common needles, with which she stitched the wound and dressed it with the white of eggs: the cure was completed with salves of the midwives compounding. In about 27 days, the patient walked a mile on foot and came to me, she frequently walks to the Market of this town which is six miles distant from her house.[152]

Mary Donally's name has been mentioned briefly in obstetric histories when the evolution of the Caesarean operation is discussed, but nothing else is known about her. Despite the eclipsing of women's voices as effective practitioners in childbirth, instances like the Donally case indicate that women did continue to subvert male definitions of female incompetence.[153] The first successful 'official' hospital Caesarean operation in Dublin was not performed until 1889, in the Rotunda, by which time suturing the uterine incision, which had been established in Continental practice, was also known here, eliminating the possibility of death through internal haemorrhage.

Dease saw the symphysiotomy as being 'still of worse consequence' than the Caesarean because 'it subjected the woman to all the dangers of the latter, without the same advantages of saving the child'.[154] The symphysis pubis is the joint made from strong cartilage that connects the two pubic bones at the front of the pelvis. The presenting part of the foetus has to move out from under the symphysis pubis in negotiating the birth outlet. The symphysiotomy entailed cutting through the cartilage and ligaments of this joint to enlarge the birth outlet and, its inventor, the French man midwife, Sigault, wrote in 1777 that he saw it as a substitute for the Caesarean. Dease rejected it because having cut one joint in the pelvis, two others were 'violently stretched', the bladder and urethra were often damaged by the incision, and even then the pelvic outlet was not always sufficiently enlarged to deliver an infant alive. Therefore, there could be no rational basis to endanger the mother's life for an uncertain outcome for the foetus. Dease concurred with William Hunter, the London man midwife, that in the circumstances of extreme narrowness of the pelvis, using the crotchet for a destructive operation was preferable, provided that the practitioner worked slowly, 'taking away one little bit after another, letting the woman rest from time to time, and taking great care that she not be wounded by the sharp bones of the child.'[155]

With the symphysiotomy, the infant was usually extracted by forceps after the joint had been severed. A similar operation in intent, the pubiotomy, became possible in 1902 when an Italian, Gigli, invented a wire saw whereby the pubic bone itself could be cut in half and although rarely used, this operation largely superseded the older approach in the first decades of this century. Women had to be supported on either side of the hips, during the operation, and afterwards they were bound with adhesive plaster round their hips for some period to prevent the hips from gaping. Three pubiotomies were performed in the Coombe in 1907 and it was also performed in the Rotunda that year by Tweedy, who became an enthusiastic proponent of it, while opposing the Caesarean as too dangerous (of 1,902 women who gave birth in the Rotunda between 1906 and 7, only three women had a Caesarean). Jellett, the Master who succeeded Tweedy, was keen on pubiotomy as a prophylactic operation for suspected pelvic disproportion and it was used this way in clinical work for an extremely brief period in 1912–13. Pubiotomy was still being performed occasionally in the Rotunda in the 1940s while the symphysiotomy was performed in the National Maternity Hospital, Holles Street in 1943–4. Browne wrote about pubiotomy that 'it has its place in the Rotunda treatment of certain cases of disproportion as an alternative to the Caesarean section'.[156]

In his 1907 clinical report for the Rotunda, Tweedy wrote that the 'new operation' of pubiotomy had been used five times, with the conjugate diameter of the foetal presenting part ranging from 6.5 cms to 8 cms. In the first case due to 'incorrect technique', there had been problems of haemorrhage and laceration of the 'soft parts' and the patient had been unable to walk for sixty-three days. Tweedy also wrote

> I have made it a point to do all these operations in the labour ward with the patient placed on the ordinary couch, as I think by doing so I press home to the students the great and educational fact that such an operation may be undertaken amidst the usual domestic surroundings.[157]

Before the problem of true obstructed labour (as distinct from medical perceptions about the extent of contracted pelves or cephalo-pelvic disproportion) could be relatively safely tackled with the Caesarean operation, which was not until this century, it cannot be denied that practitioners faced extremely difficult decisions. Fleetwood Churchill argued that craniotomy and its variants, whereby a child was destroyed to save a mother's life, were a 'sad necessity', 'to be avoided by every possible means'.[158] Nonetheless, there were clear criteria 'where one life is sacrificed to secure the other; the mother's safety being purchased by the destruction of her child, in cases where both would be lost if no interference were attempted' which the practitioner was constrained to observe.[159] Symphysiotomy and pubiotomy were alternatives insofar as they offered, in certain circumstances, the chance to get the infant out alive, without the terrible consequences for the woman which Dease sketched out (see above). But none of these interventions was without consequences. In the case of symphysiotomy and pubiotomy, they directly impinged on a woman's sexual organs.

During the first third of the twentieth century when maternal mortality with the Caesarean was still high, these operations were argued as a safer and more conservative treatment, in some circumstances, than the Caesarean. But the death rate for Caesarean sections was itself a complicated outcome of obstetric thinking because of the serious problems and additional opportunities created around puerperal fever and by the extreme tardiness of obstetrics in responding to asepsis and antisepsis. And even though these other operative interventions were sanctioned first on the grounds of safety, it was women who carried the heavy burdens of possible death or certain mutilation in absolute proximity to their sexual organs. Moreover, control over that invidious choice was not theirs.[160] It was argued in the early 1930s that the maternal death rate in Ireland had been 20.7 per 100,000 of the population in 1870, but dropped to 10 per 100,000 of the population by 1930 and septic infection, which officially had been listed as responsible for 65 per cent of maternal deaths in the former period, dropped to 33 per cent of maternal deaths in the latter (these latter figures for the Free State only).[161] By 1945, the Obstetrics Section of the Royal Academy of Medicine in Ireland was recommending increased operative intervention to lower further maternal and infant death rates.

The acceptance of teaching on sepsis and a regime of asepsis to deal with it, and the introduction of antibiotic drugs in the 1930s brought to an end a long period in which practitioners could be seen to favour the balance of the mother over the foetus, by not privileging the operative intervention with the most serious consequences for a woman, namely the Caesarean section. In the Rotunda, in Purefoy's mastership at the very end of the nineteenth century, six Caesarean sections were performed out of 11,098 deliveries. By 1940–44, the figure was 346 sections to 15,145 births carried out, or just over 2 per cent. Forceps deliveries increased from 3.8 per cent to 9.4 per cent.[162] Their field of endeavour had widened significantly to level up, as they reasoned it, their joint claims to protect both mother and foetus. However, their view of the female body had narrowed, the casualty being the school of 'watchful waiting'.[163]

By the middle years of the twentieth century, women's general levels of health and nutrition had finally slowly improved in countries like Ireland and England, so that problems like severely deformed pelves were no longer an issue. By the beginning of the 1970s, fertility levels had dropped dramatically, thus dramatically reducing the incidence of problems earlier generations of women had experienced as a direct result of the cumulative physical impact of prolonged childbearing. Then, operative midwifery really took off and it appears that we have not yet reached the endpoint of its potential. This is a development which is inexplicable only if we are not aware of the original arguments about women's bodies which underwrote this ideology of invasiveness.

Sustaining Knowledges

There are a number of points to bear in mind about the way the three pairings of natural–preternatural, error–truth, and mother–foetus were sustained. Just as lesions are created as objects of discourse,[164] so we have traced these three discursive creations which became the mainsprings of obstetric science. They assisted men midwives in new ways of looking at the female body in birth, arising from the driving intentions of obstetrics to become the principal knowledge broker about that body. Obstetrics interpreted and imbued the body with a set of significances that worked because there was ready legitimation for those meanings, the legitimation itself coming from a wider patriarchal order, which was working with newly emerging economic and political significances about the reproductive body. This is part of the answer to why obstetrics was so successful in establishing this new version of the body, while women-controlled midwifery failed to survive as a significant carrier of meanings about the body and birth.

The dyads raised many more problems than they ever answered around fact-creation and verification, not least because different preoccupations, obsessions, and emphases, on the parts of individual practitioners, contributed to these dyads. But it is also clear that no one practitioner, including Nihell, had an altogether stable and consistent system of birth management. Even the most intently interventionist model contained complex contradictions. Ould, for example, insisted that hurrying the expulsion of the foetus in the second stage could create problems with the cord and with the placenta. On the other hand, Nihell was convinced that many problems relating to post-partum haemorrhage would be avoided by early cord-cutting, before the placenta was delivered, and how odd that she did so, given her acuity of observation in other physiological aspects of labour.

Each practitioner's use of all three of these pairings indicates the absolutely social nature of knowledge formation, contingent on ideological, political and professional concerns, which lead us to interpret rather differently what Clarke referred to as a situation in 'an Hospital' where he was 'totally uninfluenced by any existing prejudices'.[165] Clarke's belief and assertions, like Ould's, that in order to confirm his theories, he made the 'strictest Examination of every Woman, which I either delivered or saw delivered',[166] are perhaps best approached through Ludwig Fleck's argument, that when considering the history of scientific knowledge, there is often no formal relation of logic between conceptions and evidence. As ever, the problem was that women paid the price for how knowledge was being built.

We can also see how knowledge forms, as they gradually build up, take on new accretions, like the category of 'natural labour' which is extended to 'tedious natural labour'. Publishing treatises, texts, articles and clinical records all helps to move this process along by keeping expert information in increasing circulation, but it often operates to exclude some possibilities around knowledge formation, while including others. This brings us to one of Latour's rules of method which is that when things hold, they start becoming true: when things are true, they hold.[167] We can see something of the process whereby things begin to hold, how the concept takes root. We can also see what Latour terms 'the disorderly mixture revealed by science in action' [though not consciously revealed by itself] in the debates on how long labour should last and when and which interventions should be carried out.[168]

This is in sharp contrast to the orderly method that science claims to command when speaking of its activities to those outside its boundaries. There is a distrust of the birth process unless it is incorporated within an obstetric scheme of management, whether of 'watchful waiting' or one which is more radically interventionist and regardless of the fact that most births come to a conclusion with no necessity for radical intervention (if we can judge by the statistics of both Clarke and Collins). Yet, although a radically interventionist model wins out over 'watchful waiting' and comes to dominate the interpretation of all three pairings, it is not as secure a black box as it intends. Nor does it entirely wipe out the opposition, for conflicting definitions of what is 'natural and normal' continue to crop up. The concept of the easy birth, abandoned when Nihell is ignored, comes back to challenge obstetric science in yet another form in the late twentieth century. Obstetrics remains both extraordinarily fluid, if not chaotic, within its own boundaries, but is always extraordinarily defensive in how it manages problems of doubt and error at and beyond its borders.

Finally, there is a problem of violence that is not resolved within any of the dyads. From within feminist theory, Teresa de Lauretis[169] has argued that the reinforcement of gender politics is dependent on how rhetoric operates. Nihell shows us one form of essentialism, which at least has the merit of concentrating on women's strength and skills – women have 'more bowels' for other women. The rhetoric of Dease, Clarke and Collins with its evident careful, caring and controlling paternalism is claustrophobic, by comparison. I find Ould, Hamilton and Tweedy brittle and cold in their writing. They are the most interventionist of the men midwives who appear in this chapter, at once the most removed and unknowledgeable about our bodies, and the most capable of a deep violence to us carefully handled as science. It is a violence about which we have all too rarely been able to speak. Gender, as de Lauretis says, has to do with history and practices, and here we see a history being built, building blocks in place and practices which are embedded with meanings about women that damage. De Lauretis urges us to peel off the scaly overlapping, to see how meanings are made. She wants us to see that there is a relationship between the rhetoric of violence and the violence of rhetoric for, she argues, the representation of violence is inescapable from the notion of gender. In other words, violence is engendered in representation and obstetric science is especially rich in its representations.[170]

Obstetrics is littered with sad footnotes and forgotten observations, amongst them this one from Joseph Clarke:

> It must be allowed that under the very best management, lacerations of the vagina generally prove fatal . . . all we can say is, that there is a possibility of recovery; we have unquestionable evidence of two successful cases, one

under Dr Hamilton of Edinburgh, the other under Dr Douglas of London. To these I think we may venture to add the case of our patient E.F.[171]

Quite apart from excluded theories like those of Nihell, for she is necessarily ruled non-scientific being a woman midwife, other knowledges get discarded and lost, knowledges that are scientific, in its sense of careful observations, like Clarke's on lacerations of the vagina and the good fortune of 'E.F.' in surviving. The consequences for women, when these knowledges become stranded, are daunting, despite the triumphs of the interventionists. The reasons why lacerations 'generally prove fatal' are related to obstetrics' most tragic controversy, before the black box of clean birth and an antiseptic regime is constructed, and this is what is explored in the next chapter.

3

Body, Power, Death: The Problem of Puerperal Fever

The Secret Revengeful Foe

Puerperal fever or childbed fever, as it was known colloquially, was the aspect of childbirth that consistently proved most troubling to the emerging science of obstetrics. The two accounts presented below are typical of how obstetrics framed this challenge. The first is a description of the fever as an enemy personified while the second is a case history in which the doctors focus, not on the fever, but on the emotional traumas of their patient.

The first one is an unusually dramatic characterisation of puerperal fever, written by Dr Hulme, a British man midwife, in the 1770s:

> The pestilence like a fierce and untamed enemy, spreads his hostile banners in open day, and feasts on carnage and destruction, till, glutted with slaughter, he himself sinks down and dies. But the Puerperal Fever, like a secret revengeful foe, stabs in the dark to the very vitals; and though he kills one only at a time, yet he is privately slaying every day, and never satiated; thus making up by length of time, what the other does by a sudden devastation.[1]

The second was written by George Johnston, a Master of the Rotunda Hospital in which he relates the story of a woman who came to give birth there in the early 1870s:

> a case of acute bronchitis, aged 25; as she was suffering from great dysponea [breathlessness], she was delivered [by forceps] when the os was 2/5 dilated; the child weighed 6 lbs.5oz. which died on the third day, the mother not being able to nurse it. She was at once put under treatment for a chest complaint. The following morning, Dr. H. Kennedy was kind enough to see her with me. She had a pulse of 130; tongue dry, brown crust – in fact all the signs of typhus fever. At noon, she was again visited when she was found crying; and on being asked why she was doing so, she stated that she had been seduced, turned out by her parents, she had nowhere to go and did not know what would become of her, that she had twice attempted suicide, but was prevented. We told her make her mind easy that we would befriend

her and get a home for her. From this, she began to mend. She was sent to No. 11 the chronic ward, on her tenth day [after giving birth], a week after which she took the place of a wardmaid where she continues ever since. This is a remarkable instance of the wonderful influence of the mind over the body.[2]

This is a seemingly hopeless case of a young woman who has been turned out of her parental home because of her non-marital pregnancy and who is in a state of dangerous ill health. The puerperal fever which she has contracted in hospital is mis-diagnosed as typhus fever, a common mistake. Nonetheless, she survives the combined physical rigours of labour and birth and the dreaded fever. The doctors pity her and offer her help; she recovers and accepts the work they so kindly offer her in the same hospital where her baby has been born and died and where she too, nearly died.

These two accounts form appropriate points of entry into the problem of puerperal fever because of the way in which obstetrics explains its own role in relation to the fever. In both accounts, obstetrics seeks to stand separate from the fever and its victims, and often denies or confuses the evidence of the fever's operations, while seemingly observing its effects in rigorous detail. The deaths of women from puerperal fever worked in such a way as to expand the knowledge base of obstetrics and thus its power. This expansion happened in spite of the criticisms and concerns about those deaths, which were expressed from outside the profession almost as frequently as different regimes of care were criticised from within. Hulme's vivid ascribing to the fever the status of a cunning vengeful killer that accomplishes its lethal work in the secret depths of a woman's body summarises the stance which obstetric medicine maintained down to the beginning of the twentieth century. During this period, its chosen position was to treat the fever as a protagonist, which it alone could challenge. The extract by Johnston is exemplary of the position of obstetrics as a defender of women, standing between women and its ravages in an effort to protect the former. In its role of defender it is kindly, paternalistic, authoritative about the woman's symptoms, intervening on her behalf to bring her back to health, even when as in this instance, the existence of the fever was denied and her symptoms attributed to another type of fever which had no direct links with childbirth.

Puerperal fever had always threatened women's health and lives. Its sudden appearance, even after what seemed an easy birth, so often ended in death, that it was the event pregnant women are reputed to have feared most.[3] According to the Dublin man midwife, Fleetwood Churchill, who republished Hulme's paper, fever and ague specific to lying-in women, which tended to be fatal, had been noted in the earliest writing on childbirth by Hippocrates and Avicenna, who attributed them to the lochia being suppressed and not evacuated from the body after birth. Thomas Raynalde, who translated and annotated the work of the German Eucharius Rhodion, published as *The birth of mankinde* in 1599, describes lying-in women frequently suffering from a fever or ague, accompanied by inflammation and 'trembling of the belly'. Churchill also quotes five medical writers in the seventeenth century, Plater, Sennert, Riverius, Sylvius and Willis, who variously describe puerperal fever as stemming from an inflammation of the uterus, suppression of the lochia, or a deficiency of the lochia, each of these arising either as a consequence of the suppression of menstruation for the duration of pregnancy, which disturbs the blood, or from an injury to the uterus. All agree that such fevers are inherently more dangerous than the 'common' fevers met with in general medical practice, whether the former are classified as epidemic, malignant, putrid or inflammatory in origin and nature.

In the 1840s, when Churchill reviewed the fever, he included the observations of a French man midwife, Peu, who in 1664 had noted the deaths of 'a prodigious number' of lying-in women at the Hôtel-Dieu in Paris. The attack 'was attributed to impure air from a ward filled with wounded, which was situated underneath the lying-in ward'.[4] That Paris outbreak marks a turning point in the history of the fever. It had always occurred in single instances and, sometimes, in a succession of cases in the same district, giving rise, for example, to the belief that there was a 'fever season' which posed a special threat to women who gave birth at that time.[5] But, as Churchill argued, there was no evidence, prior to 1664, that medical men were acquainted with the 'alarming mortality of the disease'[6] on any wide scale. Gélis argues that doctors in the seventeenth century wrote about puerperal fever as if it were a new scourge; this may be related to the fact that while serious puerperal infections were common enough for women giving birth in their homes to yield perhaps a one in four lifetime chance of contracting some form or variant during the childbearing years, the distribution of what could be identified as puerperal fever outside hospitals was so variable that many practitioners, midwives and doctors alike, might see few cases or even none at all.[7] But the fever in the form of peritonitis rapidly became identified with the institutions known as lying-in hospitals where the numbers of women affected during any one epidemic suffered high rates of mortality; in 1746, it appeared in Paris in the first epidemic recorded as such, where

> it was extremely fatal, attacking the poor, and proving much more fatal to those in hospital than to those who were delivered at their own houses. Of twenty women confined in February of that year in the Hôtel-Dieu, scarcely one recovered; they died between the fifth and the seventeenth day after their confinement.[8]

Between 1746 and 1795, men midwives reported thirty-five separate epidemics, across Europe, including England, Scotland and Ireland, and the majority of these were hospital-based. Between 1803 and 1846, seventy-one epidemics were reported, again mostly in lying-in hospitals, across the same geographical area and thus the fever became an unexpected source of contestation for the new science.[9] As we shall see, its epidemic presence undermined both the claims to greater safety, which men midwives were promising to women, and the scientific knowledge backing those claims. The table below lays out the main writers on the fever who will be considered in the course of this chapter as well as the dates and locations of their observations.

Table 3.1: Men Midwives Writing on Incidents and Epidemics of Puerperal Fever

Doctor	Year	Location
Peu	1664	Paris
Hulme	1772	London
White	1777	Manchester
Clarke	1787	Rotunda, Dublin
Gordon	1795	Aberdeen, Scotland
Labatt	1819	Rotunda, Dublin
Beatty	1834	Coombe, Dublin
Collins	1836, 1849	Rotunda, Dublin
Holmes	1843	United States
Semmelweis	1847	Vienna
Churchill	1849	Dublin
Elliott	1867	Waterford
Phelan	1867	London
Kennedy	1869	Rotunda, Dublin
Johnston	1870–75	Rotunda, Dublin
Lane	1887	Rotunda, Dublin

Body and Power

Foucault describes how, in dealing with all types of epidemics, eighteenth-century medicine did not recognise a general form of disease. The specifics, the 'special, accidental, unexpected qualities', which required constant observation to understand the nature of epidemic illness, were thought of as historically individual to each outbreak, so that it was the specific disease that was always repeated, not the epidemic. Furthermore, contagion was but one element in epidemic illness, and contagion and agents of transmission were not the focus of medicine's thinking. An epidemic was 'accidental', in the sense of a coming together in a single place by chance of a single cause that affected all people similarly, regardless of age or disposition.[10]

The problem for obstetrics, in dealing with epidemic puerperal fever, was that the lying-in hospitals were easily pinpointed as that single place and the population which was targeted was quite specific, and highly valued for their specificity as reproducing mothers. There was no public condemnation of a single individual instance of puerperal fever in the home, but an epidemic raised alarms at many levels. In Dublin, in 1820, for example, the Lord Lieutenant directed the General Board of Health, an outside body, to conduct an investigation into the frequency of puerperal fever in the Rotunda Hospital and to reach conclusions as to the measures that must be adopted to avert its high levels of mortality.[11]

The history of puerperal fever is so important because it constitutes a distinctive case study of how obstetrics has done its work as a science, producing knowledge with this gendered ideological basis which has had critical concrete effects on women. In examining this history, we will encounter how models of disease causation, which were in use just as dissection was coming into play as a clinical practice, gradually reshaped disease classification, but we shall also see how, as patterns of frequency and distribution became a crucial part of the ongoing observation of the disease, an ideology about female incompetence affected the collection and interpretation of what was considered relevant clinical data. The inability of obstetric science to accept a link between its own institution, the lying-in hospital, and epidemics of the fever, and the move to disregard that its chosen clinical practices might be implicated in the continued production of puerperal fever constituted, at times, a minor political threat to the science in Ireland, even while the fever continued to be a major threat to women's lives.

Hulme's account of puerperal fever from the 1770s poses a scenario where the new science committed itself to take up a struggle on behalf of child-bearing women. The promise was that the developing clinical skills and theoretical knowledge of men midwives would release women from this lethal foe. Hulme's work is but one early example of the many hundreds of treatises, books and articles that were to follow on puerperal fever all the way into the twentieth century. The time span itself is noteworthy because it was coterminous with the rise and consolidation of obstetrics' institutional base, the lying-in hospital. Yet it was not the case that an understanding of puerperal fever merely eluded the grasp of men midwives and that a gradual recognition of the causes came about through an improvement of scientific technique. In fact, the gendered nature of knowledge production within obstetrics played a significant role in instigating still greater numbers of deaths from puerperal fever and actively prevented the emergence of a perspective that would have protected women.

Ludwig Fleck's argument, that there is not necessarily a formal relation of logic between conceptions and evidence, comes into play with puerperal fever. Fleck himself was interested in how this problem arose in another area of medicine, the diagnosis of syphilis, another communicable disease. His concern is with how a scientific notion of syphilis gradually took shape, using the older pre-scientific notion of 'befouled blood' which Fleck refers to as a rudimentary concept or a proto-idea. As a scientific concept, syphilis makes no sense unless the history of this proto-idea, which well pre-dates the epistemological work of science, is taken into account. Crucially, Fleck argues that how syphilis presented itself as a disease might, in logic, have led scientific thinking in a number of directions in determining its aetiology, but this one particular pre-scientific idea strengthened analysis along just one line of connections only. This eventually led towards testing the blood for syphilis, in order to diagnose accurately whether a person was infected, with what became known as the Wassermann test. But the test was not conceptually possible without the deeply social notion of syphilitic blood as 'impure blood', the 'carnal scourge', that was the result of sinful activity, and the focus on blood became the predominant mode in organising syphilis as a disease. It worked as a 'closed system' that resisted other notions, either of what the disease might be or of how the disease was transmitted. In brief, the history of the discourse on syphilis is one of many diverging views, but a growing dominance of one view which, as it gained ground, made it rare to hear an alternative viewpoint. In the long term, Wassermann proved not to be the end point, but the beginning of scientific understanding of syphilis and, in order to achieve that understanding, the science had to spread out across other fields of definition and so change substantially. But getting to the test in the first place required a base outside the objective, observational, entity science perceives itself to be, in order to open up the disease. Importantly, Fleck observes that the concept of 'impure blood' provides an example of what he terms the persistence of practitioners within any given system to dismiss or smooth away any contradictory views because there is a commitment to one logical system which cannot tolerate difference.[12]

There are similar elements of persistence and commitment to a proto-idea in the history of puerperal fever. The pre-scientific views of it as a putrid fever, chills, a milk fever, lacteous metastasis or 'milk gone astray', and the consequence of unstable emotions, all found their way into the treatises of men midwives,[13] but it was the notion of a putrid fever, occasioned by some sort of miasmatic contagion, originating in a putrid or poisonous atmosphere, which emerged as the most powerful logic in the eighteenth and early nineteenth century.

A current definition of puerperal fever today would explain that the single term covers a wide range of infections which can affect the newly delivered woman because of the raw surfaces of the genital tract and uterine areas, including the placental site, as well as lacerations and incisions, changes in the urinary tract, and the lochia discharge itself which is seen as an ideal medium to promote the growth of micro-organisms with pathogenic potential. These micro-organisms can be endogenous, existing normally in the body, but becoming infective where there has been tissue damage; there are also exogenous, micro-organisms, coming from birth attendants, from the environment, and from another infected individual, which can include the virulent Group A beta-haemolytic Streptococci and contaminants common to hospitals like the *Stapholococus aureus*.[14]

In order to examine the contribution of the fever to maternal mortality rates in the last few centuries, Edward Shorter uses a five-fold classification of puerperal fever: he begins with peritonitis, an inflammation of the peritoneum which lines the abdominal and pelvic cavities; bacteraemia, where hostile micro-organisms have spread into the general bloodstream from infected veins in the uterus, creating toxins; septic thrombophlebitis where a vein becomes inflamed and subject to clot formation; pyaemia, where pus-forming bacteria invade the bloodstream and the resulting blockage of small blood vessels creates abbesses; and pelvic cellulitis where the connective tissue becomes infected and pus-filled abbcesses form.[15] Shorter also draws attention to the overlapping nature of these infections.

These infections may or may not come into play parallel to one another and some, like peritonitis, are more lethal than others. Localised manifestations, like erysipelas, where hard red patches appear on the skin, swelling and gradually spreading, and *phlegmasia alba dolens* or 'white leg', in which the woman's leg swells and is extremely painful due to the presence of a thrombophlebitis, can be traced back to a bacterial invasion of the uterus where the organism most usually implicated is the haemolytic streptococcus. But aerobic bacteria, like the streptococcus, and anaerobic bacteria can flourish simultaneously, the latter often detectable by smell. It is now common to describe puerperal fever or puerperal sepsis as a unitary whole, one which has in effect been organised by the science of bacteriology which developed the techniques to identify pathogenic agents in the late nineteenth century.

That renaming and reorganising of puerperal fever suggests confidence in how the theories of medical science in general have come to be built; it suggests a process of continuing improvement and refinement, a progressive account of how obstetric science has evolved towards greater accuracy and understanding, dropping the notion of a putrid fever and moving towards a recognition of infection. There is a need to be cautious, however, for this was not a process which occurred in a mythical scientific space of careful observation and theory-building.

Fleck warns that although the doctrines of modern medical science are supported by far more sophisticated techniques of investigation, 'the path from dissection to formulated theory is extremely complicated, indirect and culturally conditioned.'[16] Historians and philosophers of science, Canguilhem, Foucault, and Jacob for example, have observed that although it is characteristic of sciences to want to argue an ordered progression in the development of concepts, what Foucault terms a 'continuous accumulation of knowledge', towards truth or an 'increasing rationality',[17] the history of all sciences is discontinuity, not continuity, subject to breaks and sudden terminations of concepts, which are then not easily accounted for when each science attempts to explain itself and its evolution.[18] Fleck sees this almost as a rule of the formation of scientific knowledge, in which 'the tenacity of self-contained systems of opinion' has a major impact on 'the operation of cognition'.[19] In relation to puerperal fever, we can say that obstetric science has worked at the level of the irredeemably social in constructing its theories, as all sciences must do. It might also be said that the complexity of puerperal fever, its pervasiveness in lying-in hospitals, and the many forms it assumed – reflecting the many possible points of entry by different sorts of bacteria – was to require a form of cognition that could tolerate less certainty, one that could be more reflexive because it was less committed to the view that there is a single 'causative agent'.[20]

Threatened by what epidemic puerperal fever implied about its status as a science, obstetrics often found itself reacting erratically to puerperal fever. On the whole, the clinical science was less certain and less responsive when an explanation of the fever's patterns turned to look back towards its own operations; it behaved with greater certainty when it could reach for explanatory factors like a miasmatic contagion which was spread by women themselves, one to another, either in the lying-in hospitals or in their homes where they helped one another give birth. Those women who came from the surrounding slums to the doors of Dublin maternity hospitals were thought to bring the fever with them. Thus, gender itself proved a valuable organising concept to explain causality. It took almost the whole of the nineteenth century for obstetric science to stop searching for the causative agent that seemingly lay outside its control and to reframe the problem of puerperal fever in terms of its own operations. Even then, it was never to accept responsibility for its own non-recognition of the role it played in epidemic puerperal fever.

Describing the Phenomenon of Puerperal Fever

With the expansion across Europe of lying-in hospitals from the end of the eighteenth century and with increasing numbers of epidemics, written accounts of puerperal fever rarely had to resort to devices of metaphor and personification like Hulme's to achieve dramatic impact. A recitation of numbers alone accomplished that. Indeed, as in all other epidemic illnesses, it was the knowledge of great numbers of people dying which contributed to a collective dread at the appearance of the disease entity.[21] This acute sense of dread on the part of men midwives comes through in the following description by Joseph Clarke, when he was sixth Master of the Rotunda, at the start of the third major epidemic that occurred in Dublin in the eighteenth century:

> 20. During spring, 1787, the temperature of the air was in general very cold, with sharp winds from the east and north-east. Inflammatory diseases were more prevalent among our patients than usual; particularly acute rheumatism. Some were affected with severe pains in the thorax, and difficult respiration. In consequence of these complaints, we were obliged to have recourse to venesection more frequently, during February and March of this year, than during the preceding twelve months.
> 21. It was a general observation, that our patients recovered slowly; or, to use the language of the nurses, it was much more difficult to get them out of bed than usual. This was peculiarly distressing, as the admission of poor women was now very numerous, probably on account of the severity of the weather. Contrary to our established custom, we were sometimes obliged to put two in a bed, rather than refuse admittance to those who solicited at our gates.[22]

Clarke then explains that he had been waiting for funds to have the wards repaired and whitewashed and was now growing anxious that this work be undertaken lest 'these circumstances might contribute to the slow recovery of our patients'.

> 23. While we were thus waiting in expectation of repairs, the puerperal fever began to make its first appearance, and in a very treacherous manner. The first woman was attacked on the 18th of March, and the second not until the 31st; the third on the 3d of April; the fourth, on the 7th; the fifth, on the 10th; the sixth on the 11th; on the 14th, two; on the 15th, two more; and one on the 17th. It was not then till the middle of April that its progress began to be rapid, and its nature as an epidemic clearly ascertained.[23]

The details in Clarke's entries are immediately arresting: during an acutely cold late winter, the hospital is constrained by its status as a charity from giving anything more than minimal time and assistance to women who are already weakened by the effects of poverty and continuous ill-health – note that there are two occupants in each bed; then the steadily increasing rhythm of numbers falling ill to the fever asserts itself. Having described the external conditions preceding the epidemic, Clarke moves on to describe the symptoms of the disease:

> 24. The symptoms of this fever corresponded so nearly with what Dr Hulme has well described, that a very few remarks will suffice on this subject.[24] It always began with a distinct chilliness or shivering. The pain in the cavity of the abdomen was not more frequent in one part than another, nor was the tenderness so great as to be much affected by such trifling causes as the pressure of the bedclothes. Little or no vomiting appeared in any stage of the disease, no delirium, no unequivocal marks of putrescency in any part of the system. The pulse, in general, beat from 120 to 140 strokes in a minute. The lochial discharge and secretion of milk were not subject to any general law. Sometimes they continued regular for a short time, and sometimes were suppressed from the beginning. They have never appeared to me more deranged in this, than in other disorders where the circulation of the blood is equally disturbed.[25]

Some of the elements Clarke describes were part of the already circulating discourse on the fever used by men midwives in an attempt to build up a scientific notion of the disease: fever; the shaking fits called ague; inflammation of the abdomen; the condition, either suppressed or otherwise, of the milk and lochia; and the relationship between the lochia and other disturbances to the circulation of the blood. Clarke adds observations on the very rapid pulse rate, on the even distribution of abdominal pain, the lack of vomiting, the absence of delirium, and the absence of any discernible putrid festering on or within the body.

This punctilious recording of observations is an outstanding feature of Clarke's account which is, above all, a clinical account of puerperal fever. The account is written during a transitional phase of knowledge formation within medicine, where the scanning of facts across a multiple number of cases helps to make medicine more certain of its operations.[26] Clarke speaks of several dozen cases in his account. The Scottish man midwife Alexander Gordon[27] uses seventy-seven cases in his 1795 treatise on puerperal fever, and Robert Collins, early in the nineteenth century, submits collected facts on 103 cases of puerperal fever.[28] Clarke's account is compiled with the implicit assumption that in detailing the presence of the fever, and its usual mode of functioning, an explanation of the disease can then emerge. For example, in relation to the lochia, he is searching for a regular pattern of occurrence, a 'general law' and finds none. He accepts, however, that the 'proximate cause' of the disease is an 'inflammation of the peritoneum'; and hence, Clarke writes, the 'nosological name of peritonitis' has been given to it by Dr Forster, its elevation to this scientific classification a sure indication that it is becoming a disease of merit.[29]

Audrey Eccles argues that humoral medicine was displaced far earlier in obstetric practice than in general therapeutic medicine,[30] and her contention fits in with Foucault's analysis of how the medical gaze developed. It is highly probable that men midwives 'gazed' with greater intensity, using 'sight, touch and hearing',[31] upon a greater wealth of similar clinical material, pregnant women's bodies, at an earlier point than in general medicine. The phenomena Foucault enumerates of order, time, hour, the problem of localisation, watching disease travel from one part of the body to another, were so thickly recorded in respect of puerperal fever that the descriptions quickly assumed a regularity of their own, even if there was no agreement on what constituted the reasons for each of its signs.

Time and intervals were significant. Gélis notes that miliary fever, milk fever, or weed fever (which from the frame of reference eventually provided by bacteriology were all similar post-partum infections) were thought to do with the milk coming in after delivery and were noted to last for around a fortnight.[32] By contrast, puerperal fever was seen to begin suddenly, ending in death between the fifth and seventh day.[33] Gordon argued in 1795 that the 'time of attack' was important in that the earlier it began, the more likely it would prove fatal. His chart indicated two women dying within twenty-four hours of the fever's symptoms being observed; in all, more than half the fatalities occurred on the fifth day of the fever, making the fifth the most critical for clinical care.[34]

Clarke's account was first published in 1793. We have seen that he referred to Hulme. Clarke also referred to the arguments and observations of a number of other men midwives, which points to another dimension of obstetric science, the continuous circulation amongst men midwives of views, opinions, theories and treatment regimes. Journal science[35] was already well in train by the 1780s across Europe, enabling knowledges to be built up alongside the personal and institutional reputations which were also set in train by this process. But it was not a process without strife, as Foucault reminds us about science in general:

> devotion to truth and the precision of scientific methods arose from the passion of scholars, their reciprocal hatred, their fanatical and unending discussions, and their spirit of competition.[36]

This was as relevant for obstetrics as for any other science and hence the vast number of treatises and accounts which entered into circulation. In addition to these stakes, however, there was a remarkable sense of apprehension in the writings on puerperal fever which, I think, was expressed so forcibly because these men midwives could analyse puerperal fever in so many particulars, but not prevent it. This accounts for both their reaction of frustration and their personification of the fever, so that, for instance,

Clarke referred to its 'treacherous manner' whereas for Gordon it 'promiscuously seized women'.[37]

Alexander Gordon was one of the few writers who dealt with puerperal fever outside a hospital context, although he had worked in Westminster and Middlesex lying-in hospitals in London before returning to Aberdeen to run a dispensary there. He published a treatise in 1795 on his observations about puerperal fever, covering exactly the same period as Clarke, the late 1780s. They differed in their accounts of the origin of the disease, Clarke suggesting that the fever was putrid in nature, while Gordon saw it as an inflammatory disease that arises from the 'commotion excited by labour'.[38]

Gordon is writing during a period of transition when inflammatory diseases are still widely assumed to be a single disease entity that can move from one space to another in the body but which do not have a single place of origin or specific causation. But alongside the older classification, there was emerging a theory of local irritation, of which the French doctor, Broussais, became the most famous proponent when he published in 1816. This theory of local irritation was built on knowing where the disease originally began and from there being able to predict its future; it was not possible to achieve this interpretation of the local source of the disease without pathological anatomy.[39] Gordon also captures the element of local irritation and, working with that in relation to puerperal fever, sees puerperal fever and erysipelas as 'concomitant epidemics':

> The analogy of the Puerperal Fever with erysipelas, will explain why it always seizes women after, and not before delivery. For, at the time when the erysipelas was epidemic, almost every person, admitted into the hospital of this place, with a wound, was, soon after his admission, seized with erysipelas in the vicinity of the wound. The same consequence followed the operations of surgery: and the cause is obvious; for the infectious matter, which produces erysipelas, was at that time, readily absorbed by the lymphatics, which were then open to receive it. Just so with respect to the Puerperal Fever; women escape it till after delivery; for, till that time, there is no inlet open to receive the infectious matter which produces the disease. But after delivery, the matter is readily and copiously admitted by the numerous patulous orifices, which are open to imbibe it, by the separation of the placenta from the uterus.[40]

This is the 'nature of puerperal inflammation' and its connection with erysipelas is further proven by the fact that

> a very frequent crisis of the disease is by an external erysipelas; which is a proof that there is a metastasis, or translation, of the inflammation, from the internal to the external parts.[41]

The issue of the external or causative agent, 'infectious matter' in Gordon's terms, entering and irritating the local organ, which is open to being irritated, is the heart of Broussais' work. From the vantage point of that analysis, it becomes possible for medicine to determine *which* organ is sick by interpreting the symptoms and how the organ has been open to an external agent.[42] The problem in respect of childbirth is the way in which the medicine of sick organs is reintroduced into the ideological fray about women. It has to be noted that Peu in his account of the 1664 epidemic in Paris cites the proximity of the wounded bodies of soldiers to the women giving birth or in the puerperal state (see above). Gordon, as we can see, also cites evidence of erysipelas developing from those who are wounded, and goes on to describe the 'patulous surfaces' which constitute wounded tissue for women in the wake of childbirth. Importantly, Broussais' commitment to a theory of localisation of disease and causative agents issued from his work as a military doctor, dealing with soldiers during the Napoleonic wars of 1805–14.[43] Yet, despite these near connections or analogous possibilities around open wounded tissues, no matter what the origin of the wound, puerperal fever continued to be seen as a malady to which women were especially subject almost by virtue of their reproductive organs and processes and this, along with the notion of a causative agent, complicated the obstetric view of the disease for a very long period.

Gordon described the onset of the fever as including 'a violent rigor or shivering fit', followed by fever, pain 'so excruciating that the miserable patients described their torture to be as great, or greater than what they suffered during labour'; a pulse rate of 'uncommon velocity'; 'considerable tumefaction of the abdomen'; a white, soft, moist tongue in the early stages, but if the fever became protracted, the tongue turning dry and rough, resembling the appearance of typhus; muddy, 'turbid' urine 'passed with pain and difficulty'; blood with a 'thick inflammatory crust'; hot and dry skin but often covered with 'partial sweats', themselves announcing 'the approach of death'; crimson colour in the cheeks which was also listed as a 'mortal symptom'; bile, frequently vomited, either green in colour or black, and resembling coffee grounds; lochia often diminished and in only a few suppressed; no secretion of milk; and diarrhoea, the only 'symptom rather to be desired than dreaded' for 'without a spontaneous or artificial diarrhoea, very few recovered'. He also states that 'in general, the patient retained her senses to the last'.[44]

Death was seldom easy:

> the pain of the abdomen, already excruciating, was aggravated by the act of respiration, and by the smallest motion of the trunk. The miserable patient, therefore lay on her back incapable of turning on either side, and unable to breathe. Death, in such circumstances, was an event much to be wished for.[45]

Early Theories on Causation

Clarke accepts Hulme's description of the fever, as we have seen, identifying the fever firmly with the symptoms of peritonitis. But what is its nature and what are its causes? He gathers together all his evidence, first suggesting that the season itself, the severe cold of the winter, contributes to the epidemic.[46] He reports that the patients have more 'inflammatory diseases' than usual, including 'acute rheumatism'; he also reports breathing difficulties. Gordon, eight years later, sees these manifestations as indicative of puerperal fever which he considers to be a complex of a number of disease entities, hitherto considered separately. Gordon is by far the most precise in his system of classification; he divides his evidence into symptoms, nature, seat, cause (and thus his approach to classification begins to resemble how Broussais will come to write). Clarke cites the rigours of childbirth as causative. He attempts to categorise the type of labour, whether it is a first labour, whether the fever has taken hold before the child is born, as he believes he has seen; and when precisely after birth women are falling prey to it:

> 27. Most of our patients attacked in the year 1787 were admitted in a weakly state, or had tedious and fatiguing labours. Four of those who died, were cases of first children. Two appeared to be ill during labour, and continued so, without intermission, after delivery. One of them died in thirty-six hours, and the other lived till the sixth day. Three were attacked on the second day after delivery, and died on the seventh, or of five days' illness. One was attacked on the fourth, and died on the tenth. One was very distinctly attacked on the ninth day, as she was sitting by a good fire, and died on the twelfth. Notwithstanding the short duration of this patient's disease, from five to six pounds of a yellow fetid fluid were found floating in the cavity of the abdomen, and a great deal of adhesive inflammation.[47]

The tradition of identifying the critical days of an illness extends back to Hippocrates and a 'numerically fixed duration' is part of the essential structure of disease.[48] This emphasis on the crisis period, on periodicity, that is how soon women were stricken with symptoms of the fever after delivery, was carefully noted. Gordon, for example, in his chart on the seventy-seven women whom he attended in Aberdeen, who contracted the fever between 1789 and 1792, lists their names (or at least the names of their husbands as in 'John Low's wife'), age, residence, who delivered them, the day the disease appeared, whether they were cured, and, if not cured, on what day they died, counted from when the disease first appeared. Indeed Gordon argued strongly that few diseases were as uniform and regularly identifiable as the fever, and, based on his observations, one expected the fever to make its appearance on the second or third day after delivery.[49]

The preoccupation with the problem of interval and periodicity became a long-standing one. Robert Collins, Clarke's son-in-law, generated a series of tables on recorded deaths from puerperal fever during his mastership in the Rotunda. He tried to construct a meaningful ratio between the time of the onset of the disease and death, and the numbers so affected. This exercise suggested that the fourth day of onset was the critical day, with the greatest number of fatalities.[50] Collins dismissed an assertion from other writers, including Hamilton of Edinburgh, that a significant variable in the disease's presence was whether or not women had 'suffered tedious and fatiguing labours', exposing them to a greater probability of the disease occurring.

There are still other factors to be considered. Clarke examines the distribution of the disease in respect of the local space of the hospital, linking it to the theory of miasmatic disease. All deliveries in the Rotunda were done in the top or attic storey, which was divided into four areas, each with one large ward of seven beds and two smaller ones of two beds each (and if two women were put to each bed, as Clarke suggests, a total of eighty-eight women could be accommodated in any one period). Clarke is puzzled by the fact that

> one of these divisions did not lose a single patient by the puerperal fever, whereas the mortality among the other three was nearly equal, though, upon the whole, there was a greater number of women sick in two of these divisions, which have a southern aspect.[51]

He concludes that a completely 'local contagion' in the hospital ward was at fault rather than the atmosphere at large:

> 29. Such partial distribution of disease, joined to circumstances already mentioned (waiting for the wards to be repaired) . . . rendered it probable that this fever derived its origin from local contagion, and not from anything noxious in the atmosphere.[52]

Gordon reached a similar conclusion to Clarke's, that 'the cause of Epidemic Puerperal Fever . . . was not owing to a noxious constitution of the atmosphere.'[53] Yet they divided on the issue of its being putrid or inflammatory.

Charles White, an English man midwife working and writing in Manchester in 1777, nearly twenty years before Gordon, sees the fever as a putrescent one, caused by a putrid atmosphere directly attributable to the customs surrounding pregnancy and childbirth: the tightness of stays and petticoat bindings, during the early months of pregnancy, obstructs the lower intestines creating constipation, which is further exacerbated by a sedentary, inactive way of life, all of which leads to a 'putrescent acrimony'. The profuse sweats of labour, taking place in a small room with a great fire, crowded with friends, renders the air unfit for breathing but all too able to generate putrid fevers that are infectious in nature. After birth, the fear of a woman catching a chill is so great that her entire chamber is stopped up, even the keyhole, leading to profuse sweats and a condition in which the lochia would stagnate and the effluvia from the vagina and the womb turn the atmosphere putrid.[54]

White is describing the circumstances of well-off women, 'those of condition or such as effect to live like those of condition above labour'.[55] In his account women are made culpable for the appearance of the fever, by their way of life, their dress, their 'sedentary' habits and their social modes of conduct around birth, including the presumption of involvement of numberless women 'friends' whose very presence pollutes the atmosphere. But White is well able to extend his arguments to cover lower-class women 'who live in cellars and upon clay ground floors' where 'the air is still made worse by the dampness and closeness of their houses', by 'the want of clean linen, and cleanliness in general'. Should they live in garrets, 'the putrid miasmata of several families, inhabiting the lower part of the house ascend to them.'[56]

In other words, the arguments about causation flowed in a number of directions. The principal modes of classification and features seemed to be these: whether the fever was inflammatory or putrid; whether it was localised only as peritonitis in or around the peritoneum, with the folds of the omentum more especially affected or not; whether it could be 'translated' to the external parts of the body as with erysipelas; whether it was accompanied by typhus or typhus-like symptoms; whether it was a contagion or not; whether shivering fits denoted the fever or were ephemeral, lasting only briefly and unconnected. Gélis lists a 1782 table, dividing symptoms into 'permanent', like the rapid pulse rate, distended abdomen, shrinking breasts; and 'intermittent', including violent shivering, nausea, or vomiting of green or yellow matter.[57]

White concluded that whether the fever was attributed to the milk, an inflammation of the womb, suppression of the lochia, or whether it was a symptom of hysteria, 'all have agreed to its fatality, and the uncertainty of every method of cure, both in the rich and the poor'.[58] The abdominal pain associated with peritonitis that Clarke mentions was long seen as the clearest indication of puerperal fever, so much so that the two were considered synonymous. Their task as scientists was first to describe the fever, attempting to isolate it from the many contagious fevers of the period. The symptomatology of typhus and typhoid fevers, for example, were similar enough to puerperal fever that early commentators conflated the two, considering puerperal fever a variant of typhus,[59] or, even at a later point, chose to see typhus rather than puerperal fever, as with Johnston, in the passage at the beginning of this chapter. Many of the descriptions of puerperal fever report that the tongue was dry and brown and the pulse quickened, similar to symptoms of typhus.

When Fleetwood Churchill, the Dublin man midwife, put together an edited collection of papers written in the eighteenth and early nineteenth centuries on puerperal fever in 1849, he explained that he had chosen them on the basis of differing descriptions and opinions of the disease, to illustrate 'the variations of the disease in different eyes'.[60] He compiled a chart, listing the localities of all reported epidemics between 1664 and 1846 in which the disease entity connected with the fever was variously described as peritonitis, hysteritis (an inflammation of the womb), uterine phlebitis, and inflammation of the omentum. Churchill observed that there was much written about in earlier times which could now be seen 'to be erroneous, both physiologically and pathologically'.[61] For him, progress in understanding the nature of the disease entity could be judged by the fact that 'each successive treatise' fitted into a pattern whereby it contained fewer and fewer 'hypothetical statements . . . more strictly confined within the domain of experience'.[62] In reading this we are not to forget the importance of that validation of knowledge whereby obstetrics argues that it progressively moves towards a position of truth, nor Fleck's caution about evidence conforming to conceptions, conceptions which operate more and more as a closed system.

There are two possible therapeutic approaches with puerperal fever, how to prevent it and how to cure it, both dependent to an extent on what the practitioner argues is the cause of the disease. Churchill reprints extracts from most of the writers we have encountered thus far, and their prognostications on each of these aspects. One way to prevent the fever relates to the buildings of the lying-in hospital.

So Clarke, for instance, following on his conclusion that the cause of the disease was a 'local contagion', ordered that two of the great wards in the Rotunda be closed off entirely. Walls and ceilings were whitewashed, bedsteads painted, any bedding that could be was scoured, the rest hung out to the open air. A fire was set in the wards by day and by night; all the windows were kept open. These measures to halt the progress of the disease in lying-in hospitals had already been written up by Young of Edinburgh and White of Manchester. Clarke was convinced of their arguments that local infection in the part of the building where women were dying was always the source of the fever, and such activity seemed to him to largely defeat the epidemic. When a new epidemic occurred in the winter of 1788, he repeated the steps of whitewashing the walls and scouring the ward floors with lime solutions and, despite the expense, sought to make permanent a system for ventilating and purifying the wards:

to prevent the generation of such infection, I have no doubt that lying-in hospitals, whose beds are in constant use, ought to undergo annually a refit, such as already described, excepting only the article of painting. The bedding of every woman who dies should be instantly carried out and scoured, before it is replaced.[63]

Rotation of the wards in use at any one time, leaving one empty to air, and a system of air holes drilled in the frames of all windows and doors completed his general hospital regime.[64] This appeared to lower death rates in Dublin when compared with the Viennese Lying-in Hospital and the Hôtel-Dieu in Paris, for example, where rates of mortality ran to 10 per cent of all patients. The mortality rate in the Allgemeines Krankenhaus in Vienna fluctuated between 7.8 and 9.8 per cent of all women giving birth there in the early nineteenth century,[65] and, for the years 1829–49, the figures for the three institutes indicated that the Rotunda was the lowest:

Table 3.2: Death Rates of Patients in Major European Lying-in Hospitals, 1829–49

City	%
Paris	41.8
Vienna	5.35
Dublin (Rotunda)	1.34

Source: T.D. O'Donel Browne (1947), *The Rotunda Hospital, 1745–1945*, p. 123.

So the English, Scottish and Irish approaches did result in lower mortality rates compared with the Continent where sanitary and quarantine-type measures were not in use, presumably increasing the scope of operation for some forms of micro-organisms. White had proposed an even more individualised preventative regime, directing that a newly delivered woman should have clean linen at once. She should be left to sleep in a large lofty room which had a northern aspect, with no fire in summer and little in winter; if in hospital, the wards, with unglazed windows, should lie alongside lofty galleries and a system of air pipes should be installed throughout the hospital to circulate fresh air as an antidote to a miasmic atmosphere. White also argued in favour of putting a light binding around the belly, once a woman had given birth, and then sitting the woman up in bed to prevent the lochia from stagnating; also, using emetics to produce stools, and the woman rising from her bed as soon as possible, not deferring this any later than the second or third day.[66] He argued that while he had observed these rules, he had never lost a single woman at the time of her lying-in, due to the fever, hastening to qualify that he was speaking only of 'natural parturitions'; he could not include 'preternatural' cases or those which required the use of instruments or instances of floodings and convulsions when speaking of not losing patients.[67]

His recommendation to sit the woman up in bed was the measure that drew adverse comment from Churchill, editing essays some seventy years later. The latter wrote:

> As a general rule, I have preferred that the theoretical and practical errors of each essay should be corrected by the increasing information of the succeeding; but the directions in these 3 paragraphs are so pernicious and so purely theoretical, that I must enter my protest against them. Precisely the contrary is the practice of the present day: a careful presentation of the horizontal posture as much as possible for several days, both when nursing, taking food and effecting the necessary evacuations may be regarded as an axiom in the management of women in childbed.[68]

This passage raises disturbing issues of control. Why, of all White's recommendations, should one relating to women being kept bedridden for a short time be critically rejected, while the exact opposite practice of keeping women bedridden for as long as possible achieves the status of an 'axiom', a scientific principle? Physiologically, its detrimental impact slowed circulation in the legs. The 'management', that is, the control of women is the only clear answer, itself an axiom related more to the growing ideology of the hysterised woman of Foucault's analysis. Or, as Mary Poovey puts it, it is a matter of how the institutional practices of medicine do the 'ideological work of gender' in order to reinforce women's social subordination through control of their reproductive experiences.[69] Churchill's editorial comment is also a perfect example of a narrowing logical system which cannot tolerate difference but seeks to dismiss it.[70]

Clarke contended that there were two types of puerperal fever, accidental and epidemic. When the fever arose from 'accidental causes', inducing inflammation, there was 'reason for better hope of success', but when the fever was epidemic in form, there was no regime guaranteed to cure it, although one could work to relieve symptoms.[71] Forms of treatment varied in accordance with these complex beliefs on accidental and epidemic causes, with how a link could come about between the two escaping the eye of almost all observers.

As to treatment, Gordon wrote that if one accepted a link between erysipelas and puerperal fever, and one believed that bleeding and purging were an incorrect treatment regime for erysipelas, then one might prescribe instead cordials and tonic medicines (although this latter was a useless therapeutic regime, he hastened to add). For not the 'highest authority upon earth' could persuade him to 'admit a doctrine, which disagrees with my own experience'.[72] Wines and cordials were fatal; the answer lay rather in bleeding and purging. Of his seventy-seven women, forty-nine recovered and twenty-eight died. They owed their recovery to what might be termed a theory or regime of evacuation of blood and bowels, the 'two great twin hinges, upon which the cure of the Puerperal Fever turns'.[73] Friends of the particular woman or women objected to this treatment, believing that it stopped the discharge of the lochia, and made their objections heard to the woman herself, to whom access could not be restricted in the domestic setting. Gordon concluded from these experiences that 'scientific practice and popular opinion very seldom correspond'.[74] But he persevered, advising that too little blood resulted in fatalities:

> when I took away only ten or twelve ounces of blood . . . she always died; but when I had courage to take away twenty or twenty-four ounces at one bleeding, the patient never failed to recover, as was the case with Nos. 23., 28., 33., 35., 36., 40., 41., 52., 53., 54., 56., 58., 60., 61., 62., 67., 70., &c in the foregoing table.[75]

The assertion should stand out because here Gordon argues that he is making a purely scientific observation, based on his own results, and he even records his results from which he draws this conclusion. So he is proceeding in a recognisably scientific manner, from a series of descriptions to a postulate. If he were called in soon enough after symptoms commenced, he argued that profuse bleeding and the administration of a 'brisk purgative' – he preferred calomel, a mercury compound and jalap taken orally – to produce five or six strong motions daily, and an opiate to encourage sleep, brought the disease to a 'remission' by the third day or a conclusion by the fifth day, if it did not end it at once.[76] The time intervals whereby to judge the efficacy of the regime are once more noteworthy. But the actual therapeutic elements are still more interesting, combining, as they do, elements of the older medicine of humours and the tentative gropings towards what would become a medicine of microbiology and the need for asepsis. Bleeding and purgatives were part of this older system of treatment, in which it had been considered vital to keep the body fluids well regulated. For the body itself was fluid, subject to innumerable processes and shifts, and the female body most fluid and labile of all.[77]

Nevertheless, it is possible that Gordon's treatment could have helped the body rid itself of associated toxins through the production of copious diarrhoea. Part of Gordon's compound, mercury, encouraged exactly what he was aiming towards as did jalap, a drug derived from a tuberous plant grown in Mexico, and another strong purgative. The two combined would have had a dramatic effect in this regard. Mercury also had an antiseptic action, when used as a caustic, irritant or purgative; it was highly poisonous to bacteria (and to humankind as well).[78] So, even if the principles of microbes and antisepsis were not so named, the effects of mercury were, and, because Gordon was so careful in recording his observations, he noted where precise improvements occurred. Additionally, the opiate-led patterns of sleep might well have proved beneficial in preventing more minor forms of infection from having a more major impact leading to death.[79]

On the other hand, another strong component of humoral medicine, that deep inflammation could be countered with surface irritation, leading to treatment with caustic substances to raise blisters on the surface of the skin, was a practice Gordon rejected, on the basis of his observations. He found that blisters, when applied to the abdomen, irritated and induced sweating with uncertain results, and fomentations where flannels were wrung in hot water and applied, quickened the pulse still further, and so he discarded what he considered these useless forms of treatment.[80]

Clarke mentions carrying out blood-letting, or venesection, on his patients before the first epidemic in the Rotunda, but he did not consider it a treatment for puerperal fever. He had read the arguments other men midwives had advanced in its favour but he judged it to have only the effect of alleviating the symptoms and remained unconvinced of any curative properties, where the fever was present.[81] Clarke did use purgatives however, and his entry on those and what influenced him to choose that mode of treatment also points to this network of communication amongst medical scientists across Europe. Enormous increases in deaths from puerperal fever in Paris in the 1770s, rising to 9.6 per cent in 1778, led to the serious concern of the French government and the medical professionals who were searching for solutions. In 1781, a man midwife, Doulcet, concluded that the fever was a sort of gastric fever and on that basis, in order to induce vomiting, began administering grains of ipecacuanha, another plant of Latin American origin, whose roots had an emetic effect, to newly delivered women in the Hôtel-Dieu. Initially, it was hailed as a 'miracle cure' and instructions on the regime were circulated throughout France in a government-sponsored promotion of a curative programme. But after all, it appeared that what Doulcet had cured was a milk fever and not puerperal fever at all and the cure was abandoned.[82]

Before ipecacuanha was discarded, though, it was employed in Ireland, on the basis of the French example. Clarke comments that during the 1788 epidemic, he used a combination of tartar emetic and ipecacuanha 'as lately recommended by the Royal Medical Society of Paris', along with clysters of senna leaves and tobacco meant to irritate and thus stimulate evacuation. Once more, there is the important circulation of possible interpretations and treatments through scientific journals. Clarke commented that there were 'very unusual degrees of insensibility' to this regime and the inability of women's bodies to respond was accepted as meaning an extremely poor outlook for recovery.

By the late 1820s, the therapeutic regime of bleeding and purging, the latter especially relying on the use of mercury, was seen as the treatment which had proved most reliable. But it had numerous additions. In the Rotunda, Collins used a draught of castor oil and oil of turpentine for emptying the air secreted in the intestines; three or four dozen leeches followed by a warm bath to remove the blood, both leeches and baths to be repeated at intervals of four, five or six hours; stuping, the 'fomentations' of which Gordon had disapproved, with the cloths wrung out and spread across the entire surface of the abdomen 'as hot as can be endured'; mercury, in the form of calomel, and ipecacuanha powder, four grains each, administered every second, third or fourth hour; and a mercury ointment applied externally to the whole surface of the abdomen until it blistered, opium to ensure rest, and wine, whey and chicken broth as desired by the patient.[83]

The strategy was one of dealing with the fever as a local inflammation, wherever it was thought to take hold; hence the concentration on the abdominal area, both internally and externally. Thomas Beatty, first Master of the Coombe Lying-in Hospital, characterised the regime as one of 'counter irritation' and 'local depletion' accompanied by the 'judicious use of stimulants'.[84] Beatty wrote up case notes on the impact of this therapy in his first annual report on the Coombe, like the following:

> The other case occurred in a woman aged 30 years, who was delivered of her first child on the 18th February, after an easy labour of eight hours. She complained of pain in the uterine region extending to the right side, on the second day after delivery, pulse 120. She was leeched freely, purged, stuped, and slightly mercurialized, under which treatment the urgent symptoms subsided, but never entirely disappeared. The pulse continued at 100, and the skin hot; however, she appeared to be getting better until the 25th, just ten days after her delivery, when she was suddenly seized with violent pain in the belly, rigor, vomiting; pulse 140, weak; she sank rapidly and died in twenty-four hours.[85]

Collins presents similar notes on his 103 cases which ended in death. Both scientists are still aiming at an inclusive description of the case in hand, searching for the common components which might explain under what circumstances the fever proves exactly fatal and, equally, under what combination of symptoms, treatment appears most successful. The sense of complete confidence in the regime, despite the fatal outcome for these 103 women, is marked.

In his first report, Beatty also includes the case notes by Dr Houghton, his colleague, for Margaret Grant, who gave birth in the Coombe Hospital on 31 October 1834. Within three days, she had developed 'symptoms of inflammation of the uterus'. Treated with the customary regime, she was moved after ten days to Sir Patrick Dun's hospital from where after almost a month she was discharged as well. Three weeks after she had returned home, still 'complaining' of a swelling and soreness in her right side,

> her father came running into the hospital, South Cumberland-street, at half past ten o'clock, earnestly requesting that medical aid should be instantly given her . . . I went with him to their dwelling in Grand Canal-street. She lay screaming with agony on her left side, with her knees drawn towards her belly. She threw her arms to me supplicating some relief, not moving, however, any part, except the upper extremity and thorax . . . she related to me with difficulty, that about half past nine o' clock . . . she was all at once seized with a pain of excruciating intensity at the right side of the belly . . . she was placed on the bed immediately, in the opinion of the people present, dying. She vomited and fainted. On proceeding to examine her abdomen, she screamed to keep off my hand from touching her; it was swelled up in a round form.[86]

Margaret Grant then went through this regime for a second time, being bled 'ad deliquium', that is until she fainted; likewise, she was blistered, treated with calomel, opium, turpentine, salts, jalap and so on. A week later, she was much improved; by the 27th, 'now decidedly advanced to recovery' although there were ongoing symptoms and after-effects, pain and tenderness.

> May 2nd. I called to see her to-day. She is grown full and strong, but the belly is somewhat swelled, and some tumour still remains in the region of the right ovary . . . she has never menstruated since, although the milk was stopped at the time of the accident.[87]

Beatty adds as an afterword:

> The recovery is worthy of record, in as much as it shews the efficacy of bold and scientific practice. The quantity of opium, and calomel administered was very great and I think it is very likely that either of them alone would not have been successful.[88]

Gordon, writing up a similar case, probably of cellulitis, judging by the description of purulent matter that burst through the woman's umbilicus, had treated her primarily with opiate in large doses, for in the first instance, he assumed there was no hope and sought only to relieve the pain. The opiate-induced sleep itself may have done much good and he continued in the same vein, and wrote: 'I was now in hopes that nature would provide a cure'. A month later, the woman was much recovered:

> Thus we have a very singular and uncommon termination of a very dangerous and deplorable case, which shews the wonderful powers of nature, and what she is capable of performing, even in the most desperate and hopeless cases.[89]

However, Shorter points out that in such instances, recovery, which for men midwives meant not dying, most probably entailed 'abscesses, adhesions, or chronic tubal infections . . . an enduring, painful souvenir of her infection'.[90] and, with this legacy, women had to face pregnancy and the threat of puerperal fever again. Gordon mentions women who are several times pregnant following puerperal fever.[91]

Preventing the Fever: Using Death and Dissection

Foucault reminds us that Hippocrates presented an early codification of medicine in which experience, the process of linking, seeing, and knowing, became dominated by the latter so that seeing ceased and metaphysics and philosophy held sway. The challenge of seeing and creating knowledge from what was seen, of developing theory from the less visible rather than the more visible surface of the body, became possible once dissection was part of pathological anatomy in the eighteenth century. After death, the body could yield up its knowledge about disease, leading to death.[92] Obstetric science was in an excellent position to use dissection to extend its clinical knowledge in the lying-in hospitals. In the Paris outbreak of puerperal fever in 1664, Peu had already used dissection to find that the bodies of women were 'full of abscesses'.[93]

Dissections, and the information gleaned from them, were regularly recorded in Clarke's registry, the registry itself an indication of how rapidly women were inserted into a clinical routine of surveillance, dividing up the day according to when observations were made and clocked in, as distinct from women's individual rhythms. Clarke is unequivocal on the importance of dissection:

> The Registry, from which the preceding abstract is taken, was kept by my assistant in the hospital, and for the most part under my own inspection. The occurrences of every twenty-four hours were noted daily, at an early hour. Patients who died, labouring under doubtful symptoms, were examined by dissection, whenever permission to do so could be easily procured from their friends.[94]

His comment on seeking permission points to a fundamental issue for obstetrics. Gordon wrote that he was often prevented by 'friends' from undertaking dissection.[95] But it must have become less easy for friends to object to dissection as time went on because the medical strategy of identifying causes of death established itself as a quasi-legal practice of great authority, indeed a practice integral to interpreting what was happening in the wider society, that might or might not require levels of surveillance.[96] As part of a science in the making, Clarke saw his registry as a way to establish authoritative truths:

Of every death and dissection a short note was made in the Registry, generally by myself. Upon the whole, therefore, I am inclined to consider what is here offered to public notice as a collection of matters of fact, or at least as near an approximation to truth, as the nature of such subjects will permit.

With the view of rendering these facts more useful to the inexperienced, I have subjoined some short practical remarks – By these means, it is hoped, accurate ideas will be conveyed to the reader, of what actually passed in the hospital, during the period it was entrusted to my care.[97]

The definition of what constituted puerperal fever or in Gordon's words where 'the seat' of the disease was located emerged from dissection. Clarke, during the 1787 epidemic, recorded these observations:

25. The appearance, on dissection, of the bodies of six patients who died of this fever, were not materially different from what have been described by writers who have seen the disease in hospitals. In all our subjects, the omentum appeared inflamed, and wasted in substance, but in no instance mortified. I am inclined to think, from numerous observations, that those writers who have described mortification of the omentum, and some other parts of the abdominal viscera, allowed the dead bodies to remain too long after death before they inspected them. In all our dissections, the peritoneum appeared everywhere unusually vascular and inflamed. Next to the omentum, the broad ligaments of the uterus, the caecum, and sigmoid flexure of the colon seemed to suffer most by inflammation. We always met with more or less a turbid yellow, and sometimes fetid fluid floating among the intestines; coagulated purulent-like masses, adhesive inflammation, glueing the intestines to each other, &c. In no instance did the appearances of inflammation seem to penetrate deeper than the peritoneal coat, on any of the viscera of the abdomen or pelvis.[98]

There followed a lengthy aside, in which Clarke pondered why the omentum was so greatly affected with this disease, Clarke then accepting Forster's conclusion that the disease was usefully identified by the nosological name of peritonitis, that is, inflammation of the peritoneum.[99]

Gordon argued that to understand the fever medical men urgently required observation, rather than theory, and that dissection was essential to this process:

I am fully persuaded, that if practitioners had observed more and reasoned less, there would have been little dispute, either about the nature or seat of this disease . . . the doctrine which I propose to deliver, concerning the nature of the Puerperal Fever shall be grounded on the cases which I saw and the dissections which I made.[100]

Dissection anchored the medical gaze, extending the boundaries of medicine and, along with record-keeping, became the instrument of instruction, transmitted from doctor to student doctor.[101] What Foucault writes about dissection is precisely relevant to the stance taken by both Gordon and Clarke, that if life hides the truth and death reveals it, 'death is the great analyst that shows the connections by unfolding them'.[102]

Tragically, in relation to puerperal fever, what operated was a curiously lethal inversion, in which revealing the truth accumulated death for women, who were already overburdened with its presence at birth. We see Gordon and Clarke move towards the science of the clinic that is above all an 'oracular' science,[103] with dissection the key that enables medicine to speak with confidence and even authority. There is a sense in which dissection became part of the strategy of immortality for obstetrics, substantiating the claim of the science to guarantee maternal and infant life on sure and certain principles. This is how Gordon writes of it, that the 'established facts and incontrovertible truths', which dissection revealed, were the basis for his 'doctrine of the Puerperal Fever'.[104]

A crucial moment in his understanding of the disease comes with dissection. Isabel Allan, 'No. 17' of Gordon's cases, was a thirty-six-year-old married woman, to whom he was called in some twenty-four hours after delivery, when she had been attacked by a shivering fit and acute pain in the right side of the abdomen. He attempted his usual treatment of bleeding and purgatives. But she died within five days of the disease first appearing:

> Leave being given to inspect the abdomen, I went on that business on the evening of the 28th, attended by Mr Harvey, Mr John Gordon, and Mr Joseph M'Rae. Upon opening the abdomen, I found the peritoneum, and its production the omentum, mesentery, and mesecolon, in a state of inflammation. The omentum had lost about half its substance by suppuration; the mesentery and mesecolon, and that part of the intestinal canal, with which they are connected, were very much inflamed. But the disease appeared more especially to the right side; the right ovarium had come to a suppuration; the colon from its caput along the course of the ascending arch, was much inflamed, and beginning to run into gangrene. A large quantity of pus and extravasted serum appeared in the cavity of the abdomen, which when taken out and measured, amounted to two English pints. The peritoneal coat of the uterus was inflamed, and the organ itself not so compact and contracted as it ought to have been. Upon opening it, the cavity was found covered with a black coloured substance, which at first sight had the appearance of mortification, but when wiped off, was found to be, nothing else than the membrana decidua, in the state in which it naturally is about this time.[105]

For Gordon, the dissections provided the incontrovertible facts of the existence of puerperal fever, or peritonitis, along with Allen's case notes.

Robert Collins worked in a similar manner some thirty-five years later. In his case notes, Collins catalogued the time each woman became ill, the interval after birth, whether this was a first birth or not; the sorts of symptoms each woman exhibited; the treatment regime of each; when she died in relation to the onset of the illness; and, finally, the appearance of her body when dissected, most especially where the disease had attacked. The state of the peritoneum, the omentum, how much bloody serum was found in the abdominal cavity, were presented for each case. But because all these cases were presented sequentially, with the dissection of each, we can read in two directions, back to the previous dissection and forward to the next and thus we have a clue about the reason for the death of each succeeding woman. This tracing of changes and symptoms led to a concrete and accurate account of the disease known as puerperal fever, although the accuracy remained limited to its description under dissection only, and not to a linking of causes, most especially not to a linking between contagion and the practice of dissection itself.

Gordon asserted that 'the cause of this disease was a specific contagion, or infection' for which contention he had 'unquestionable proof'.[106] The disease 'seized such women only, as were visited or delivered, by a practitioner, or taken care of by a nurse, who had previously attended patients affected with the disease.'[107] His observation was that the infection that caused the disease was more quickly communicated than smallpox or measles, and worked more rapidly than any other infection he could identify. His chief argument was this:

> With respect to the physical qualities of the infection, I have not been able to make any discovery; but I had evident proofs that every person, who had been with a patient in the Puerperal Fever, became charged with an atmosphere of infection, which was communicated to every pregnant woman, who happened to come within its sphere. This is not an assertion, but a fact, admitting of demonstration, as may be seen by a perusal of the foregoing table.[108]

Using his table, he then tracked how the midwife, Mrs Blake, who delivered James Garrow's wife, 'carried the infection' to James Smith's wife, 'the next woman whom she delivered'. He himself attended both these women and carried the infection to 'No. 5. and 6., who were delivered by him, and to many others'.[109] He traced the infectious spread of a fever through an entire country parish, whence it had been carried by a midwife who had delivered the fifty-fifth woman of his table.

His account of how infection is transported becomes quite literal: a man servant carries it from his sister in Aberdeen to his wife, six miles distant (although it is not clear whether he has helped deliver her or what the physical contact is); the midwife who is present to deliver his wife infects two other women both of whom die. The key to Gordon's being able to make these connections is that he conceives of puerperal fever as being similar to that of synochus, a non-specific but unremitting fever or typhus, another class of acute fever. So his initial organising category is that these are all contagious fevers, infection from which is common for pregnant women. He argues that puerperal fever acts like these other two fevers, with the difference that it affects the peritoneum so immediately. A second difference is to do with the times of onset: typhus 'always' takes place before delivery whereas puerperal fever only occurs after delivery. Thus, whatever circumstance makes infection from puerperal fever possible seems to prevent typhus. Timing in the onset of a disease becomes a second important distinguishing feature.

The third feature has to do with contagion itself; the contagion that produces typhus is not the same as puerperal fever. Therefore the diseases have quite different symptoms, the chief one in puerperal fever being pain in the abdomen, and of typhus, pain in the head with no abdominal complication. Interestingly, he quotes Kirkland who sees typhus as a miasmatic fever, a term more usually associated with this notion of a putrid fever, which Gordon otherwise rejects.

Clarke, for his part, was content to rest with the notion of puerperal fever as a local contagion which affected the peritoneum. He limited his preventative measures to the wards and the individual bedding whereas Gordon said that, to prevent the fever, fresh air and cleanliness were insufficient for its destruction:

> The patient's apparel and bed-clothes ought to be burnt or thoroughly purified; and the nurses and physicians, who have attended patients affected with the Puerperal Fever, ought carefully to wash themselves, and to get their apparel thoroughly fumigated before it be put on again.[110]

The critical emphasis is on the necessity of washing hands *after* attending women with puerperal fever, and before attending another patient. This is the first time the notion that a birth attendant might carry the disease and that the chain can be broken by hand-washing, along with Gordon's other measures, appears in print as both observation and intervention against the fever's scourge. Like the initial value of the Wassermann test, in the development of scientific thinking about syphilis, the usefulness of Gordon's method and results were not immediately clear for what they might represent, even for Gordon himself, who continued to search for a curative treatment.

Gordon writes that he settled on his regime of treatment, purging and bleeding, after he was convinced of the nature of the disease by the evidence of his dissections:

> If the cure be early attempted, and conducted according to the method which I propose, only one in ten will die, if we calculate according to my

success in the above-mentioned fifty cases. And it deserves to be remarked, that all these five died before the third dissection, from which I discovered the certain method of curing the Puerperal Fever. The time when the third dissection was made, may be reckoned the era from which we are to date the discovery of the cure of the disease; for, after that time, of thirty patients who were treated in the manner to be afterwards mentioned, not one died.[111]

This was his third dissection, his fourth case of puerperal fever, a twenty-five-year-old married woman, whose name Gordon appears to deliberately leave blank in his chart; she appears as No. 38 only, with not even her husband's surname to identify her. From December 1789 to December 1790, when this woman was delivered, thirty-seven women had died in Aberdeen from puerperal fever, leading Gordon to keep his records about this epidemic. She fell ill after an 'easy labour' and Gordon purged her and bled her, but less vigorously than he came to recommend thereafter. Her subsequent death 'afforded a lamentable proof of the imperfection of our art' for, when he carried out the dissection, he discovered 'but a slight degree of inflammation' in the abdominal cavity compared with the usual ravages of the fever. He concludes, therefore, that 'we lost our patient for want of courage to carry out evacuations to a proper extent', and, the 'truth' of his conclusion 'which I formed from the dissection . . . was confirmed by my success in all the succeeding cases to which I was called'.[112]

Between 1790 and 1792, Gordon's results in diminishing death from puerperal fever were partly due to a combination of hand-washing by attendants, disinfecting clothes of attendants and the woman giving birth, and burning bed linen, in order to prevent 'carrying' the contagion. These measures tackled two major sources of infection, the examining hand and the septic environment in the form of the clothing of the attendant, carrying the contagion from an infected woman to one not yet infected. It did not deal with infection after an obstetrical operation necessarily, nor did Gordon's regime indicate that attendants were, as a matter of course, washing their hands before and after each delivery, where suspected contagion with puerperal fever was *not* yet an issue. But even the measures he did take would have reduced women's exposure considerably.

Yet it is possible to trace the exact point in Gordon's investigations at which he inadvertently lifted from women the most virulent epidemic source of the fever. It involves his belief that he had found the cure for puerperal fever, on the heels of that third dissection. He relates that, thereafter, only nine deaths resulted amongst thirty-nine women, compared with nineteen amongst thirty-eight in the first part of the epidemic. It appears that he carried out *no further dissections*, once he was convinced of his grounds for treatment, and it is therefore in a double sense that 'the loss of this patient was the means of saving others.'[113] For, in ceasing dissection, he ceased to infect women as a result of that work. Hence it was that of seventy-seven women who contracted puerperal fever, forty-nine survived.

Gordon wrote candidly that 'It is a disagreeable declaration for me to mention, that I myself was the means of carrying the infection to a great number of women',[114] and he found it a 'consolation' that he had discovered a cure, knowledge which diminished his uneasiness that his attendance had caused deaths. As an aside, Gordon notes that in the course of dissecting a woman's body, where puerperal fever has been the cause of death, if the surgeon scratches his finger, the wound 'festers', 'inflames and suppurates'. He offers this insight as proof that the fever is inflammatory at the outset, and then turns putrid in its effect.[115]

Gordon's is the most complete regime of preventative care to guard against puerperal fever until the publications of Oliver Wendell Holmes in the United States, in 1843, and Ignaz Semmelweis, in Vienna, in 1847. For our purposes, we must ask why the notion of contagion, as outlined by Gordon, did not go 'downstream', and why his methods of analysis, especially the tracking of cases, and his results did not get picked up by men midwives of his era. It may be related to his not having been part of the emerging teaching structure located in the hospital, given that the hospital was the special and preferred site in the politics of sustaining emerging rationales and systems of thought in obstetrics.

But it may also be that which Oliver Wendell Holmes referred to as 'the painful subject which has come before us',[116] – the issue that puerperal fever was spread by contagion touched on nascent sensibilities within the science, which grew rather than lessened over that fifty-year period, and were further strengthened with the tightening of logical arguments around female frailty. So often, these gendered arguments doubled back on a woman, her frailty making her responsible in effect for her own death.

Fleetwood Churchill, for example, was curiously ambivalent on this theory of contagion in his introduction to collected essays on the topic in 1849. For him, it was a 'very important question' which remained unproven either way:

> So far as the weight of opinion goes, it is in favour of contagion, among practitioners of the present day, but I think we are scarcely yet in a position to speak quite positively.[117]

And yet he had little difficulty in accepting that women could spread it to one another in the lying-in ward. Churchill listed some authorities who denied the notion of contagion but a majority who affirmed it, including Gordon, and, moreover, several of whom, like Gordon, argued that a third person could transmit the contagion. He quotes a Dr Campbell, writing in 1831 from Edinburgh in reply to another practitioner, Dr Lee, on the subject of the fever's contagiousness, in which Campbell recounts carrying out a dissection of a woman in October 1821 and then pocketing the pelvic viscera and, without changing clothing, going to assist some of his students deliver another woman by forceps who dies, many others whom he delivers also dying in the next few weeks. In June of 1823, he finds himself assisting at a dissection and 'for want of accommodation' is unable to wash his hands with 'that care which I ought to have done' so that arriving home and finding two patients requiring his help 'without further ablution of my hands or changing my clothes', he delivers them. Both women die of puerperal fever.[118]

Even with this evidence, Churchill is not altogether convinced, saying that '"Post hoc" is not always "propter hoc", however, and we must not forget that puerperal fever was epidemic in Edinburgh in 1821–2'.[119] Discussing practitioners who quote similar cases, Churchill then writes:

> The Evidence and proofs thus adduced are of extreme importance, and I fear we must conclude, however reluctantly, in favour, not merely of the contagiousness of puerperal fever, but of the possibility of its contagion being carried by an intermediate party.[120]

Churchill quotes the advice of a Dr Copland that any doctor engaged in obstetric practice, where puerperal fever occurs, should relinquish care of women who are giving birth while tending to cases of the fever or of erysipelas or else 'he should change all his clothes and carefully wash his hands, after seeing cases of either of these maladies, before proceeding to a puerperal female',[121] and should not carry out autopsies in the same period of time. Churchill mentions in a cautionary fashion that

> the practice of midwifery is doubly distressing during the prevalence of an epidemic, and ought deeply to impress us with the necessity of the utmost care and caution.[122]

And yet in 1869, on the still vexed issue of whether practitioners themselves could be instrumental in spreading the fever, Churchill stated unequivocally that

> a doctor could not carry infection from one patient to another. Having first explained that his precautions were the same as those practised by [Evory] Kennedy, he added that he was satisfied that he himself had never carried infection from one woman to another, or of being himself a carrier.[123]

For all his careful review, Churchill's resistance was entrenched.

Holmes and Semmelweis are the two doctors most usually associated with proving the basis for contagion in puerperal fever. In the mid-1840s, when they published their articles on puerperal fever, both doctors were hospital-based, Holmes as a professor in the Harvard Medical School and

136 *Reading Birth and Death*

Semmelweis as assistant professor in charge of several of the wards in the Vienna Lying-in Hospital, yet the work of neither was happily received. The rejection of Semmelweis's work is especially intriguing. He was convinced that the autopsy was the lethal source of epidemic cases in the lying-in hospitals. But the reaction of absolute hostility on the part of his fellow professionals to his findings included an outright rejection of the depth of his clinical data on rates of morbidity and mortality before and after he issued his edict to his students to wash their hands in chloride of lime 'to destroy the cadaveric particles'.[124]

One response to Semmelweis' publications came from the seventeenth Master of the Rotunda, Denham, who stated that 'With respect to the opinions put forth by Dr Semmelweis . . . I feel it would only be a waste of time to dwell on them.'[125] Denham quoted a German man midwife who declared that the fever was caused by a 'poison' taken up before labour sets in:

> on which basis Denham concluded that the fever was 'epidemic' rather than infectious. He also quoted the American Meigs, who had been vitriolic in his dismissal of Holmes' account of the same principles. Meigs was reputed to have said 'Still, I certainly never was the medium of its transmission.'[126]

Edward Murphy published a paper on puerperal fever, in the *Dublin Quarterly Journal of Medical Science*, in 1857, in which he acknowledged for the first time, in Dublin obstetric circles, Semmelweis' 'valuable observations', but yet he continued to personify the fever and make it responsible for the deaths of women, rather than the obstetricians, by declaring that 'puerperal fever selects its victims'.[127]

This confused and confusing resistance lasted despite the fact that the notion of contagion was not novel. Fleck mentions a very early Greek definition of micro-organisms;[128] and in the fifteenth century, a theory of contagion based on the existence of 'particles our senses cannot see', began to circulate as popular knowledge.[129] The existence of contagion was accepted by lay people long before it was accepted in scientific medicine. During the great European plagues of the late Middle Ages, people were using this notion when they reacted by either isolating plague victims, in special hospitals away from the uncontaminated population, or when the population removed themselves from the immediate vicinity of contaminated individuals.[130] By contrast, obstetric science was absolutely reluctant to accept contagion, and its own responsibility in spreading the fever, even when the data became quite solid and convincing. It was easier to retreat to a system of beliefs about women, rather than accept the unhappy conclusions that resulted from the theory of contagion. Yet none of this is to say that while Gordon, Holmes and Semmelweis were more correct, others were staggeringly incorrect, occupying the wrong end of the conceptual scale. For instance, there was an effort to deal with a distinction between 'accidental' puerperal fever and epidemic puerperal fever, the former occurring on a seeming once-off basis, with no clear link to contagion, while the latter was obviously spread through some route or other. As Fleck reminds us, 'there is probably no such thing as complete error or complete truth.'[131] So we must rather argue that science in the making is an irredeemably social act which in this instance of epidemic puerperal fever had lethal consequences for women.

Accounting for Puerperal Fever by Social Class and Geographical Location

Unwilling to accept the theoretical possibilities which the notion of contagion offered, obstetrics had nonetheless to develop rationales to explain the fever, which continued to haunt the hospitals in epidemic form, a problem for men midwives which was above all a political problem. Robert Collins, who became the twelfth Master of the Rotunda, in his book *A Practical Treatise on Midwifery* wrote about puerperal fever:

> No subject has given rise to a greater diversity of opinion, or has stronger claims on our attention than puerperal fever. It is a disease, which when met with in Lying-in Hospitals, is singularly alarming, proving fatal to a vast majority of those attacked under every mode of treatment as yet recommended.[132]

Collins' sense of alarm was well justified. During his mastership in 1829, the Rotunda was threatened with closure by the Lord-Lieutenant of Dublin because of the rate of death from a puerperal fever epidemic. Collins had already limited admissions to the hospital and attempted to stave off the epidemic, using the same measures advocated by his father-in-law. During the epidemics of the 1780s, Clarke had cited the wretched circumstances of working-class women coming into the Rotunda as a contributory factor and always maintained that the fever was absent from the homes of upper-class women. He was quoted by his son-in-law as saying: 'I have never lost a patient by it in private practice and that no "malignant low fever" had appeared amongst that class of women for thirty-five years.'[133] But Clarke's remarks reflected a series of distinctions which he thought meaningful, between the 'character' of epidemic puerperal fever in hospitals and elsewhere, a distinction Collins picked up and also employed. Collins asserted that in private practice, puerperal fever was never accompanied by the 'low typhoid symptoms' that presented in hospital and even though the fever was the cause of fatalities amongst upper-class women in London and Edinburgh, the same variant of the fever did not appear in Dublin in those circles.[134]

Why might these different forms of the fever attack women differently by class, as was maintained in the Rotunda writings? There were other positions that could have been argued. Gordon, for instance, had been clear that the fever was not a feature of lower-class women only, but this was tied to his argument about contagion:

> Women in higher walks of life were not exempted, when they happened to be delivered by a midwife or physician, who had previously attended any patients labouring under this disease.[135]

The Rotunda was investigated and closed in 1820, 1829, and, a third time, in 1856, because of the high rates of maternal mortality during epidemics of puerperal fever.[136] What now occupied centre-stage in the debate among men midwives on the reasons for epidemic puerperal fever was the impoverished state of the women themselves, which transformed the locus of concern into an entirely different discourse.[137] An early example in the nineteenth century comes from one of Collins' predecessors, Labatt, who closed the hospital in 1819 when an especially severe epidemic occurred. Labatt had followed Clarke's regime of cleaning and purifying,[138] but to no avail:

> On the 15th of October I was much alarmed on finding seven women complaining, and from this time until the beginning of December, there was scarce a day that two or more were not attacked. Early in December, with the concurrence of several governors, I sent notices of the unhealthy state of the hospital through the city, in order to prevent those from coming in who could provide themselves with accommodation at home, to whom, at the same time, I offered our gratuitous attendance at their residences. This had the effect of lessening our numbers; but many wretched creatures still continued to present themselves for admission at our gates, saying that they would run the risk of fever in the hospital, where they would have food and attendance, than remain at home destitute of both.[139]

Under such circumstances, how far could the hospital regime itself be held liable? The social relations surrounding the issue of widespread poverty made culpability for illness intensely personal and class-related. By the early nineteenth century, the contagion notion was inscribed in the discourse of public-health medicine through what has been termed the 'geographical spaces of quarantine',[140] and the regime of sanitary medicine which then held sway relied on a distinction between local climates which induced illness and those which sustained health. It was a discourse bound up with a critique of slum conditions that insisted on containment of the threat of disease, so that it would not break out from its place of origin (and threaten the non-poor), but it was written in the seemingly neutral language of science.[141]

Essentially, the theory of miasmatic or zymotic (infectious) disease stated that disease was spread through a sick person's exhalation of her own noxious matter onto another body nearby. It was not necessarily exclusive to lying-in women. Nightingale adhered to this belief in enforcing her sanitary regime in military hospitals, and the concept was part of the thinking on public health for all epidemic illness, which was perceived as always being worse in the poorest and most overcrowded localities.[142]

Quarantine was the public-health answer to the threat of widespread epidemics like influenza, but the obstetric approach to puerperal fever was resistant to this notion, a predictable reaction, since obstetrics needed its hospital space to maintain its legitimacy on a number of fronts. Yet during an epidemic outbreak, exclusion from the hospital meant greater safety for women.

It was in the interests of all men midwives to keep their private practices as clear as possible from the charge of epidemic puerperal fever and to sustain the notion of the disease as one of miasma or local contagion, and not in the least dependent on or connected to men midwives and their practices. Poor working-class women were thus seen to embody their own self-inflicted threat in the nineteenth century, by virtue of their poverty, and the issue became how best to respond to that threat, given the grudging acceptance by medical men that maternal mortality rates were much higher in hospitals.

By the 1850s, there were two major lying-in hospitals in Dublin, and a series of smaller hospitals like the Western Lying-in Hospital associated with Fleetwood Churchill. There were also the lying-in wards attached to the workhouse and fever hospitals. The latter were in various locations around the country and were meant to provide an additional service, in the person of a trained medical doctor, for local midwives as part of the local dispensary system, for difficult lying-in situations.[143]

The numbers of women handled by the workhouses were far smaller than that handled by the two Dublin lying-in hospitals. By the middle years of the nineteenth century, the latter were experiencing, at least in the public perception, a considerable increase in the levels of maternal mortality, and a decrease in absolute numbers entering their doors. A challenge to the large hospitals was formally thrown down in 1867 from the medical officer of the Waterford Lying-in Hospital. John Elliott wrote that the increase in the Dublin institutes' maternal mortality figures was as 'undesirable' as it was 'unexpected', and such a development was scarcely consistent with the hygiene and sanitary precautions which had become common practice for them. The question of whether they ought to be closed down, 'magnificent' as they were, was provoking keen discussion amongst professionals and members of the public. Though their resources were 'extensive', their record simply was not as good as that of the smaller establishments. Elliott argued that their local facility in Waterford had never been forced to close in its twenty-nine years as a consequence of puerperal fever, and of 3,409 women who had been delivered over that time, only five had died of the fever.[144] Elliott quoted figures: in the first six-and-a-half-years of the hospital's existence, 753 women were delivered:

> of these, six died, three of the deaths being the result of puerperal fever in one or other of its forms, thus giving a total mortality of 1 in 125½ being a per centage of 0.79 or 4-5ths nearly; and a mortality from puerperal fever of half the amount viz. 1 in 251 or .39 per cent.[145]

Schedules of mortality, with similar calculations, had been a conventional part of presenting practitioners' work to one another since Clarke and Gordon's time. But if anything, the play on numbers intensified during this period, as the stakes in respect of reputation increased. Elliott's argument was that the small institution was less subject to puerperal fever. Because it was often empty for periods of time, the chance for the disease to mount its attack amongst women massed together was diminished. He did not claim that the poor of Waterford were any less subject to 'zymotic' diseases than elsewhere, and he even stated that the fever was known amongst women who were delivered at home, but not in epidemic form. But to him, the small cottage hospital appeared safer. Of course, even if cases of puerperal fever were being recorded in Waterford as either accidental death, or death from typhus fever and so on (as was the practice of the period), there are two further possible explanations for the much lower death rate Elliott discusses: early discharge of women from the small hospital, so that their deaths occurred elsewhere and were attributed to some other cause; and the absence of the practice of dissection because facilities were so limited.

A London doctor writing from a public-health perspective, Denis Phelan, had already pursued the problem that the large lying-in facility posed, drawing together many of the published reports on mortality figures, including those of John Simon, the medical officer to the English Privy Council, and a keen protagonist in this widening debate. The figures compared the Coombe and the Rotunda with published figures from larger Continental institutes in Vienna, Paris and St Petersburg, as well as London and Liverpool.[146] The cumulative figures for the best maternal outcomes, Phelan suggested, made Liverpool the model to follow if there were to be lying-in hospitals.

Table 3.3: Deliveries and Deaths in Major European Lying-in Hospitals

Lying-in Hospital	Year(s)	Number of Deliveries	Number of Deaths	Ratio of Deaths to Deliveries
Vienna Krankenhaus	1838	4,453	179	1 in 25
Paris	1862	2,204	166	1 in 13¼
St Petersburg	1844–59	8,036	306	1 in 26⅔
York Road, London	1836–56	4,960	146	1 in 31
Glasgow	1861	2,705	13	1 in 54½
Liverpool	1855–62	1,092	11	1 in 99
Rotunda	1857–64	8,224	252	1 in 32⅔
Coombe	1857–64	3,142	45	1 in 70
Coombe District	1857–64	4,473	20	1 in 223
Rotunda District	1857–64	617	10	1 in 62

Source: D. Phelan (1867), 'Comparative Advantages of Attending Women in Lying-in Hospitals and their own Homes', *Dublin Quarterly Journal of Medical Science*, vol. xliii, February and May 1867, pp. 73–5.

Phelan wrote:

> It would be reasonable to ask how it happens that a greater relative proportion of women die in lying-in and other hospitals on which great attention is paid to ventilation and other hygiene conditions and over which highly educated and experienced medical men preside, than die at home, in residences many of which are completely wretched and ill-ventilated and with far less comfort to carry them through their confinement.[147]

The argument that either home-based or small-institute confinement was safer than the large maternities hit at the crucial teaching and accreditation functions of the large institutions. It also brought into question the hierarchy of professional competence on which they were based, with the gradual ascent to the posts of Assistant Master and Master. The figures also destroyed the original rationale for institutionalising women, for they revealed the levels of danger to which women were exposed in the hospitals set up to rescue them. On this, Phelan quoted Simon who had written in his Sixth Report on Public Health:

> 'it is of course, possible that certain circumstances, may (as in Dublin) render a lying-in hospital like a workhouse a matter of necessity and it is also possible that certain cases in which special dangers are to be apprehended at the time of delivery would be safer in an institution where they could be carefully watched than at home'[148]

So the contradiction emerges that women who are confined in institutions, because of the social organisation of poverty, may be safer in their homes.

However, implicitly protecting the all-important dimension of teaching and the development of clinical science, Simon introduces the notion of balancing off one set of dangers, exposure to puerperal fever, by another set, 'special dangers', which require the hospital location in spite of the first set of dangers. This would provide fertile ground in the future development of the discourse about maternity hospitals.

For the time being, doubts and disquiet were expressed by those not immediately involved in sustaining the reputations of the large institutes, and this public disquiet undermined those professional credentials. Phelan's comments were especially damaging, for he saw the Rotunda as the most commodious and well-funded lying-in hospital in either Britain or Ireland. Yet when he examined the records of the Rotunda, he looked at the range of deaths before and since 1854. In the latter period, the lowest annual mortality rate was one in sixty-four, the highest rate one in thirty-seven-and-a-half, 'facts', he assured his readers, 'which can only be ascertained on a careful examination of the statistics of the institution'.[149]

The protracted arguments would later deepen to crisis level for the Rotunda when a former master, Evory Kennedy, entered his judgement. What stands out is that throughout this debate, women were still trapped within a construct that was costing them their lives, even if they themselves chose, for whatever set of reasons, to engage with the larger institutes or were constrained to be there, as in the instance of those sent to the large workhouses in Dublin. Phelan's argument that more women died in hospital, under professional male attendance, than at home without that attendance was a serious blow to the practice and legitimacy of the large lying-in institutes, which were responsible for teaching, transmitting and extending the authority of obstetric science.[150]

Women as Perpetrators and Victims: Another Way to Account for Puerperal Fever

Foucault has stated that the principal problem for medicine in the classical period was to do with how knowledge was shaped or encoded; what needed to be shifted was how the doctor actually 'saw' things, and this was the epistemological break in its system of thought that occurred towards the end of the eighteenth century. So, for example, Pomme's way of 'seeing' the body was no longer valid. Medicine was no longer seeing the body through the patient's symptoms, but through the signs and meanings of those signs, as revealed by pathological anatomy.[151] The impact of this transformation on how the female reproductive body was seen was arguably different to the global shift in medicine, for embedded in it was the deeply gendered account of the female body, in all its weakness, along with the production of the 'hystericised' woman.[152] This account came to play a useful role in relation to puerperal fever also. If one way to implicate women in the problem of puerperal fever, displacing responsibility directly on to them, was to draw on class-related detail, making the fever a concomitant factor of poverty, a second way was to implicate the female sensibility, drawing once more on the fertile and unceasing imagination of male medical discourse.

Amongst other elisions in the discourse, this entailed a blanket denial of women's perceptions of themselves, of their realities, and of their ways of dealing with the fever, as if they had neither the competence nor strategies. It entailed denying women's active awareness in a situation where death was not an infrequent outcome.[153] It also seemed to be a phenomenon of the nineteenth-century writing on childbirth, rather than the eighteenth.

Gordon, for instance, wrote about women's awareness of what was facing them. He recorded that the woman who was No. 38 on his chart 'thought herself secure' because he would attend her. But her 'easy labour' was followed by the characteristic shivering fit the following day. Her state from that point to her death five days later was open for family and friends to witness. This is how Gordon described her death:

> The remainder of life was one [of] continued conflict, painful to the patient, and distressing to the spectators . . . alarming symptoms seemed to increase every hour; the intellectual faculties began to suffer by a temporary delirium: convulsions were frequently interposed; the pulse became weaker and weaker, till at last it ceased altogether; the extremities grew cold; the sight failed, and death closed the melancholy scene.[154]

The medical historian, Roy Porter, has argued about death that it was an 'obvious shaper of social modalities' before the twentieth century in the way, for instance, that early deaths disrupted marriages.[155] Porter also argues that the doctor's position in relation to all deaths he attended was changing in the nineteenth century. If, up to then, the role of the doctor had been to fully inform his patient of her fate and then withdraw to allow her to ready herself for her death, this began to shift more towards the task of alleviating pain and soothing mental anguish. By the beginning of the nineteenth century, one consequence of this move was that the person dying was rather less in charge and the doctor, with the family's agreement, rather more so. The courage to face death that was seen as necessary in the seventeenth and eighteenth centuries, a courage requiring all one's faculties, faded from the scene to be replaced by 'the first golden age of stupefying drugs', and the notion of an 'easy' death, which looked as 'natural' as possible, meaning that people were more often dying an 'insensible' death.[156]

Some aspects of this shift in the medical reaction to death do begin to appear in accounts like Gordon's, at least in respect of treatment. We hear of Gordon's use of opiates to alleviate pain and procure sleep for the woman with puerperal fever, and also of a closely observed movement into death, by family and friends as well as the doctor, as his account of his unnamed patient indicates. Yet, although opiate drugs were beginning to be used for women, when they were dangerously ill after birth, it seems improbable that women had the 'insensible' and passive deathbed role of which Porter speaks, not only because the fever itself did not permit that, but because women were never insensible to the possibility of death in birth.

There is an acute problem in locating women's own stories in relation to the growth of obstetrics, but nevertheless, there is some evidence even in the medical treatises themselves that women clearly knew childbirth was a challenging undertaking, in which they might die. In relation to puerperal fever, women expressed considerable fear about their diminished chances of surviving it. Thus Semmelweis, in his account of the spread of the fever in the Krankenhaus in Vienna, wrote that women entering the hospital begged 'in terror' not to be sent to the First Division, that part of the hospital which was 'devoted exclusively to the instruction of accoucheurs' and which was known to have the highest death rate.[157] The argument about the doctor's role, including soothing mental anguish, had far more to do with the creation of that role and the power of the man midwife to define and record it in his own terms of reference rather than with women remaining unaware of what they were facing.

Hospital accounts of women's deaths tended to be anonymous and usually quite brief. In his registry for example, Clarke refers to women like 'A.B. admitted on the 30th of March, 1787' and 'C.D. Admitted and delivered on the 12th of April, 1788; of a ninth child, a boy dead'.[158] The doctor in hospital was not in constant attendance, of course. Collins tells us that when a case with puerperal fever was diagnosed, it was the invariable rule to see the woman every six hours rather than the customary twice daily rounds.[159] What was meaningful during the doctor's rounds – what he recorded – was what he saw in the space of these brief visits, along with whatever information might be gleaned from nurse tenders.

The movement is towards a more recognisably contemporary 'clinical' observation of encroaching death, where the person's knowledge of death is largely irrelevant to the clinical sign which the doctor sees (though this is being challenged now by the hospice movement). And, in the case of a childbed death from puerperal fever, the circumscribed space that remained for the woman could be interpreted as one where she almost brought her own woes upon herself because of her fears. Clarke, for example, noted a number of 'general' fevers in the Rotunda during the 1787–88 epidemic.

These 'febrile disorders' he attributed 'to the fears and apprehensions naturally excited by the numerous deaths produced by puerperal fever'.[160] He also noted that 'some patients, during this epidemic were affected with delirium before death',[161] a point we shall return to shortly.

Collins was concerned that women often reassured their attendants that they felt no symptoms at all, and were free from any complaint of puerperal fever, when in fact the disease had already taken hold. Note his phrasing about this, the reduction of the woman to a 'female': 'In hospital, the female, (perhaps from fear) will at times insist that she is quite easy and free of pain.'[162] Collins suggested that this insistence reflected a woman's fear of discovering the truth of the matter, and thus facing the likelihood of death. Yet, as we learned from Labatt in the 1819 epidemic, women continued to see the asylum of the hospital as a risk worth taking, preferable to wherever else they might have to give birth.[163] Both comments suggest that working-class women who entered the Rotunda, with good reason, feared puerperal fever, but were dealing with their realities as best they could.

Descriptions, like this one below, from Beatty in the Coombe Lying-in Hospital, were commonplace in eighteenth- and nineteenth-century urban accounts and underlined the deep poverty and corresponding ill-health with which many women struggled:

> The sixth case of death was that of a wretched female, who was found by one of the pupils of this hospital, lying on a clay floor, in a damp cellar, in labour, and apparently dying of pneumonia. He had her conveyed to the hospital, where she was delivered, and died on the second day after. Both lungs were found extremely affected with pneumonia in the third stage.[164]

Amongst other things, such accounts contributed to the notion that miasmatic or zymotic diseases, that is infectious disease locally generated, were the special privilege of the destitute.

But even if men midwives generally accepted that puerperal fever was a form of zymotic disease, with the added dimension of women's capacities to impede their own well-being, the disquiet over lying-in hospitals and the ways to deal with puerperal fever continued to range freely outside the hospitals. In 1854, a House of Commons Committee on Dublin Hospitals formally heard about the admissions policy of the Rotunda and the only precondition for admission, that a woman be in labour, was exhaustively interrogated. There were large numbers of women giving birth in the Rotunda, regardless of marital status. The Commons Committee heard that there was no way the hospital could refuse a woman whether she was poor or not, whether she carried an illegitimate child or not. All women were accepted, 'the abandoned, as well as the virtuous'.[165] All women were treated as married women whether they had a husband or not. No rule existed to prevent the entry of 'that immoral class' of unmarried women, much to the dismay of the Commons committee. This theme of the immoral woman was about to re-emerge in a truly perverse form within obstetric practice itself, as a result of this kind of public pressure.

In 1867, Evory Kennedy, who had been Master of the Rotunda from 1833–40, published an open letter to the governors of the Rotunda Hospital, in which he laid out his argument that the objectives of the hospital's charter, ones which had been fulfilled in the past, were no longer being fulfilled. Labour admissions had diminished to nearly a quarter of the numbers admitted to the hospital in 1818, and puerperal fever, Kennedy contended, was the sole reason for the decline. He proposed that the hospital should be remodelled along the style of Swiss chalets, with small detached dwellings, to lower the rate of contagion, for such an arrangement was least favourable to the spread of zymotic disease. Of course the hospital had to continue as a teaching hospital. He was perfectly aware, he said, that observation of case numbers in the fifties could not replace observation in the thousands. But an extension of the wards given over to gynaecological and therefore non-contagious diseases, and an extension of the home attendance scheme, where pupil male practitioners attended women who lived nearby in their homes, would fulfil the criteria that a great teaching hospital like the Rotunda should possess.

Kennedy's proposal was overwhelmingly rejected by the governors. Returning to the attack, he then delivered a paper on 'Zymotic Diseases' to the Dublin Obstetric Society in 1869 in which he continued to assert that puerperal fever was endemic in the large lying-in institutes, to the point that 'they stand in relation of cause and effect'.[166] He set out his evidence to prove thirteen propositions on puerperal fever, the principal ones being that puerperal metria or fever was 'due to the absorption of a poison by the parturient female'; that the poison was contagious; that the 'generation and absorption of this contagion' was 'in a direct proportion to the number of parturient females cohabiting' during that period; and that only the separation of women from one another would prevent the disease from arising. There was good evidence of 'traceable contagion in which the contagion was carried from another case similarly affected by the medical attendant or nurse-tender',[167] raising once more that 'painful' subject of contagion and men midwives. Kennedy supported his propositions with a range of figures culled from the Rotunda, from other Irish institutions, from the reports of Registrar-Generals in England and Wales, from the reports and writings of medical men in Ireland and on the Continent. Quoting from the figures for his mastership and from his own private practice, he drew a sharp contrast between mortality outcomes. In the latter, he claimed to have lost only three women to the fever out of 3,500 deliveries:

Of the patients delivered under my own care, and for whom I was responsible to God and man, ten and eight-tenths, or almost eleven died of those in my charge in hospital for one in private, or in their own homes.[168]

But significantly, Kennedy was moving away from the labelling of working-class women as responsible for their own deaths. It was not class but hospital which was doing the damage. He examined the death rates of the Rotunda from 1757 to 1868 and confirmed for his listeners an 'alarming rise in mortality' in the most recent period; the Rotunda's best year had been 1757, when the ratio of deaths to deliveries was one in 227, followed by one in 220 in 1822, whereas in 1862, the figure was one in fourteen. Kennedy forcibly rejected the argument of many Rotunda men that because the hospital had to accept all who came, no matter what their condition, complication or stage of labour, it had begun to experience a higher proportion of deaths from puerperal fever.

All these 'casualties and peculiarities' could not possibly account for the increasingly high death rate. Based on the annual returns of births and maternal deaths from puerperal fever to the Census Office for 1864–68, for all women and the figures for the lying-in hospitals for 1862–63, he assumed that the numbers of deaths outside the hospital would have been broadly similar in those same two years. Hence, he concluded that:

> in the City of Dublin alone 7½ women die out of every 9 from being cofined in hospitals; in other words, that in all the deaths that have occurred in Dublin for the last seven years in parturition, out of every nine deaths, 7½ women have died, who would in all human probability be at this moment alive had they been confined in their own homes, or in isolated cottage hospitals.[169]

In reviewing the returns from British and Continental hospitals as well as smaller establishments around Ireland, Kennedy was quick to point out that the Rotunda's mortality rates had never been as woeful as lying-in hospitals elsewhere. But the only reasoned answer to this level of 'mischief', to 'something so defective and objectionable in the system of the hospital itself' was to close down the 'great institution' and create in its place a different system, and 'not a moment should be lost in correcting it in the manner that experience, science, and observation best dictate'.[170] This comprehensive paper, coming from a former Master, an eminent obstetrician before and since his mastership, produced uproar amongst Kennedy's colleagues. The Dublin Obstetrical Society was forced to hold a series of lengthy and extremely heated debates on Kennedy's paper, the published results of which ran to almost 200 pages.[171] There were several overlapping issues: whether doctors could see that their own practices were dangerous; whether women were simultaneously responsible for and victims of this disease; the slowness to accept asepsis as a principle and the constructs which lay behind that principle. Emphases and points of debate differed from one practitioner to the next, but what remained constant was the necessity of a teaching hospital, for it was the institutional base of obstetrics which would sustain and advance the discipline.

In this prolonged debate, statistics were curiously helpful for moving *away* from the issue of responsibility, as was the concept of zymotic disease, for the notion of a concentration of poison was still being used by practitioners to avoid their own contributions to mortality. Some concluded that a reliable statistical picture of deaths in childbirth was impossible to obtain, because all deaths from a lying-in hospital, which were listed by the state's officer, the Registrar, were considered by this official to be the hospital's responsibility, a judgement which gave an utterly false picture. Lists of deaths registered from the Coombe were produced at one of the Society's meetings in 1869 to prove that the hospitals were not so 'culpable' for 'we know that in the first child women are more liable to metria', meaning that all deaths of women giving birth for the first time could be discounted as not having meaning in this debate. Surely the disease had to be 'charged with the crime, not the hospital'.[172]

The debate itself ended inconclusively but the concept of miasma and filth in people's homes continued to be helpful in avoiding the issue of the lying-in hospitals themselves. Johnston, Master of the Rotunda from 1869–75, felt personally under attack by Evory Kennedy's proposal, to dissolve the hospital as constituted, and declared that the hospital's open-door policy was what was required of it. Whether women arrived in a weakened state which allowed the disease to take hold, or whether they brought the diseases in with them, spreading it to one another, the source of the disease had to be first found and it was not in the hospital but

> in the narrow, filthy, unswept streets, the courts and alleys in too many instances reeking with the pestilential effluvia of half-putrid offal and ordure, which by imperfect sewage or no sewage at all, allows the noxious gases escaping therefrom to pervade the overcrowded, small unwashed, ill-ventilated apartments, their bedding if possessed of such a luxury, saturated with filth and dirt; the unfortunate occupants frequently in a weak, emaciated state, from want, penury, starvation and disease.[173]

Johnston soon let this argument about the geographical location of the disease lapse in favour of an argument about women's emotional frailty being the principal contributory factor to the disease:

> The victim of seduction, the houseless stranger, the famished wretch, all seeking admission may enter at any hour, night or day, without either note or ticket of recommendation, their only requirements being that they stand

in need of our assistance, a circumstance which, so far as I am aware, is peculiar to this institution. The modest girl, who, having been led astray, and acutely insensitive of her fallen state, flying from the observation of her family and friends, in order to avoid the scandal and opprobrium that she would be exposed to were she to remain in her own home or neighbourhood, seeks the shelter of the Rotunda, where unknown, among the multitude, she hopes to elude observation. Women deserted by their husbands, or who have been left destitute by their partners having fallen victims to the many diseases always so prevalent in large cities, but particularly within the past year, leaving the widow in a state of mind often bordering on distraction, themselves and families being in a state of penury, not knowing where to look for succour.[174]

This was the Rotunda's special constituency, according to Johnston, and also the reason why the hospital's mortality rates were so high. He pushed this notion of women 'afflicted with anxiety or despondency' to a new level, pinpointing acute emotional distress as the factor which provoked tedious slow labours and then too quickly led to both puerperal fever and mental illness. From here, it was but a stepping stone for Johnston to reach the novel conclusion that the prophylactic use of forceps on women whose labours seemed to be slow and whose cervixes were only partially dilated would save them from the rigours of labour and possible death:

But as soon as we find the natural efforts beginning to fail, and after having tried milder means for relaxing the parts [the cervix], or stimulating the uterus to increased action, and the desired effects not being produced, we consider we are justified in adopting prompter measures, and by our timely assistance relieve the sufferer from her distress and danger, and her offspring from an imminent death. Why, may I ask, should we permit a fellow-creature to undergo hours of torture when we have the means of relieving her within our reach? Why should she be allowed to waste her strength and incur the risks consequent upon the long pressure of the head on the soft parts, the tendency to inflammation, and sloughing of the vagina, or the danger of rupture of the uterus – not to speak of the poisonous miasm that emanates from an inflammatory state of the passages, the result of tedious labour, and which is one of the fertile causes of puerperal fever and all its direful effects, attributed by some to the influence of being confined in a large maternity, and not to its proper source – i.e., the labour being allowed to continue until inflammatory symptoms appear, and the patient worn out by the fruitless efforts of labour pains and the evils consequent therefrom?[175]

This passage indicates that Johnston's practice is not in any way casual, and in that sense, arbitrary or impulsive, but part of an obstetric model of management with some attempt to set criteria, although they are far from clear criteria, around efficient uterine action, related to both length of labour and the emotional state of the woman. It is also consummately a model committed to overriding the woman's body rather than working with her. The obstetricians find that the woman's labour is going slowly, according to their judgement, and their response is to try mechanical techniques, like sweeping the cervix with the fingers or administering an enema, to stimulate the uterus, and what pharmacological techniques are available to them in that period, either sedating the woman or giving her stimulating medicines or diet, until her labour recovers the rhythm which is considered sufficient. Approaches like walking in labour, as Nihell had suggested, are not employed not least because it is part of the Rotunda style of management that women are strictly confined to bed during labour. They are patients, not equal players and joint negotiators in their regime of care. If Johnston is working with a model, it is a closed system in the sense that he or his colleagues are its purveyor. But it is also a closed system because the issue of the inflammatory symptoms that so often precede puerperal fever, how and why they appear, is caught up in Johnston's urgent need to define the large maternity hospital as a safe institution, blameless in relation to the fever. If there are other ways to query why these symptoms occur, beyond what Johnston suggests (in relation to the growth of anaerobic bacteria and consequent damage where a foetal head is stuck in the birth canal for a period of time, his observations tally with subsequent deaths of women from puerperal fever), he excludes them. For example, he records one woman's death after the sloughing of the vagina as attributable to the 'too frequent examination of the patient',[176] but does not pursue that any further. Instead, he is committed more than ever to a model of intervention to prevent their deaths ever arising.

Johnston employed this 'timely interference' with special care on unmarried women, or women who were '*innuptā*', a category, he declared, who suffered from remorse and fretting because of their 'seduction' and as a consequence, fell prey to the fever in greater numbers than their married counterparts. The actual result of his extraordinary intervention was an increase in deaths from puerperal fever, which ensued in the wake of infections that took hold after this operative delivery. By the conclusion of his seven years' mastership, Johnston had used the forceps on fifty-nine women whose cervix was only two-fifths dilated, forty-four of whom were first-time mothers. The intervention led to severely torn cervical and vaginal tissues as a result of the application of forceps, which could give way to the sloughing off of perineal, vaginal and cervical tissue. It also led to the deaths of six of these women. Of the total 752 cases of forceps use in his seven years, 554 were first-time mothers, of whom forty-eight women died. Twenty-eight of them were unmarried. Johnston's statistics indicate that these women had a one in fifteen chance of contracting puerperal fever, compared with a one in 233 chance amongst those women who had escaped a forceps delivery.[177] And, in one of the most disturbing examples of a closed logical system, the woman's death in the wake of this operation actually reinforced Johnston in his conclusion that this was a beneficial practice for women, not least because her symptoms during labour were evidence for him that she would develop puerperal fever and that it was best therefore to deliver her early. Her post-mortem revealed that her cervix had become completely detached and had been sloughed off.[178] Johnston argued that:

> we did not allow the labour to be prolonged so far as to produce any of the symptoms indicative of vaginal inflammation, considering it safer to interfere before such should appear.[179]

If they did not die from the fever they contracted, the symptoms they exhibited as a result of the fever were organised around the category of 'mania'. The delirium common to pyaemia, the blood poisoning that was one form of puerperal fever, along with other symptoms of high fever, prostration, an increased feebleness of the heart and raised pulse rate, was interpreted as a further indication of the emotional instability of women in birth and was not seen as part of the body's reactions to infection at all.

The consequences were that women who were 'attacked with violent mania', but who survived the onslaught of puerperal infection, were declared mad and sent to the insane asylum. Johnston reports on the case of C.D., who had been 'seduced' and had been delivered with the aid of forceps, who then 'became quite maniacal on the 4th day, sent her to the Asylum on the 14th.'[180] Compared with this account, we can better understand the good fortune of the woman whose details are presented at the beginning of this chapter, whom Johnston encouraged in her illness by offering her a job as nurse tender in the Rotunda. She too had puerperal fever (which Johnston ascribed to typhus), as a result of her extremely premature delivery by forceps, and luckily enough did not develop delirium but was offered work instead. Reports on mania continue to appear in clinical notes into the twentieth century, being accepted as an inevitable outcome of the natural process of birth. Lane includes case notes on a woman who contracted puerperal fever, after her admission and delivery on 1 June 1886: 'Became maniacal. Died 19th June, 1886 of septicaemia.'[181]

Puerperal fever rendered the maternal body threatening, both a 'dangerous space' and endangered.[182] Medical discourse quarantined this body – Clarke, Kennedy; savaged it – Johnston; and sequestered it – Johnston, Lane. Obstetrics' management of puerperal fever, a management which expressed the incontestable power that medicine, in general, had come to wield,[183] significantly remade the individual identities of women who had to confront the fear of contracting the fever, and the realities of dealing with and dying from it.

Accepting Antisepsis; Receding Threat

The same year that Kennedy's letter to the Rotunda governors was published, 1867, Lister's paper on the 'Antiseptic Principle' appeared as three separate articles in the *Lancet*, describing the mortality from infection after compound fractures and the usefulness of carbolic acid in reducing mortality, especially for hand-washing before treatment as well as for dressing operative sites after treatment. His proposals made a tremendous impact on the medical community and were put to the test by the Prussians during the Franco-Prussian war in 1870.[184] In the Rotunda, the routine use of carbolic acid for hand-washing began to infiltrate practice in 1875–76 but it was not until 1882 that the following notice, signalling the effective commencement of an aseptic regime, was posted throughout the hospital:

> NOTICE.—Rule.— No one shall make a vaginal examination without having first washed the hands in carbolic acid solution, using a nail brush carefully. By order, Arthur V. Macan, Master of the Hospital, November, 1882. The Master feels confident that the Pupils of the Hospital will assist him in seeing that this rule is strictly carried out.[185]

In its own histories, obstetrics is keen to ensure that its account of itself is one of always moving towards a more refined and accurate science, the 'continuous history' that is a history with a 'continuous accumulation' of knowledge, the purpose of which is to avoid or deny radical discontinuities.[186]

A pertinent example of continuous history is found in a conventional account of obstetric history in Ireland, where we are told that

> Holmes and later Semmelweis, thus laid the sure foundations upon which others strove to build a defence against puerperal fever. Unfortunately, progress was slow, largely due to prominent members of the medical profession.[187]

What exactly can this mean? In 1664, the French man midwife, Peu, observed the similarity between the fevers of wounded soldiers and women in childbirth. In 1795, Gordon published his results, hypotheses and prerequisites for preventing puerperal fever, which he defined as a contagious disease spread from woman to woman by her attendants, both midwives and medical men. He left aside the problem of dissection, although he noted its ineffectiveness, but inadvertently reduced his death rate by no longer feeling obliged to dissect women's bodies because he had found a successful treatment. Numerous practitioners from the 1820s onwards commented on the circumstantial evidence of contagion being spread by birth attendants, including doctors, and queried the wisdom of carrying out dissections while being responsible for delivering women at the same time.

In 1843, Oliver Wendell Holmes published his essay on puerperal fever, his contentions largely the same as Gordon's, but with the important addition that infection was carried from dissecting rooms to the live bodies of women in labour and with the absolute rule that no doctor should 'take any active part in the *post-mortem* examination of access of puerperal fever' if he were to assist a woman in labour. If he did take part in a dissection, not only must twenty-four hours elapse, but 'thorough ablution', and an entire change of clothing was essential to protect the life of the lying-in woman.[188] This article was reprinted in 1855, 1861 and 1883 and had a wide circulation amongst the international obstetric community. Semmelweis, working at the Vienna Krankenhaus, where the rates of maternal mortality had been amongst the highest in European lying-in hospitals, brought about a 6 per cent drop in mortality rates by insisting that students and attendants use a solution of chloride of lime to wash their hands before assisting women. For him, the link was the lower rate of fever amongst patients in wards where only nurses attended, compared with student-supervised wards where the students also participated in dissections. He first published in 1847–48, and in 1861 his complete findings and conclusions were published in a widely circulated account.

Between 1795, when Alexander Gordon published his work, and 1882, when the Rotunda instituted an aseptic regime, obstetrics had become a legitimated science, shaping the modalities of an increasing number of women giving birth. The numbers of practising obstetricians and ordinary doctors involved in attending women at birth had expanded exponentially in this period and the use of published material circulating internationally had long been established as an important practice for the science. Within that science, the scandalous puzzle of puerperal fever had given rise to continuing debate and detailed examination of all known possible perspectives from within the profession, which might provide a workable strategy. Nevertheless, almost ninety years elapsed during which their own logical system of thinking about the problem could not admit easily of acting on different possibilities, ninety years during which many thousands of women's lives were lost to the fever at the hands of men midwives and within lying-in hospitals.

By contrast, Bruno Latour points out in his study of pasteurisation, that Pasteur's work, which really only amounted to a few test results, was adopted with lightening speed by scientists who had to 'believe in the enterprise of science . . . well beyond what can be comfortably asserted by way of "hard facts".'[189] Latour links this to how successfully Pasteur's writing fitted into the agendas of public health and the discourses on hygiene: a theory of contagion which implicated the masses of poor people in the fates of the rest of the population was quickly responded to on the basis that 'the contagious poor can blow up the whole outfit.'[190]

Obstetrics occupied a different space. It claimed that the female body was its object of attention but individual bodies somehow counted less than the body as an abstract concept, counted less than the expansion of the science which needed to be achieved. Women's deaths were secondary to the expansion of obstetric knowledge claims so that even when epidemic fever posed a threat to the continued existence of lying-in hospitals, the response was that the science was learning through death. And, in one sense it did learn, but only to the boundaries of its limited model, constrained by its ideologies and institutional modes. Latour makes the point in respect of the acceptance of Pasteur's work that knowledge cannot be distinguished from belief.[191] This is exactly the problem with the method and evidence about epidemic puerperal fever. Obstetrics was unable to commit itself to believe in the knowledge about puerperal fever.

In 1887, the following case notes appeared in the Rotunda's report covering the years 1884–86:

> Case XI – B.C. first pregnancy, admitted 24th November, 1884, and delivered same day by natural efforts; face presentation. The patient was examined by a student who had not washed his hands after having examined a labour case with foetal discharge (who also died of septicaemia [an alternative name for pyaemia]). Died, 1st December, of asthenia [failing strength] and puerperal peritonitis. No post mortem.[192]

Lane listed forty-three deaths amongst 3,414 women giving birth during those years, and claimed that of them only eighteen deaths were from sepsis. Significantly, post-mortems were carried out on only eight of these women, as if there was no longer an urgent need to know the routes or forms of sepsis. Lane gave the mortality rate as .52 per cent, or one in 189.6 and added:

> but I consider a better criterion of the health of the hospital is the number of patients who had absolutely normal temperatures and pulses during the puerperal state.[193]

These years are spoken of as a 'transition' period by medical historians,[194] years in which the hospital and the science continued to be valorised over the claims of individual women as this passage indicates. In 1888, internal examinations were halted for a month 'to test the *efficiency* of antisepsis' and thereafter the numbers of student examinations were limited to '*one student only on each occasion a woman was examined*' (italics added).[195]

Between 1903 and 1910, the Rotunda experienced its lowest mortality rates ever. The Master during that period, Tweedy, instituted a new regime on hand-washing and disinfecting, and the use of rubber gloves. He also concluded that it was necessary to halt the early discharge of patients recovering from puerperal fever, where their symptoms were not being recorded. He noted that 'any careless probationer nurse might record the pulse and temperature wrongly whenever it suited her to do so.'[196] The old demarcation line was still being carefully maintained, of responsible, professional doctors in training on one side, and the irresponsible 'careless' women midwives on the other.

Shorter estimates that the risk of death from puerperal fever after a hospital birth fell by six times between 1870 and 1939, after which time the risk of infection in hospital evened out to the same level as a home-birth setting, if sepsis from abortions was excluded.[197] Shorter also argues that the adoption of antiseptic principles was rapid, after Lister's 1867 paper, and that from the 1880s, antiseptic measures along with a growing recognition of asepsis, guarding hands with gloves and faces with masks, brought about a drop in rates of death from puerperal fever in the hospital setting with the biggest drops occurring in the decades of the 1880s and 1890s.[198] The historical demographer, Irvine Loudon, is not convinced of this thesis and cautions that infection leading to puerperal fever did not come just from unclean hands, clothes, or instruments, for the streptococcus was also carried asymptomatically and spread via throat and nose. Hence, he argues that the final dramatic downturns in maternal death from puerperal fever required the input of laboratory science and the response of the pharmaceutical industry in favour of a cheaply produced drug, introducing the first sulphonamides into hospital practice by 1936.[199] Loudon also raises the possibility that the virulence of the streptococcus virus varied widely from period to period, and that both peaks and fall-offs in deaths could be related to the dominance of a particularly virulent strain, followed by its diminution or even disappearance altogether.[200]

But it is also arguable that, compared with the notion of deaths from the wounds of war, the 'naturally occurring' death of women in childbirth was infinitely more difficult to reframe for a male profession. Latour speaks about the 'enthusiasm' of surgeons to adopt the notions of antisepsis and asepsis because it extended their territories. By contrast, obstetricians were caught up with a deeply rooted sense of a gendered body which required the notion of vulnerability, the vulnerability for which obstetricians argued their necessary presence, and this appears to have created a hostile indifference to the notion of infection after it had become accepted as a commonplace in general surgery. On this point, Gélis argues that there is direct culpability of obstetric medicine in the deaths of three generations of women because the microbial origin was denied by 'great obstetricians' who refused to wash their hands.[201]

However, as we have seen, the problem is not just that of the great or prominent obstetricians, but the way in which the science built itself on a number of interlocking elements that seemingly could not be jettisoned, without bringing the whole into jeopardy. Obstetrics required an institutional base to teach and legitimate, to continue to accredit and reward; therefore it required the use of dissection in death to further its ends as a teacher and builder of science. It also required an ideology about women which overtly refused them agency, while covertly holding them responsible for their deaths, one which concentrated on women's weaknesses, for then obstetric practitioners could assume their stance of the defenders of women against the foe of puerperal fever.

The subject of maternal mortality as a result of infection during delivery remained controversial. J.A. Musgrave noted in 1931 that deaths for puerperal sepsis in the Irish state were still running at 1.1 per 1,000 births but that a 'trained controlled midwife service' could reduce these rates.[202] The old theme of controlling the 'dirty ignorant midwife' was still in currency despite the fact that there was a serious problem with student doctors. In 1935, Bethel Solomons wrote that the root of the continuing problem of infection was the training of the aspiring doctor, and the General Medical Council regulations governing 'him'. After his five years' training,

> there should be a rule that he is not allowed to do private midwifery practice – that is, to work without supervision – until he has 'done six months' postgraduate work in a maternity hospital. Then the maternal morbidity and mortality rates will drop with a bump.[203]

Jellett, another Rotunda man, published an entire book on the subject of maternal mortality, in 1929, in which he proposed a way of interpreting obstetrics' past and present responsibilities:

> I am inclined to think that there are two conclusions at which we can arrive in regard to maternal mortality. The first is that it is mainly due to 'personal' as opposed to 'impersonal' causes. The second is that it is largely preventable.[204]

He defined these terms thus:

> Let us take septic deaths as an example. A woman is unavoidably confined under conditions which makes it, humanly speaking, impossible to avoid the possibility of infection. She becomes infected and dies. I regard such a death as, under the circumstances, unavoidable, and the 'personal' factor had little or nothing to do with it. Another woman is confined in a properly constructed maternity hospital, in which it is possible to prevent the passage of infection from one patient to another. She too gets infection and dies. Her death is due to a 'personal' cause, which originates either in herself or in some one else and is capable of correction.[205]

His argument that an 'impersonal' cause could become 'personal', because of increased knowledge, subsumed any notion of culpability, while making the further growth of the science the principal factor in preventing maternal deaths. The tendency was to move towards greater knowledge which meant that deaths would become 'personal' and therefore preventable.

Jellett described explicitly the problems that obstetrics was creating for women, problems which were contributing to their deaths. He wrote that 'civilisation' had 'forced' women to have their babies in abnormal attitudes, where being sent to bed in the first stage of labour 'and her position and mental anxiety make labour tedious'. Then, the 'nurse' thinks labour is going too slowly, presses down on the uterus, and when that movement is released, fluid lying near the opening of the vagina, fluid which has been infected by an 'unsterilised' wipe, is taken in to contaminate the vagina. The continuing slow labour ends with a forceps delivery and the manual removal of the placenta. The 'patient' has signs of sepsis within thirty-six hours and is dead three days later.[206] Jellett argued that this death was preventable through a 'radical alteration' of her regime of labour (without ceding obstetric control of the labour), and was therefore 'personal' because 'we are beginning to know enough to make such an alteration. A generation ago we should not have done so, and the cause of the woman's death would rightly have been termed "impersonal"'.[207]

The question is not whether we are discussing a move from 'impersonal' to 'personal' causes (although Jellett's conceptualisation opens obstetrics to further hubris, that all deaths are preventable), but whether knowledge formation within obstetrics will always be premised on a closed form of rationality which excludes women yet operates at the expense of women. One can also take Musgrave's line, and indeed this is what obstetrics has always done. He wrote of public-health officers that their role was:

> to combat that apathetic and somewhat heroic attitude of many poor and other mothers concerning the sicknesses suffered with childbearing. This carelessly stoic frame of mind is somewhat akin to that of men who follow perilous callings, and curiously enough, the tendency to balance this matter actually exists in the minds of many people 'Men go to battle, women bear the children.'[208]

In this sense, the science acted exactly as sovereign states have always done, building itself on death.

4

Calculating Life and Death: The Risk–Death Pairing

Taking Statistical Readings of the Body

In the lengthy controversy on puerperal fever and its supposed causes, women were divided into numbers and fractions, in order to argue the value of one or another treatment regime. This is why Robert Collins, in his *Practical Treatise on Midwifery*, presented summary figures so that he could state confidently that mortality in the Rotunda from puerperal fever was the lowest ever recorded, once his measures had been implemented:

> Of the 10,785 patients delivered in the Hospital subsequent to this period [after an epidemic in 1829], only 58 died, which is nearly in the proportion of one in every one hundred and eighty-six; the lowest mortality perhaps on record, in an equal number of a similar class of females.[1]

Another way of viewing this passage is that through his statistics, Collins was concerned to demonstrate that with his regime the *risk* of dying was radically reduced. The notion that risk is statistically measurable is now a commonplace one. Risk itself is a statistically derived mode of perception which has had growing salience in modern society, one which is linked to and dependent on the emergence of the doctrine of 'probability', that the possible occurrence of events does not arise out of subjective circumstances so much as from objective data, which are measurable and which thus permit mathematically stable predictions. At the beginning of the nineteenth century, how long a person would live was reckoned on a wholly subjective basis, whereas by the end of the century, predictions about length of life were based on these so-called 'laws of chance'. The notion of probability had a strong relationship with the related concepts of 'normal' and 'abnormal' or 'pathological'. Nowhere did this complex of probability, the normal and the pathological, have greater meaning than within medicine, where to be able to measure who might live or who might die, to measure the cumulative impact of epidemic death, became critical to the expanding work of medicine during the nineteenth century.² In this chapter, I want to examine how these concepts grew within obstetric medicine, and what the impact of them has been in modern obstetric practice.

There are several conventions in the presentation of Collins' data that deserve comment. The first, which is self-evident only to our retrospective view, was the creation of a 'population' of pregnant women about which to collect data. The creation of subsets from the general population, in this instance of pregnant women, in order to make them the focus of attention of a medical social apparatus, is precisely what Foucault means when he refers to the formation during this period, of a *biopolitics of the population.* Nothing was to be left to chance any longer; laws about fertility, illness, disease, death and population decrease and increase, all came into play through the careful regulation and monitoring of subsets like the reproducing woman.³ The second convention which Collins uses is the practice of producing aggregate numbers, abstracting the characteristics of his population subset in mathematical form. This was a practice which greatly intensified in medicine from the beginning of the nineteenth century, and it became the marker for proving one's claim to having an expert opinion.

The third interesting convention, captured by the phrase, *only 58 died, which is nearly in the proportion of one in every one hundred and eighty-six,* was the use of ratios to support one's argument. The practice of fractioning women's bodies mirrored the increasing use of dissection, and permitted the production of an orderly mathematised rationality about their labours and deaths. The fourth convention, the judgement on the probability of surviving or dying from puerperal fever, was the critical endgame for obstetrics of these statistical practices on puerperal fever. In the debate by members of the Dublin Obstetrical Society in 1869, on zymotic disease and puerperal fever, Evory Kennedy stated that,

> in all the deaths that have occurred in Dublin for the last seven years in parturition, out of every 9 deaths, 7½ women have died, who would in all human *probability* be at this moment alive had they been confined in their own homes, or in isolated cottage hospitals [italics added].⁴

The term 'probability' referred to the notion that there was a predictable, quantifiable chance of death from puerperal fever in certain circumstances. That is what statistics like these sought to prove, down to the fractured half-woman of Kennedy's '7½'. The acceptance of Kennedy's approach, if not his conclusions, was really the acceptance that death was due not so much to whatever individual cause was involved, but to a cause that could be predicted through the laws that were considered to be implicit in the empirical data of numbers and frequencies, presented in series like the above.⁵

An early and important expression of probability was contained in the actuarial tables produced in the late eighteenth century for the growing business of life assurance and even though these tables were seen more as a descriptive summary of facts, rather than a statement of causality, of why death happened, they indicated how to open up the field of numbers about the population.[6] This new mode of expression soon enough bore fruit within medicine, which was itself working with a new set of definitions in this same time span, as it discovered that 'uncertainty may be treated, analytically, as the sum of a certain number of isolatable degrees of certainty'.[7] The way was opened to a calculation of facts and events which had less to do with the individual sick person than to a population of sick people, about whom the facts of sickness could be recorded, measured, and compared. This, for Foucault, is what the work of bio-politics looked like, creating populations, bringing 'life and its mechanisms into the realm of explicit calculations',[8] and in this work, medicine had a specific role in the 'supervision' of 'propagation, births and mortality, the level of health, life expectancy and longevity'. These were the issues on which the science of public health was based.[9]

To William Farr, the first British Registrar-General, this supervisory work turned on the success of its methodology, especially in relation to epidemic illness and death; there was an urgent necessity, Farr wrote, 'for an instrument capable of measuring the relative duration of and danger of illness'[10] and he was convinced this could be accomplished by the formula: 'the *force* of mortality at any period of disease is measured by the deaths of a *given* number *sick* at a *given* time.'[11] The philosopher, Ian Hacking, has argued that for medical practitioners like Farr, such formulae could work only if there were a new way of cataloguing death. Thus the nineteenth century had not long progressed when Farr set up a definitive list of the causes of death, which became a model for the Western world and which continues broadly unchanged even now.[12] Farr termed his methodology 'nosometry', using the nosological classification of diseases, and counting their impact in terms of morbidity and mortality, for which he depended heavily on hospital records over the previous hundred years to set up his classification. Hacking argues that Farr's systematising tied together the process of enumeration with the classification of disease and death and hence, for us, when considering how the mechanisms to calculate normality and risk became possible, we need search no further than published works like Farr's. Farr made his initial forays during a period between 1820 and 1840, which saw an explosion in the use of numbers, which was perceived, Hacking argues, as 'statistical law . . . on the march, conquering new territories', able to quantify with 'numerical regularities' what were now seen as the laws of sickness and death.[13]

The growing perception of the scientific importance and validity of this type of statistical information explains the force of Hamilton's position in his debate with Collins, which we examined earlier. In a relatively short space of time, the concept of aggregate statistical information on illness and death became a standardised technique within obstetric medicine, making it possible for Evory Kennedy in 1869, when he reviewed the history of puerperal fever in the Rotunda and elsewhere, to use both Robert Collins' figures on maternal mortality and the classifications Farr had prepared for his reports as Registrar-General. Obstetrics was beginning to feel confident in arguing its case, exactly as Farr did, using a series of numbers over long periods of time, to tie together quite disparate practices and their outcomes, and thus further augment their bundle of theories about the female body.

Statistics was not the only technical mode open to obstetrics in practising 'continuous history', treating its work as a science which always progressed towards greater and more complete and significant truths, but it was to become its most enduringly successful technique. But also, with its use of statistics, obstetrics was participating in a general deployment of statistics, which became one of the critical technologies for the 'technology of power in a modern state'.[14]

Possibly the most essential aspect of the technology of statistics has to do with the commitment to the doctrine that you cannot know something unless you can measure it.[15] However, there are problems with the instrument of measurement itself, which go largely unacknowledged when the notion of measurement is taken outside the discipline of mathematics. Hacking also argues that a transference of a mathematical model that is dependent on a tradition of constants with fixed parameters, of variables and of boundaries, in order to produce a description of the world, often produces a vulgar notion of what constitutes a law of nature, vulgar in the sense that counting itself and its resulting profusion of numbers are taken to be sufficient proof of the existence of a law. There is no recognition within this process that the mushrooming of numerical series and equations still raises significant problems to do with the meaning and definition of those constants being used.[16] Commenting on the problem of how you know what you are measuring, Thomas Kuhn has observed that, between 1800 and 1850, everything was measured with a view to establishing ordered regular intervals as laws and concludes:

> The road from scientific law to scientific measurement can rarely be travelled in the reverse direction. To discover quantitative regularity one must normally know what regularity one is seeking and one's instruments must be designed accordingly.[17]

The search for regularity, and the way it was conducted, was an approach that, in the hands of the positivists, too frequently resulted in their producing 'laws' about areas where they had failed to develop any deep theoretical understanding, with the result according to Hacking, that what were proposed as laws were 'any equations with some constant numbers in them'.[18]

It was in this same under-theorised space that an applied science like obstetrics positioned itself, taking the fluidity of an individual woman, her body, her labour and pinning her down to a pattern of regularity, essentially a form of invention in respect of its chosen constants and equations. There was much more at stake with this than 'the power of the practitioner' to control the pace of labour, as James Hamilton of Edinburgh had phrased it. The multiple rewards of a discipline, believing that 'statistical laws' could be used to predict, organise and explain phenomena,[19] were, for obstetrics, the reduction of maternal mortality, alongside the production of axioms, systems and approaches that afforded statistical proof of having achieved a reduction of maternal mortality.

The logic of creating an enforceable regularity for women in labour, and from there, producing a series of statistical laws, permeates a mid-nineteenth century textbook on midwifery, published by two assistant Masters of the Rotunda, who were keen to prove the effectiveness of the Rotunda's approach to childbirth. In *Practical Midwifery*, Edward Sinclair and George Johnston presented maternal mortality statistics divided into three separate categories: deaths from 'accidents' of puerperal fever, meaning the fever was beyond their control or power; deaths which were not from the 'effects of labour', meaning deaths which were not accidental but which had nothing to do with labour; and finally deaths which they attributed directly to the 'effects of labour'. In all, the pair surveyed 13,748 women who gave birth between 1847 and 1854 in the hospital, of whom 163 had died. Working through their numbers, this yielded a proportion of maternal deaths to deliveries of 1:184⅓. Their next step was to subtract the 'accidental' deaths from puerperal fever from the total, bringing the ratio of death to labours down to 1:48¾. Then, subtracting deaths 'not from the effects of labour', which they otherwise attributed to women's general weakness and ill-health, Sinclair and Johnston arrived at the 'true' rate of maternal mortality, which they calculated as 1:295⅔.

This very respectable outcome was achieved, they argued, by the application of midwifery principles which included surveillance of dress, diet, length of bed-rest and timing of discharge, in addition to monitoring the stages of labour and position of birth.[20] The exercise in numbers (although for the authors it was a serious bid to prove their claims scientifically) is a good example of Hacking's vulgar mathematical model. What was measured, maternal mortality, and the way the measurement was carried out – by setting up supposedly discrete categories of constants, like 'accidental death' – bore no direct relationship to the realities of maternal death and why it occurred, let alone to the regime of care to which they attributed their final calculation of 'true' maternal mortality. But the system of classification, of maternal deaths into 'accidental', indirect and direct categories, had all the plausibility of a statistical law.

Although this significant play on numbers, frequency and intervals was a seriously flawed one, in which at least a minimum of 15 per cent of all puerperal deaths were misclassified before 1930,[21] the principle of statistical laws and the need for classification in order to build up a profile of the impact of the disease were not called into question. The problem of classifying puerperal fever as an 'accidental' death, for example, was just that, a problem of classification, which over time could be refined and corrected, rather than a failing on the part of obstetrics. Indeed this was exactly what Jellett argued, when he spoke of the science being able to move from the knowledge and identification of causes which were impersonal at an earlier point and which became personal as the science refined its views and progressed towards greater understanding.[22]

The early nineteenth-century view held by men midwives like Collins, in which 'accidents' of labour were perturbations of nature, and midwifery was an art which could help diminish these effects, gave way to a much firmer conceptualisation of obstetrics as a science which was predictive and reliable, and which, on the basis of its predictions, could effectively intervene to reduce maternal mortality. It was far closer to the model of the science that James Hamilton had promoted in his debate with Collins. One aspect in the discourse on puerperal fever was shifting ground. Similar to the thinking about epidemics in general, which moved them from being conceptualised as a 'deterministic scourge', over which doctors had little or no control, to a 'probabilistic contagion', in which doctors could predict, calculate and safely evaluate,[23] puerperal fever was being transformed within obstetric medicine to a phenomenon on which obstetrics could comment extensively, with all the authority lent to it by statistical reasoning.

Evaluation is exactly what the forthright George Johnston offered in his summary study, presented to the Dublin Obstetrical Society as a paper in 1878, a *Clinical Report of 752 Cases of Forceps Delivery in Hospital Practice*.[24] The devices of bio-politics, statistics, enumeration, classification, and the creation of difficult and deviant sub-populations, were all there in this report, in which Johnston promoted his notion of the prophylactic forceps operation as a 'timely interference' in labour, in order to circumvent the danger of contracting puerperal fever that arose from the prolonged pressure of the foetal head on the maternal 'soft parts'. We have seen that this physiological rationale Johnston presented about the need for forceps deliveries was extended to include a psycho-social reading of the sub-group he created, women who appeared to him to be distressed and extremely nervous, and therefore who must not be allowed to go through a long labour, especially unmarried women, or '*innuptâ*', as each was classified in his records. By his reading, they were the most vulnerable to puerperal fever, and he recommended for them, if their labours appeared to be slow, the application of forceps to deliver the baby before full dilatation of the cervix.

The most detailed table in his 1878 report, 'Showing the Number of Cases in which Delivery was effected by the Forceps before the Os Uteri was fully Dilated', has twenty-six categories for each of three sub-divisions, 'where the os uteri' was dilated at two-fifths, three-fifths, and four-fifths respectively, when the forceps were applied. The eleven 'causes of interference' of labour, which Johnston cites, including that of 'extreme nervousness, great exhaustion', mark an expansion of the grounds for forceps use, over and above even that recommended by James Hamilton, on curtailing the first stage of labour after fourteen hours with manual dilatation and the forceps operation. We are moving towards a regime of management in which prophylactic measures to deal with what might happen begin to predominate, and the table and its categories themselves are an indication that a statistical profile, however simple, is considered vital to the logic of obstetric arguments.

Johnston's table is conveniently accompanied by a line drawing of the 'degrees of dilatation of the uterus', the four inches of concentric circles representing the cervix, overlaid by the width of the two-inch blade of a forceps. Johnston writes that, after some experimentation, the forceps of choice was 'a Barnes' double-curved forceps' and asserts unequivocally that despite the lack of full dilatation

> in no instance did the patient sustain any injury of the uterus or vagina from the instrument, either by the passing of the blades or in the process of extraction; laceration of the perineum sometimes did occur, but not to any serious extent, nor was it attributable to the forceps.[25]

This is more evidence of the closed system at work and the anxiety to get evidence to conform to theory. Of the fifty-nine women who have the forceps applied to them when they are only two-fifths dilated, Johnston states that eighteen have the operation when the foetal head is still above the pelvic brim; seventeen when the head is 'in the brim' and twenty-four when the head is 'in the pelvic cavity'. In other words, for a significant number of these women, in addition to a cervix which was only partially dilated, the baby's head was not yet engaged and had to be brought a long way down the pelvic cavity to the birth canal. Similar to Roussel's fantasy about the absence of a woman's sexual attributes exactly where her sexual organs are, Johnston invents a chiasma, an inversion of events, in his description of his forceps operation under such conditions. Despite the actual damage done to the cervical and vaginal tissue, at such an early point of dilatation, it is rendered invisible.[26] It is a mercy that he uses chloroform in the vast majority of cases, for the operation lasts from fifteen to twenty minutes, with one operation continuing for three-quarters of an hour, and it is something of a miracle that a mere six women of this group go to their deaths as a result of 'timely interference', all of them unmarried.

The categories under which their deaths are classified are: convulsions, gastro-enteritis, sloughing, peritonitis, uterine diphtheria, and distress of mind. With the possible exception of 'convulsions', which might be attributed to eclamptic fits, where hypertension has reached a critical point, they are evidently the result of puerperal infections. This includes 'sloughing' of the cervix, which has become completely detached as a result of untreated sepsis, but they are defined by Johnston as deaths 'not from the efforts of labour', and therefore as causes of death independent to the labour and subsequent obstetric operation. This mode of reasoning is applied to the summary statistics of the 169 women who had the forceps applied to them before full dilation, whether two-fifths, three-fifths, or four-fifths. Of the eight instances where there was sloughing of the vagina, cervix, or perineum, Johnston has a useful rationale in all instances. Of the last condition, he wrote that it occurred to women who were already in bad health, which he attributed to their distress of mind as a result of their seduction. Only three of the women in this last group lived.

Johnston's analysis of the cause of death is another striking example of the extent to which medicine excludes the density of its own history, choosing instead its account of progressive betterment. In this instance, Clarke's caution about lacerations to the vagina has long been lost to view, as has his category of 'vagina ruptured by efforts of art'.[27] This is a different era in which Johnston's 'ardent love' for the forceps[28] equals the enthusiasm for numbers. To use Elaine Scarry's terms, both the enthusiasm and Johnston's marshalling of the evidence to support his notions suggest a 'referential activity',[29] in which the discussion and approach to puerperal fever is no longer bound by the original context of a woman's personhood. She now only exists as a potential number to be slotted into a pre-determined category.

These features dominate the debate which follows the paper's presentation, Johnston is praised by his colleagues for his data, which is presented with 'care, clearness and candour' in their eyes.[30] He does not escape criticism, however. His colleagues are concerned about whether this obstetric technique has quantifiable provable benefit for both mothers and children. If the former gain some advantage from it, the latter seem to lose out, 'the saving of children by the use of forceps' being not 'very great' when Johnston's outcomes are compared with those of earlier masterships.[31] One colleague, Dr Kidd, attempts a critique of comparative statistics. He wonders if the frequent use of the forceps is as 'favourable to the mothers as the more moderate use of that instrument', which can only be addressed by examining available summary statistics from the Rotunda. It would appear that tedious labours, during Dr Clarke's mastership, amounted to 1.79 per cent of all births; under Dr Collins, 1.32 per cent; and under Dr Charles Johnson, 3.90 per cent, while under Dr Johnston's recent mastership, the percentage was 9.56 per cent of all births. Dr Kidd's query is whether that constituted the former regimes as 'negligent midwifery' or Dr Johnston's as 'meddlesome midwifery'. The mortality statistics from 1757 to 1847 record that of 156,100 women delivered, 1,903, died while under Dr Johnston's mastership, in 7,862 deliveries, there were 179 deaths, a percentage of 2.27 per cent compared with 1.21 per cent for the first ninety years of the maternity hospital. Whatever the answer, Johnston's use of the statistics from previous masterships is criticised by Kidd who sees Johnston's main 'sources of error' as a reinterpretation of the term 'tedious and difficult labours', which has contracted in its time span. What was once a term applied to labours longer than twenty-four hours is now an unspecified shorter space of time.[32]

Interestingly, what is pinpointed as the key problem in this shift in time is that it violates the criterion 'that the cases compared shall be similar'.[33] In the debate in the Dublin Obstetrical Society, this difficulty raised by Dr Kidd of the lack of 'parallel cases' persists, so that efforts to determine retrospectively whether a series of cases delivered by forceps under one practitioner 'would have delivered themselves unaided' under another practitioner cannot be resolved: 'It is obvious that the results of the two modes of practice cannot be compared.'[34] In the course of the debate, it also becomes clear that Johnston has raised the use of forceps to a new level of sophistication with the fine-grained statistical detail he presents on the degree of dilatation. In using this data, he makes an implicit claim about the reliability of observation and recording of these precisely regularised intervals of dilatation of two-fifths, three-fifths, and so on. Obstetrics is learning to take on the applied science of statistics, with the apparatuses of comparability and serially recorded numbers and cases, in order to extend its own boundaries and authenticity. As Hacking argues, no one person opted for this 'new style of reasoning' but it appeared a form of enquiry which could unproblematically solve practical problems.[35] Statistical enquiry sets up the fertile ground on which arguments about risk schedules will proliferate but in real terms, the fertile ground is composed of women who are now transformed into a further kind of objectification, the statistical schedule. Women's deaths are a practical problem to solve, and both the techniques of obstetrics and the demographic, technical work on maternal mortality, are brought to bear on this problem.

At the close of the debate, Johnston is quite undeterred by his critics, declaring that:

> the most influential agent in the production of the mortality among women is puerperal fever. When it is absent the mortality is small, and vice versa; and unless Dr Kidd is prepared to prove that the use of forceps strongly favours the development of puerperal fever, his line of argument is fallacious. I maintain, therefore, that the practice I have set forth is a favourable one, as is proved by the following statistics.[36]

Throughout the debate, the underlying argument is still the material of the Hamilton–Collins altercation: whether interventionist practice constitutes 'meddlesome midwifery' or whether its absence is 'negligent midwifery', a black box which never quite resists being reopened. What has been completely accepted, however, is that statistical practice alone can accomplish the work of classifying, proving, and hence predicting whether a particular obstetric approach is worthwhile or not. Hence Johnston exhorts one of his critics, Dr Kidd, to marshal his proof with figures. It is the same Dr Kidd who observes that to play this new game requires new sorts of rules, not just distributions of numbers, but of 'like' numbers. These 'irreducible statistical laws' that the sociologist, Émile Durkheim, tells us exist at the end of the nineteenth century,[37] are going to be difficult to handle. The convoluted statistical discourse about the evaluation of claims for the effectiveness of different care regimes to predict and eliminate risk is just beginning.

Normality, Pathology, and Risk: Introducing the Notion of Avoidable Death

So we have the tool of statistical probability more or less in place. Establishing a scientific use of normality is the next step in pairing risk and death. In his study of probability, Hacking argues that normality is a 'vastly important' concept in our culture.[38] The word 'normal', as we have come to understand it, first came into use in the 1820s. Our feel for its usage is derived principally from medical discourse, where the range of meanings for normal has been extraordinarily diverse. But the root of the distinction within medicine is the comparison of the 'normal' with the 'pathological'. Clinical medicine, as it developed, was dominated by the experience of the structure of pathological reactions, observations which were based on pathological anatomy.[39] In this context, normal was the opposite of pathological. A significant contributor to the notion of how pathology worked was the Frenchman, Broussais, whose duties during the Napoleonic Wars enabled him to establish the doctrine that Gordon had begun to evolve in relation to puerperal fever some twenty years beforehand, namely that the inflammatory nature of fevers arose from an outside agent which created a local irritation.[40] Although Broussais' 'axiom of localisation' in clinical medicine,[41] that disease had a local seat as its originating point which could be determined by autopsy after death, was not fully connected to the problem of puerperal fever for many decades, his view of pathology, that 'Nature makes no jumps but passes from the normal to the pathological continuously',[42] was a notion which obstetrics was able to take on with ease.

According to Ian Hacking, 'normal' became the 'inverse of pathology' in general medicine, in the sense that 'something was normal when it was not associated with a pathological organ'.[43] But if 'normal' was the starting point from where deviation took off,[44] and pathology was removed from normal only by degree, then normal was also the *beginning* of pathology, a potential always there to be activated. It is this set of meanings which came to determine the use of normality as a retrospective concept, one you can only be certain about after the last possibility for a pathological symptom has been eliminated. This retrospective approach fitted well into obstetric thinking, where the interventionists increasingly appeared to have the imaginative edge in describing how symptoms of pathology arose suddenly in birth, without warning. However, over time, the discourse on normality was not limited just to the nexus of normal-pathological. If normal is the point of measurement for the absence of pathology, Hacking has identified at least three other clusters of meaning for normal, a 'benign and sterile-sounding word' which 'has become one of the most powerful ideological tools of the twentieth century'.[45]

In a second cluster of developing meanings, normal became synonymous with the 'average', the middle point, literally, an averaging out of intervals and numbers. Georges Canguilhem writes that it can be observed from the nineteenth-century work of Quetelet on anthropometry how a problem arose with these two concepts.[46] In his experimental work measuring height, Quetelet determined that the average could be taken to express a mathematical law, in which all divergences are purely accidental and the number which occurs most frequently thereby is the marker or definition of the average. In the case of Quetelet's work, this was the basis for his creation, *l'homme moyen* or 'the average man'. The problem was whether it could be argued that the norm or normality behaved in a similar way to a mathematical law of chance, and therefore whether every divergence was in that sense abnormal, as Quetelet also argued. Additionally, there was the related problem of whether there could be a purely biological fact, of physical growth, for example, based on a calculation of probabilities and clearly separate from all the socially derived effects leading to variability, like tradition and habit.[47] But despite the fact that this debate continued on some levels within science into the twentieth century, it also appears, according to Hacking, that the notion of an average had special meaning within medicine, but without questioning the links between average and norm, to the point that a medical reading accepted that the average of a species, its 'central dense mass', could be represented by a single number.[48] That belief in the capacity of the average number to carry the burden of representation has been a potent instrument in organising and interpreting populations and sub-populations, so much so that the production of figures like the average family size, or the average age of a woman having her first baby, creates a form of reality to which we all relate, measuring our personal situations. However, in the associated idea or use of normality, it is *only* an average, a marker which can either be met or a marker which we have not met. Once more, however, there is a lack of clarity between average as a mathematical representation and average as a concept of what is 'normal', but which we relate to as if it has a concrete reality. The average length of labour, for example, is a measure of a central tendency, derived from a data-set about a given population of women. Whether it is expressed as an arithmetic mode or a mean, it is a form of data which as a mathematical average cannot necessarily be conflated with 'normal', not least because of the variability and divergence of the phenomenon of labour which reflects not a 'pure' biological environment but one which is always socially derived and affected.[49]

Bound up with extensive medical usage, it has become more common for us to think of normal as a fact, 'what is', derived from the averaged 'dense central mass'. We can also think of normal as a value, 'what ought to be' (as in the belief that every birth 'ought' to end in the delivery of a 'normal', healthy baby). A gap should be distinguished here, between what the single number represents and what is an idealisation, yet in practice a gap is seldom, if ever, acknowledged. And although we think we understand normal as a 'what is' category (without being aware of the history of that category), we need it and use it as we also need and use 'normal' to mean 'what ought to be'.[50]

Thus, the concept of normal is never clear-cut nor even especially stable, despite its reputation of being a critical conceptual tool. In everyday usage, it has often been used in conjunction with abnormal. The word 'abnormal' was first used in 1835, tellingly as a 'deviation from a rule or system' (*Oxford English Dictionary*), a distinction which marks out the Foucauldian territory of disciplined, normalised populations, about whom abnormality could be precisely determined. As the concept of normal/

abnormal took hold within obstetric medicine, the older distinction between natural and preternatural – to try to distinguish those situations in birth where the woman was unable to give birth unaided – decreased in value and, as an explanatory scheme, it was gradually discarded. At the same time, the newer concept was far from straightforward, carrying all the nuances discussed above along with it, even if their anomalous status was rarely identified as such.

What were the risks attached to the individual female body deviating (as it surely must) from this confused plurality of propositions about 'normal'? 'Risk' itself is the starting point for answering this question. Coming from the Italian 'risco', meaning 'that which cuts', it took shape as early as the sixteenth century and was used to describe the hazard or danger of losing a cargo at sea in the insurance plans against this eventuality, so not surprisingly, risk is seen as the bedrock notion of insurance.[51] The everyday meanings about risk still have to do with danger, with measurable threats, all of which should be avoided, if possible. If avoidance is not possible, insurance is used to finance the risks one runs, including the risk of illness.[52]

But risk-taking is also seen as essential to the spirit of entrepreneurial capitalism[53] and by extension to the undertaking of heroic deeds of all sorts, which are usually male defined (including the practice of heroic medicine). François Ewald argues that in the business of insurance, risk 'is a specific mode of treatment of certain events capable of happening to a group of individuals' for although nothing is a risk in itself, 'anything can be a risk' depending 'on how one analyses the danger'.[54] That analysis is how the insurance business is created, using a kind of 'calculus' dependent on the combined formula of probability and accident. The task of the insurer is to produce schedules of chance happenings that might result in loss, on which basis people buy insurance against risks, *not against reality*. The calculability of risk gives rise to the idea that all individuals of a given population of subjects, say, Himalayan mountain climbers, are equally 'exposed' to risk because each person is one part of the whole of that population, and the calculation depends on the creation of an 'average' individual, based on the average of the whole of that population or group.[55] To work with risk requires the generation of statistical tables in order to evaluate the probabilities for a given population. Ewald argues that the consequence of this philosophy of risk is that ill-fortune or blows of fate are replaced by the notion that *causality* (my italics) is something for which society 'becomes the general arbiter, answerable for the causes of our destiny'.[56]

Similar notions about causality are abundantly evident in medicine as the nineteenth century continues, where danger moves from something completely unpredictable and unpreventable to a schedule of probabilities and predictabilities. Risk develops an autonomy from danger: a specialist can confirm 'the *real* presence of a danger, on the basis of a *probabilistic and abstract* existence of risks' and in this sense, one of the principal effects of the process of abstraction is that the individual subject ceases to be,[57] replaced instead by potential pathological outcomes in localised areas of her body. In the case of obstetric medicine, this results in the fractionising of women and the production of statistical schedules, like those of Johnston's, in which the reasons given for intervention are based on the *possible risk* of contracting puerperal fever, plotted against a standardised measurement of dilatation. It is in practices like those of Johnston's that we can see the beginning of an obstetric regime based on a risk system.

As obstetrics grows more 'scientific' in its practice, it begins to pose the challenge of avoiding death, not by assisting nature, which is the relationship most frequently suggested by eighteenth- and early nineteenth-century men midwives between themselves and the birth process, but by predicting or scoring the risks faced by the body, the averaged, normalised body of obstetric statistics, and then matching that risk-scoring with an appropriate programme of obstetric intervention to avoid those risks. By the end of the nineteenth century, obstetrics has ceased to read the *individual body*. The beginnings of this can be found in the models or prescriptions on avoidable death put forward by Hamilton and Johnston. In a distinctly separate approach to the therapeutic practice of 'watchful waiting' associated with Clarke and Collins, with the aim of alleviating the effects of illness in childbirth which could lead to death, these men were generating statistical categories and populations where death was more or less likely to strike and then tailoring their overall management of cases to those categories, in advance of any actual symptoms arising. Johnston spoke quite explicitly about preventing a woman from wasting all her strength in labour so that she might not 'incur the risks consequent upon the long pressure of the head on the soft parts'.[58]

What was happening was that obstetrics created a 'population' and then proposed a scheme of management to cover all women who fell into that obstetrically created category. In Johnston's case, for instance, the population was a group of women who appeared to be in danger of a slow labour, affected in particular by their mental state. A number of misconceptions were thus set in train about risk, including the mistaken perception that data on a given population could be applied to an individual and still produce a reliable indicator. This is a point to which I will return in greater detail. For the moment, it is worth noting that these misconceptions about risk entered into clinical practice, with a forcible impact which continues to affect women whenever they engage with contemporary obstetric science.

Johnston's mode of intervention fell into disuse (the masters who followed in the Rotunda immediately after Johnston were disinclined to pursue his policy), but it was nevertheless part of the general drive towards intervention which became stronger over time, gathering its credibility from the notion of identifiable risk factors and the hope that obstetrics could prevent death, all deaths, maternal and infant alike, by responding to those risk factors. Johnston's rationale for a prophylactic high forceps delivery before full dilatation was the forerunner of a view of the woman's body commonly found in twentieth-century obstetric texts, in which pregnancy and birth were seen as an obstacle course, littered with increasing numbers of risks.

The American obstetrician, Joseph de Lee, for example, produced a complete scheme of labour management in 1920, based on a prophylactic forceps operation, which influenced American obstetric practice over several decades. De Lee wrote that birth was a 'decidedly pathological process' from which only 'a small minority of women' ever escape without damage.[59] He was dismissive of any notion of a 'normal' birth, arguing that the reality of labour was 'a painful and terrifying experience' that often left 'permanent invalidism' because of the tearing, injury, rupture, distraction and displacement of the maternal soft tissues, all of which was highly abnormal:

> If a woman falls on a pitchfork, and drives the handle through her perineum, we call that pathologic-abnormal, but if a large baby is driven through the pelvic floor, we say that it is natural and therefore normal.[60]

De Lee's birth-management policy centred on a prophylactic forceps operation for every woman once the foetal head had moved down to the pelvic floor. This was combined with a fiercesome pharmacological regime, using morphine and scopolamine (so-called 'twilight sleep'[61]) every one to two hours, then 'sodium bromide and chloral given per rectum to aid the morphine', followed by gas and air. He argued that it was essential to obtain 'complete spontaneous dilatation of the cervix', though 'spontaneous' was interpreted with unusual latitude given that the woman was so drugged she had to have a special bed with safety railings put round her. After the forceps, which required an episiotomy, the placenta was removed manually. So under this regime, a woman had administered to her five drugs plus two operations, episiotomy and forceps, followed by manual removal and another two drugs to counter post-partum haemorrhage. It was to prove so successful from the viewpoint of doctors, that in the Chicago Lying-in Hospital, where de Lee had first practised, the rate of forceps deliveries between 1946 and 1951 was 68.2 per cent.[62]

The regimes of Hamilton, Johnston and de Lee permit us to see how, as soon as obstetrics has discarded one mode or technique on the grounds that it has proven non-productive (although the measurement of success or failure has often been as laden with misconceptions as the technique itself), it has searched for another, always using the argument that more refined technologies and schemes of management can reduce risks and ultimately bring down the mortality rates of both mother and child. At first glance, this sounds a plausible and even commendable line of approach. A closer examination, however, reveals a number of problems. There is firstly a problem of how far one can reduce risk. Can it be reduced to nil? To achieve its own immortality, obstetrics must argue that this is an attainable goal.

But in fact, despite its immortality strategies and its assertion that greater obstetric knowledge can control death, obstetrics does face an irreducible problem. There are women who, however it has come about for them, are undeliverable by ordinary means and who require extraordinary means to try and prevent their deaths and these means may not be successful, and, for these women, the proximity to death increases. Johnston describes a fortunate instance of this where he delivers a woman with forceps who, on her ninth pregnancy and either thirty-nine or forty years old, arrives at the hospital in labour, three-fifths dilated, and with the foetal head unable to move down through the pelvic cavity because of the presence of a bony tumour on her sacroiliac joint. The forceps are applied only with great difficulty, he writes, and 'after a considerable amount of traction and time', he delivers a

> female child – left frontal bone being greatly depressed for a space of 3½ × 1¾ inches. It was some time before child could be resuscitated, the depression decreased, and both mother and child went out well on the 12th day.[63]

He is lucky in this instance that the woman and baby live. Johnston and every other obstetrician continue to face circumstances where intervention is vital for women, as distinct for expanding the boundaries of obstetric knowledge. The issue is how they see the body. Can they distinguish when intervention is vital? Do they have the conceptual skill to use the potential of the female body, and the skill to construct and collect sufficiently sensitive data which is accurate in how it reads each woman's body and every woman's individual circumstances, and thus be able to predict risk and act accordingly? The woman who has a bony tumour needs the forceps or some equivalent and effective birth technology which perhaps obstetrics is not able to conceptualise, so that she will not die as the result of an obstructed labour. But does the woman who has been seduced require the forceps? Is the extreme nervousness and fretting Johnston claims as an intrinsic part of her incapacity to labour really the result of her seduction and amenable to no other solution or is this yet one more chimera of the obstetric imagination? We never hear from the women directly and we have no knowledge of how they construct their own situation. To construe them only as victims of their bodies and their circumstances fits in with the obstetric agenda, as does the notion that data about outcomes can actually constitute proof about causation, as distinct from description.[64]

The search to defeat death with obstetric techniques, aided by a pre-set bundle of predictable risks, has become the equivalent of the philosopher's stone for obstetrics, to the extent that the whole of the current system of childbirth management is determined by this frame of reference.[65] In theory, a schedule of predictable risks, if it worked, could have been a positive benefit coming out of the drive to systematise the female body, to the advantage to women, providing them with an assessment of whether they fell into a life-threatening category or not. But in addition to the problem of a basic misunderstanding of what is description and what proves causation, there are two further reasons why this advantage was never going to materialise in practice. Firstly, the categories themselves were shot through with a view of women that concentrated on their frailty and their tendency to emotional lability and madness. Secondly, the categories were based on an abstracted averaged account of the female body. As a result, the presumed causal relationships arising out of the process of categorising are suspect, because they have absorbed individual physiological patterns and differences while overlooking any other version of what woman is.

This has been particularly striking around the issue of the timing of labour and its various phases. As modern clock time increased its influence and with it, the notion of productivity, which was quite divorced from individual circadian rhythms, obstetrics carefully recorded the time each phase of labour took. How long the entire labour took became an important indicator *in itself* of when things were going well or badly. Observations like that of Fleetwood Churchill's, in the 1840s, that in 143 of his cases where the first stage of labour (when the woman's cervix is dilating) ranged from sixteen to 176 hours, not a single mother died,[66] were no longer meaningful to a science which was becoming committed to the notion of intervention to secure the lives of both mother and child, investing in the idea of predictable risk to help bring about this dual success.

What Sally Inch terms the 'assumption of pathology'[67] gradually won out during the nineteenth century and the perception of normality as being the potential of the normal to turn abnormal without warning became a major determinant of obstetrical management of birth. With an ever expanding armoury of technologies and an expanding application of categories which make up the risk system, obstetrics has hedged its bets, for it simultaneously argues that the risk of death will always be there and therefore every woman must be treated as if she might be at risk.

A typical contemporary schedule of obstetric risk factors comprises: a woman who is thirty years of age or more, expecting her first child; a woman thirty-five years of age or more expecting her second child; a woman expecting her fourth or subsequent child; low social class; disorders of maternal growth – women who are less than 158 centimetres or grossly overweight; a woman who has rhesus problems or has experienced isoimmunisation; a woman who has had a uterine operation, including a Caesarean section; a woman with previous problems in the third stage of labour (which is the expulsion of the placenta); a woman with a 'bad obstetric history' including previous forceps deliveries; a woman who has had previous low birth-weight babies; pre-existing maternal illnesses such as diabetes or renal disease; a woman who has had no formal medical antenatal care and therefore has not been screened for any risks; and finally any condition which arises in the course of a pregnancy which puts the woman into a risk category such as pre-eclampsia, antepartum bleeding, foetal growth retardation, malpresentation, and poor maternal weight gain.[68]

Very few of these categories are as precise as they might first appear. Will all first-time mothers over the age of thirty have the same health profile? Will their bodies respond to pregnancy in exactly the same way? If the factor of low social class stands as a proxy for poor long-term maternal health, how does that interact with the category of age? Viewed this way, could it mean that the first pregnancy of a professional woman will be unaffected by age (which indeed available evidence on perinatal outcomes appears to suggest[69])? Will the same apply to all women thirty-five years of age or more and those with four children or more? Will all these women encounter difficulties because of these factors alone, or will many be fine while some will develop problems? How accurate is antenatal screening as a way of picking up possibly risky conditions? How many conditions does it catch as distinct from all it misses?[70] If foetal growth retardation ultimately turns out to be associated with the use of ultrasound, as is now being suggested,[71] what will that mean for its inclusion as a risk factor? Is malpresentation now listed as a risk factor because fewer and fewer doctors are being taught the skill of delivering a breech baby vaginally, rather than by Caesarean section?[72]

In reality, this schedule can only represent the 'central dense mass' of an averaged body, reading risks, not the bodies of individual women and certainly not the body which is caught in a crude trap of obstetrics' making, for example, when the maternal body is subjected to forceps or Caesarean section which as a consequence leads to the body being defined as risky. Yet these schedules determine schemes of care for women, often to their detriment, not least because the risk system, for all that obstetrics has invested in it, is not predictive of who will develop a life-threatening complication because the complexity of the personal and the social for each woman cannot be captured.[73]

At some remove from the efforts to valorise this kind of categorisation, Mary Douglas and Aaron Wildavsky have developed an anthropological perspective on risk in which they argue that there is no single acceptable notion of risk because complete knowledge does not exist.[74] And, even if it did exist, there would still have to be agreement on the ranking of risks. They see risk as an expression of knowledge, with the addition of consent about the options that might be undertaken in relation to that knowledge. The statistical relationships which have generated risk schedules within obstetric thinking, like the one above, or like those on the need for hospital confinement rather than birth at home,[75] must produce standardised risk factors to make their various cases. They do so on issues where there is often intense disagreement between the professionals themselves about meaning and causal links.[76] But when these same schedules are presented to child-bearing women, they are meant to inspire confidence and end in agreement, that is the woman agreeing with the medical position. This is not a negotiated agreement, more an acquiescence. If active disagreement arises, then, as Douglas and Wildavsky point out, coercion is introduced into the equation of what constitutes risk.[77]

And coercion in this instance means that a woman is not free to raise her objections to a particular form of treatment, to a particular regime. She is prevented from taking an active role as a responsible agent in determining her own well-being because negotiation with a woman over what constitutes risk and over what is an avoidable death is unheard of within the obstetric domain. Marsden Wagner has defined the medical use of risk as the probability of an undesired effect which medicine believes can be measured empirically and statistically. Within those narrow and flawed parameters, medicine refuses to concede that the importance of what is considered an undesirable effect or outcome for the individual involved is a 'social value judgement'.[78] Such judgements can only be made by the persons who might suffer from that negative outcome.

To see how this has worked, I want to examine how a possible life-threatening problem was converted into a risk category. In the pre-obstetric period, women giving birth could voice their concerns and their decisions about the problem of post-partum haemorrhage. But this was gradually made into a problem where decisions were no longer theirs.

Avoidable Maternal Death: Post-partum Haemorrhage

Ian Hacking argues that there is a common feature in the presentation of risk, one which is in line with the creation and tracking of population and sub-populations and with the creation of expert knowledges or discourses which claim complete authority about those populations. In this configuration and, as part of what can be termed the 'risk portfolio', polarised extremes are defined and presented as 'dire perils'.[79] The 'dire perils' of maternal and foetal death have been the twin poles of the obstetric risk portfolio. This is the spirit in which Thomas Beatty, first Master of the Coombe Lying-in Hospital in Dublin, wrote about 'the train of symptoms indicative of danger' for a woman during birth. In his account of how death could be seen to enter the scene for a woman, he fastened on women's emotional responses: 'an anxious and disturbed mind; a disposition to sing in a plaintive and wailing tone of voice has in particular been considered a very frightful symptom.'[80] Beatty defined the principal obstetric dangers as the death of the mother or child or both before delivery; the death of the mother after delivery;[81] and 'inflammation terminating in abscess or sloughing of the soft parts ... producing effects fatal to the future comfort of the patient', that is long-term morbidity and illness for the mother as a result of giving birth.[82] These 'fatal accidents' and injuries were fitted into the obstetric premiss that maternal death was avoidable, if the right intervention could be found.

Post-partum haemorrhage is a case in point. The most dangerous factor in causing post-partum haemorrhage arises because of the incapacity of the uterus to contract (other factors causing haemorrhage are vaginal or cervical lacerations and episiotomy). The major difference in how contemporary obstetric practice responds to this threat, compared to the pre-obstetric and the early obstetric era, centres on the notion that it is possible to intervene in the birth process in such a way as to prevent post-partum haemorrhage, or at least substantially reduce the incidence of occurrence, by treating all women as being at risk of post-partum haemorrhage.[83] But obstetrics has moved to this position with a specific model of what happens to initiate haemorrhage and this model has profoundly influenced its methods of treatment.

In one sense, the possibility of haemorrhage is faced by every woman, although not in the way obstetrics has come to see it. A dramatic moment in the birth process comes after the baby has been born, when as the woman's uterus contracts, the placenta peels off the uterine wall and is pushed out of her body by uterine contractions, while blood vessels in the uterine wall supplying the placenta are clamped down by uterine muscle tissue. If the blood vessels are not clamped down, women can die rapidly. If the placenta does not peel off or only partially peels off and breaks into pieces, all of which are not expelled, this can initiate haemorrhage and infection which can also end in women's deaths.

Always aware of the threat of post-partum haemorrhage, women have responded to either the specific event or to the early few days after birth as a potentially dangerous time. In the pre-obstetric period, in France, a woman was thought to have 'one foot in the grave' until after the placenta was expelled. Within the Bolivian Andes, the concept of *sajt'ay* expresses a woman's vulnerability to death in the first few days after giving birth and the need to be especially mindful of protecting her well-being.[84] In Greek medicine, in the writings of Hippocrates and Plato, the uterus was seen as an organ which had independent powers of movement, rather like an animal. The uterus could become discontented and angry, especially if it remained unfruitful, wandering through the body, closing up the passages of breath, and obstructing respiration, which provoked the extremities of disease.[85] It is perhaps this idea of an organ which wanders and can cause damage to a woman that was reflected in the belief of women in seventeenth- and eighteenth-century France that once the baby was born, the placenta would travel up, rather than down, and choke the woman. It led to the custom of tying the umbilical cord to a woman's thigh to keep the placenta from wandering, once the baby's end of the cord had been cut.[86] And, whatever about traditional practices like this one, in settings outside the scientific domain, men midwives, like women midwives, were affected by fears about the placenta not being expelled at all. There was a widespread notion in early obstetric writing that the neck of the uterus would contract so quickly after birth that the placenta would be trapped inside, resulting in the routine practice of manual removal of the placenta by the man midwife.[87]

Elizabeth Nihell quotes a famous instance of post-partum haemorrhage from the treatise by Guillaume de la Motte, a French man midwife writing just at the end of the seventeenth century. De la Motte had delivered the wife of a 'glover' in Valogne with 'all the facility imaginable' and left her to the attentions of a nurse. Shortly afterwards, he is asked to return in haste, and he finds the woman dead, the cause of which is instantly apparent to him, a 'stream of blood which ran about the floor ... after soaking through the bed itself'. Nihell reports to us that de la Motte explains:

> ... these melancholic accidents are not without example, since such ladies as the princes of – and madam la Presidente de – with numbers of others, have, on the like occasion, undergone the same fate, as her he here treats of. These are, according to him, proofs that all human science and dexterity often cannot prevent the like misfortunes, since these great ladies had been lain by the most celebrated men-midwives.[88]

De la Motte was clear that the proper handling of this potential problem was to get the placenta out as quickly as possible, by pulling on the 'navel-string', which we now call the umbilical cord, to hasten the placenta's exit, and then to reach in and manually remove the placenta, if need be.[89] This implies that the umbilical cord was cut almost at once after the baby's birth to enable the man midwife to have something to pull on which he did. What is noteworthy here is the construction of the delivery of the placenta as a problem in itself which led to 'melancholic accidents'. Practitioners' fears of sudden death from 'flooding' or haemorrhage, or from a 'morbidly adherent' or retained placenta, and therefore the consequent incitement to intervention remained long after notions like a wandering placenta faded. The continuing problem obstetrics created for itself was that the event of post-partum haemorrhage was posed in isolation to the overall physiological and social context of birth. Each element in the series of events leading to placental separation, as it became identified: uterine contractions, the placenta peeling away from the uterine wall, the intertwined action of contracting muscle fibres and constricted blood vessels; uterine blood being pumped through the umbilical cord, came to be seen in a hierarchy of importance, with separation from the uterine wall as the most important element. This model of a hierarchy of events in turn influenced the obstetric mode of response. For, even though the explanations became more scientifically dense over time, and in that sense, more detailed and more accurate, the initial tendency to see separation as important, and to discard the other elements as unimportant, led to a situation where risk was identified with separation itself. On the basis of this model, which only partially realised all the interconnected elements, obstetric emphasis settled on the need to get the placenta out quickly.

In the early obstetric period, there was already dissension about whether the expulsion of the placenta could be regarded as a natural process or was one which must be aided. De la Motte chose to pull on the umbilical cord, with care, in order to facilitate expulsion in every case. One of the conditions that Henrik Deventer, the Dutch man midwife, laid down to define a 'natural' birth was that the 'After-birth is presently to follow the Infant, without any remarkable Hindrance'.[90] This was at least an admission that it was possible that the physiological work of birth could complete itself without intervention but, as we have already discovered in Chapter 2, Deventer had a very limited definition of natural. He advocated manual removal of the placenta as a matter of course to forestall any threat of haemorrhage. Fielding Ould disagreed with Deventer and argued that the commonplace but groundless fear amongst many 'operators' of the uterus closing and trapping the placenta inside pushed them into over-hasty action which itself caused 'fatal Accidents'. He nevertheless advocated intervention by pulling on the umbilical cord, at the same time making the woman stop

> her breath and forcing as if she were at stool which if she be not able to do herself, she must be compelled to it by putting a finger into her throat, which will cause a pressure of the Diaphragm and muscles of the belly by her efforts to vomit.[91]

Southwell, the Kildare man midwife, who disliked Ould's work, condemned this method as 'inhumane teazing' of a woman but promoted in its place manual removal as Deventer had recommended.[92]

Elizabeth Nihell argued that if 'evacuation' did not take place naturally, the problem lay in an 'over-repletion of blood' and 'a defect of the contraction of the uterus'. She recommended bleeding for the former during pregnancy; if after the birth of the baby, 'Nature' appeared 'tardy or deficient' the midwife must encourage the woman to cough and sneeze to bring about evacuation and only if that failed, should she manually remove 'all the clots of blood' and 'extraneous matter'.[93] It was Nihell's rival, William Smellie, who described the contractions of the uterus squeezing and separating 'the placenta from its inner surface'. Nihell quotes him, scornfully dismissing his argument that if there is no danger from a flooding and the woman rests a little, the uterus will complete its work unaided.[94]

In 1767, John Harvie, a London man midwife who worked with Smellie, published a pamphlet on 'delivering the Placenta without violence', in which he rejected the three common methods of management: manual removal, pulling on the navel string (umbilical cord) or forcing the woman to sneeze, cough or vomit.[95] Of the first, he said that what was considered by many practitioners 'a right and necessary measure' was attended with great pain and danger either through injury to the uterus or consequent inflammation (which he said was accompanied by often 'fatal fever', referring to puerperal fever). Pulling on the cord could too easily result in an inverted uterus, in which the uterus might end up being pulled outside the woman's body, which was 'extremely dangerous' to the woman. The third 'hurrying method' of forcing a woman to press down on her diaphragm through the action of sneezing and so on, precipitated a haemorrhage in its own right. Although nature could be trusted to complete this work, in five minutes generally or usually within an hour, if it took much longer than that, women themselves became alarmed at any delay, even though it was safer to leave it to nature: 'if not performed instantly they blame the accoucheur.'[96] This prejudice of women prevented a 'most judicious and rational practice'[97] and practitioners were afraid to leave nature alone. Therefore what Harvie recommended as a safe practice was for 'the accoucheur' to apply 'light and gentle pressure' externally to the contracting uterus bringing the hand downwards towards the pubes when 'he will feel the uterus sensibly contracting, and often will feel it reduced in size, so as to be certain that the placenta is expelled.'[98] Once the placenta was out, if the movement were repeated, any small clots left behind would also be expelled. If parts of the placenta had broken off or it was retained, then he recommended pulling gently on the navel-string. By comparison with other techniques, Harvie's is less invasive. He is the only writer in this group to attribute the pressure for a quick delivery to women's fears of haemorrhage. Whether the pressure to do something emanated from the woman in labour or her woman or man midwife, the perception of the placenta as problematic entailed some concrete intervention and hence his pamphlet. But he is interesting in his conviction that left to itself the placenta will generally come out in five minutes.

Nihell writes that 'these haemorrhages are but too frequent, especially with those women who neglect the precautionary bleeding.'[99] Yet how great a problem post-partum haemorrhage was before hospitalised birth is not clear. The effects of poverty, anaemia and malnutrition, along with unregulated fertility resulting in too many pregnancies, undoubtedly destroyed many women's health and left them open to fatal and near-fatal outcomes, if haemorrhage occurred. However, Clarke in the Rotunda records only twenty-four haemorrhages in all, from his 'population' of 10,387 women, ten of which were post-partum haemorrhages. Thus he feels justified in writing that 'the proportion of haemorrhages that proved alarming after delivery, is very trifling, not more than one in a thousand'.[100] There were no fatalities among his ten cases of post-partum haemorrhage. Retained placenta occurred after the labours of twenty-one women, twelve of them first-time mothers. He attributed these low numbers to his regime of keeping women 'very cool' and preventing any 'voluntary exertions' during labour. And, there was also the fact that because Clarke did not utilise cord-traction or any sort of cord-tugging, the cord was not cut immediately. As we saw in Chapter 2, Clarke felt there were benefits for the child in not cutting the cord at once. But this also signalled a recognition that other factors, and not just the expulsion of the placenta, were involved. Echoing Smellie's and Harvie's thinking, he concluded that the uterus must be allowed 'gradually to empty itself', but where there was an indication of 'imperfect uterine action', there was an alternative to manual removal:

> I have been for some years in the habit, not only of retarding the expulsion of the foetus in these cases, but, with a hand on the abdomen, of pursuing the fundus uteri in its contractions, until the foetus be entirely expelled, and afterwards of continuing this pressure, to keep it if possible in a contracted state.[101]

In the case of retained placenta, Clarke preferred to wait two hours and even then in 'introducing the hand' sought to stimulate the uterus to contract rather then 'forcibly extracting' the placenta.[102]

The results of manual extraction were severe, as Johnston and Sinclair wrote in their 1858 *Practical Midwifery*: 'the manual extraction of the placenta . . . may involve very serious consequences . . . but in hospital practice particularly are its results to be dreaded.'[103] They listed as possible consequences: initiating the haemorrhage manual removal was done to prevent, an inverted uterus, shock, and puerperal infection from the invading hand, all possibly leading to the death of the woman. But, if manual extraction were not to be used, then a combination of continuous external manual pressure and pressure from a binder, usually made from twilled calico, was to be applied to achieve 'command over the uterus', for the woman still risked dying.[104]

Beatty, first Master of the Coombe, stated emphatically that 'the safe course . . . is to treat all parturient women as if they were about to be attacked with haemorrhage, they are in fact all in danger of it.'[105] The notion that all women were liable to haemorrhage led to the principle on placental management, that intervention equalled prevention, and it was this line of argument which became the familiar obstetric response. Beatty favoured the binder, a version of which he designed for use in the Coombe Lying-in Hospital. He instructed that the binder be 'slipped under the patient' during labour.

> I prefer delaying it until the head of the child has entered the pelvis for its application is taken by the woman as an earnest of a speedy delivery from her sufferings, and if the labour is not terminated in a reasonable time after it [the binder] is put on, she is apt to become disappointed and despondent.[106]

Despondency might well have been an appropriate response on the part of men midwives for figures on post-partum haemorrhage began to increase in hospital births. By the time of Collins' mastership in the Rotunda, 1826–31, the number of women experiencing post-partum haemorrhage was on the rise, from just 1 per cent in Clarke's years to 3 per cent. Half of these cases Collins recorded as 'severe'.[107]

In a departure from the otherwise optimistic account he presents of the progress of obstetric science, the historian, Edward Shorter, admits reluctantly that the frequency of all haemorrhages steadily increased in the nineteenth and twentieth centuries, with the increasing numbers of women giving birth in hospitals.[108] Using composite hospital records, Shorter estimates an incidence of six per thousand cases before 1850, increasing to eighteen per thousand between 1850 and 1900, and then to twenty-two per thousand between 1900 and 1940.[109] It is possible that the increase in absolute numbers may be attributed in some part to increased diligence in recording numbers as well as to a change in the definition of how much blood a woman could lose before it constituted a haemorrhage. But when the consequences of the range of interventions are considered, it is an increase more likely to be associated with the intensified blanket application of techniques and styles of birth management in hospitals which provoke exactly the outcomes they hope to avoid.

Time and average intervals begin to weigh more heavily in the decision to intervene, and although there was evidence that waiting for the placenta produced it without trauma and without haemorrhage, such evidence was ignored in the rush to bring yet another aspect of labour within the ambit of scientific thinking. Fleetwood Churchill, for example, who set up the Western Lying-in Hospital in Arran Quay in 1836, attempted to systematically record what time intervals were involved if the practitioner waited for the placenta to come out. He produced a table on expulsion of the placenta, covering the labours of 313 'females'[110] for which time intervals were supposedly precisely observed:

Table 4.1: Time Intervals From Birth of Baby to Placental Expulsion

Time Elapsed: Number of Cases

5 min: 69	30 min: 31	1 to 2 hrs: 15	8 hrs: 1
10 min: 54	35 min: 7	2 to 3 hrs: 2	
15 min: 63	40 min: 9	3 to 4 hrs: 2	
20 min: 38	50 min: 3	5 hrs: 4	
25 min: 3	60 min: 11	6 hrs: 1	
Total Cases:			**313**

Source: F. Churchill (1838), 'Second Medical Report of the Western Lying-in Hospital and Dispensary, 31 Arran Quay', *Dublin Quarterly Journal of Medical Science*, vol. xiii, p. 238.

The logic of Churchill's distributions, indicating that 92 per cent of women delivered the placenta within an hour, was not of interest to hospital-based obstetrics, although the collection of data like this was essential to the internal debates in obstetrics. But as with puerperal fever, an incomplete conceptual model demanded that evidence conform to its dimensions and prevention through intervention, in whatever guise, became the obstetric norm, if the placenta were not immediately expelled after the baby's birth.

For a long period, the techniques remained much as they had been in Ould's time. Manual removal of the placenta was favoured by some, while others favoured external manipulations of the abdomen, and the use of strong cloth binders around the bellies of women in labour. At the extreme limits of the intervention scale, in the middle of the nineteenth century, was the clinical teaching of the German doctor, Credé: once the baby was born, the uterus was to be rubbed until the friction initiated a contraction, at which point we seize with one or two hands the fundus and when the contraction arrives at its maximum intensity we press upon the fundus and on the walls of the uterus, at the same time driving it downwards into the small pelvis.[111]

The violence of this practice was not just discursive in nature. It was terribly painful and easily sent women into physiological shock from the severe trauma, which itself could prove fatal. Credé's method (although now it is rarely used, it is still taught as a technique when there has been only partial separation of the placenta) formed part of a curious attempt at the beginning of the twentieth century to claim that the delivery of the placenta by external manipulation of the abdomen did not originate in Leipzig with Credé himself, but in the Rotunda Hospital. One of the hospital's obstetricians, Henry Jellett, published a paper in 1900 in which he argued that what he termed the 'Dublin Method' of placental management had long preceded Credé, whose procedures were an elaboration of techniques which could be traced all the way back to Fielding Ould in 1742.[112] These had 'been practised clinically at the Dublin Lying-in Hospital from time immemorial', Jellett wrote; in Ould's Treatise

is the first recognition of the great principle upon which the Dublin method of effecting delivery of the placenta is based – that *vis a tergo* [force from behind] is to be preferred to *vis a fronte* as a mean of obtaining delivery of the placenta, and also a recognition of the fact that the uterus should, if possible, effect the detachment of the placenta itself.[113]

As it happens, Jellett's case for the continuity of the method, part of building a case for the continuity of obstetric thinking, ignored the fact that in Ould's procedure, which centred on the umbilical cord, force is applied from the front, as much force as on the downward movement of the diaphragm.

It is no surprise that the notion that the placenta would detach itself moved upstream and that the woman became an involuntary and even unnamed agent in the model that moved downstream. Within a hospital-based system of monitoring and surveillance, the institutional logic of getting in and terminating a labour quickly and easily won a debate about dealing with the third stage of labour. It was simply easier to see every woman as a risk and to intervene. In fact, one of the keys to understanding the escalation in post-partum haemorrhage in the hospital setting was the obstetric insistence on using the same procedures Jellett sought to valorise. All these abdominal manipulations contributed to the likelihood of partial separation of the placenta, and where this occurred, the remaining fragments would lead to both post-partum haemorrhage and infection. Other insights about the placenta and how it came to be expelled by the physiological action of the body were abandoned: Smellie's description of which part first peeled off the uterine wall and his advice to let the woman rest and wait for the placenta to come out; Harvie's notion that if one waited, without manipulating, most placentas would come out; Churchill's list of cases to prove Harvie's point; Clarke's careful practice of not cutting the cord at once. All these were to remain untapped referents for a different model of placental action for a very long time.

Moving Towards Active Management Protocols

And meanwhile, the move towards total obstetric management of the placenta and the conversion of post-partum haemorrhage into a risk category were made possible as attention shifted from mechanical systems of intervention to pharmacological means. To accomplish this, obstetrics first had to take over ergot from the peasant pharmacopoeia. For centuries, traditional midwives had stimulated uterine contractions with ergot, derived from the fungus growing on rotten grain, especially black rye, to act as an abortifacient, to induce labour, or to slow haemorrhage.[114]

In 1807, the use of ergot was first reported in the scientific journals by an American obstetrician to bring to a conclusion 'lingering parturition'.[115] Gradually ergot found its way into clinical protocols for post-partum haemorrhage. By 1878, Lombe Atthill reported using injections of ergot in conjunction with injections of perchloride of iron (also in order to cause uterine contractions) and cold and hot water in the Rotunda to arrest what he termed haemorrhages 'of an alarming nature'.[116] Death from post-partum haemorrhage was still far from uncommon for Irish women in the 1920s and 1930s, although even then, deaths from post-partum haemorrhage amounted to less than a third of deaths from puerperal sepsis.[117] Between 1928 and 1930, post-partum haemorrhage accounted for between 22 and 24 per cent of all maternal deaths in Ireland.[118]

In 1935, four different pharmaceutical companies, in the United States, England, and Switzerland, announced that they had isolated a water-soluble and stable form of ergot. Known as ergometrine in England, this oxytocic chemical was thought to be free of dangerous side effects, including the overdosing that had made ergot so problematic, and so it became the treatment of choice for post-partum haemorrhage. However, it was noted that the placenta could be trapped inside the uterus if an injection of ergometrine was administered before the placenta was delivered.[119] Despite this caution, obstetrics argued that it was now equipped with a workable pharmacological regime, and ergometrine entered use not just as a treatment for post-partum haemorrhage when it occurred, but as a preventative measure. The literature from the 1940s onwards is filled with accounts of ergometrine as a prophylactic.[120]

These pharmacological advances were accompanied by moves to produce uniform clinical definitions of what signified a haemorrhage, as distinct from ordinary blood loss after birth. Not every clinician agreed that measurement was possible. As far back as 1909, Tweedy had said in his clinical report on the Rotunda for that year that 'we do not estimate post-partum haemorrhage by the amount of blood lost . . . in our opinion, it is impossible to draw useful conclusions from such data.'[121]

Nevertheless, by the 1960s it was standard practice to attempt to measure blood loss after each birth in hospital, along with abdominal examination for a flaccid or poorly contracted uterus, to determine if there was a haemorrhage, and a post-partum haemorrhage was deemed to exist with any blood loss of 600 millilitres or over.[122]

Problems abounded with this approach, firstly because spillages and extra fluids from amniotic liquor make exact measurements unfeasible. Secondly, the attempt to produce a set figure below which a woman might be deemed to be alright with blood loss, and above which she was not, ignored the fact that every woman who enters labour is not in the same circumstances. For a woman with poor general health and an extremely low level of haemoglobin prior to the pregnancy, a blood loss as small as 250 millilitres may prove threatening, while a blood loss up to 700 millilitres may not be particularly difficult to handle physiologically if the woman is not anaemic and is in good condition otherwise.[123] This is the problem of depending on averages and in fitting an averaged model onto the individual body.

Along with the attempts to measure what constitutes a post-partum haemorrhage, there have been concerted efforts to pinpoint who might be at risk and to develop schedules of risk in order to identify these women. Predisposing factors which obstetric literature has linked to post-partum haemorrhage are: primiparity; grand multiparity, five children or more (the more children a woman bears, the more likely she is to have a flaccid uterus unable to contract well); anaemia and poor nutritional status; multiple pregnancy; large baby; previous third-stage abnormality; prolonged labour; operative delivery; general anaesthesia; antepartum haemorrhage; placenta praevia; coagulation disorders; an intra-uterine death and structural uterine abnormalities.[124] For the purposes of effective screening, however, these risk schedules have been found to be less than workable. Like the schedule on who is at risk in giving birth, these categories are not actually predictive of outcome. The idea of predictive risk sounds as if it ought to work; when a retrospective statistical schedule claims that a previous third-stage complication creates a risk of a post-partum haemorrhage two to three times greater than that of women without this history, obstetrics feels it ought to be able to act on that information. The primary problem is a total misapprehension of the meaning of risk, that correlations composed of 'risk factors' and outcomes from broad populations or subgroups are easily applicable at an individual level, because they can at best only present evidence of outcomes, not proof of linkages between risk factors and outcomes.[125]

Doubts about the feasibility of risk schedules did not prevent a complete package for the active management of third-stage labour being put together by the early 1960s. Obstetricians had two choices: either use the risk schedules to isolate which women might be at risk from post-partum haemorrhage and seek to avoid that outcome by using a preventative package of measures. Or, using this same package, they could choose, as more and more did, to make preventative treatment for post-partum haemorrhage a routine precautionary measure for all women.

The current package of measures for what is called the active management of the third stage of labour, that is hands-on obstetric management, is underpinned by a stable oxytocic drug which can be injected at a number of points in the labour process, but in all cases before there is any indication that post-partum haemorrhage is occurring. The injection, either intravenous or intramuscular depending on individual regimes, might be injected at the birth of the anterior shoulder or after the placenta is delivered.

In the most rigorous version of active management, ergometrine or syntocinon (a synthetic ergometrine) is injected as a prophylactic, either intravenously or intramuscularly while the anterior shoulder of the baby is delivered in the case of a woman giving birth for the first time, or as the head of the baby is crowning in the case of a woman who has given birth before. Once the placenta separates from the uterine wall, it is then delivered while controlled cord traction is applied and fundal pressure is used to push the uterus, first gently upwards and then downward until the placenta is expelled.[126] The same principles, an injection of an oxytocic drug, controlled cord traction, and fundal pressure, operate in the other variants as well, where an injection might be given after the baby is born and before the placenta is delivered, or after the placenta is delivered. All three presume that the woman is placed in a supine or semi-supine position.[127] All three claim that there is a problem with time; that if the placenta under this active management does not emerge in a given time frame, anything from fifteen minutes after the birth of the baby to an hour, then further measures – massage of the uterus, additional oxytocic drugs, bimanual compression of the uterus, and manual removal of the placenta – will be required treatment.[128]

A critical variable in all these approaches is that cutting and clamping the umbilical cord before the placenta is delivered is seen, on the one hand, as a routine practice. Early cord-cutting is essential to the technique of controlled cord-traction, if that is being employed. On the other hand, when the cord is cut and clamped is seen as a process largely independent in its effects to that of the placenta separating and being expelled. One common recommendation is to cut the cord once it has stopped pulsating after the baby's birth, approximately three minutes, during which time the baby is held at or below the level where the placenta is presumed to be attached to the uterine wall. There is no notion of a related progression of events, including when the cord is cut, which would facilitate placental detachment without intervention. There appears to be no awareness that early cord-cutting means the blood drains out of the placenta which shrinks it down so that it does not separate as quickly or as completely from the uterine wall, in the way Smellie described.[129] Of course this becomes an irrelevant point if a quick-fix technological approach is to hand, which is essentially what active management of the third stage is.

Active management has not been put in place without its critics. Its sequelae for women run from mild disturbances like nausea and vomiting to significant increases in blood pressure, as a result of ergometrine, to quite serious outcomes. The midwife Sally Inch has pointed out that the cardio-vascular effects of oxytocic drugs are significant and can plunge some women into serious post-partum illness, including hypertension, eclampsia, and pulmonary oedema.[130] As early as 1962, the reported death of a young woman from intercranial haemorrhage, who had otherwise enjoyed a normal labour up to the routine administration of ergometrine, was accompanied by a warning that 'blind adherence' to 'the postpartum ritual was contributory or causative in this death'.[131]

Critics cite other risks attached to active management. If oxytocic drugs are injected before the placenta is delivered, the placenta must be delivered within approximately seven minutes of the injection before the drug induces contractions of the lower segment of the uterus and of the cervix. This is because the impact of the oxytocics is to close the uterus down, with the effect of either trapping the placenta or leading to its partial separation. This may itself lead to increased maternal blood loss or even the need for manual removal of the placenta. If ergometrine is used, one of the negative outcomes is a rise in maternal blood pressure which can be a serious complication for women who have had high blood pressure or toxaemia during their pregnancy.[132] In addition to the nausea and vomiting linked to the use of ergometrine, there are also reported side effects of ergometrine and Syntometrine, a synthetic variant (when the latter is given intramuscularly). Active management of labour, where oxytocic drugs are used, has also been implicated in a greater incidence of the uterus not contracting well and of secondary post-partum haemorrhage, that is a haemorrhage occurring twenty-four hours or more after a baby has been born.[133]

Calculating Life and Death: The Risk—Death Pairing 189

The Irish midwife, Cecily Begley, reports from her extensive study of third-stage policies in a major Dublin maternity hospital that active management will result in more women requiring manual removal of the placenta; more women having problems in the immediate two hours after birth, including pain; and more complications in the first six weeks after the birth requiring treatment, including treatment for increased instances of secondary post-partum haemorrhage and infection. Begley reported the following negative outcomes as a result of active management with ergometrine: uterine cramping, dizziness, headaches, tinnitus, retinal detachment, and coronary-artery spasm. Moreover, the time needed to complete the third stage is not significantly reduced over non-intervention.[134] Inch reports instances of inverted uterus directly attributable to active management of the third stage.[135]

For the baby, there are complicated consequences as well. Early cord-clamping is a necessary element in the active-management package, but the newly born baby will either not receive its full physiological quota of blood, possibly resulting in respiratory distress, or is in danger of being over-transfused.[136] This is because the use of oxytocic drugs before the placenta is delivered leads to much stronger uterine contractions, resulting in over-transfusion.[137] So practitioners may have to make a decision about when to cut the cord, choosing between that outcome and the value to the baby of an extra 50 millilitres of blood (if over-transfusion does not occur). It is thought that early cord-clamping can lead to feto-maternal transfusion, a complication that is especially grave for rhesus-negative women.[138] Early cord-cutting has also been associated with an increase in blood loss and a longer third stage of labour and may predispose to retained placenta and post-partum haemorrhage.[139]

It is true that when post-partum haemorrhage now occurs in Western settings, death is a rarity because bleeding can be quickly controlled with oxytocic drugs; if necessary, fluids and blood volume can be replaced and manual removal carried out with an anaesthetic. It is equally true that intervention in labour at the many points obstetrics has decreed, allied with the 'fundal fiddling' of third-stage policies, has created a further range of hazards that also contribute to post-partum haemorrhage. For instance, linked to the increasing use of oxytocic drugs, either to induce or accelerate labour by stimulating uterine contractions, there has been an increased tendency to post-partum haemorrhage for first-time mothers.[140]

This is indeed a crude trap that obstetrics has made for women. Post-partum haemorrhage has assumed the status of a chiasma, where obstetrics, working as a 'learned imagination',[141] has constructed an imaginary version of the placenta, denying its relationship with the totality of a woman's body, denying what it can be rationally held to possess, its capacity to function well, without pathology. Obstetric practice has invented risk schedules and probabilities of maternal death, to accompany its thesis of active management, denying that if post-partum haemorrhage results, obstetrics can then move to intervene, without any necessity to disrupt the process before a point when any pathological consequences have appeared.

Avoidable Maternal Death: The Obstetric Contribution

There has been and continues to be confusion within obstetrics about risk and its meanings. Often obstetrics has stated with great authority that risk of serious illness and death can be defined precisely, a position that by definition should also entail pinpointing those women not at risk. But just as often and sometimes simultaneously to this first position, obstetrics states that every woman is at risk, an argument which is advanced with the rider that all women must give birth within specialist obstetric units because of the unpredictability of risk. What is most important about these incongruous and disparate lines of argument is the notion of risk itself and the extent to which this has saturated the thinking around childbirth. This goes beyond obstetric science to include the planning and organisation of health services for pregnant women. It is extremely difficult for us to move outside this frame of reference when we think of our bodies in pregnancy and birth. The risk approach has appeared cogent and has fitted in well with packages like active management. In the many interventions obstetrics has chosen to take on board, even if only temporarily, their thesis has been that all of these have contributed to bringing down the rates of maternal death.

But what if death is often preventable for reasons which lie entirely outside the obstetric domain? The science has rarely searched for analyses and explanations that lie beyond its own territory. For example, it is generally reluctant to draw correlations between impoverished and anaemic women and the hard work of pregnancy and labour in order to seek an improvement in social conditions for women and thus improve their chances during birth. Instead, it confines itself to what it can define as purely medical actions, either prophylactic or therapeutic. In 1955, an article appeared in the *Journal of the Irish Medical Association* by J.K. Feeney, Master of the Coombe Lying-in Hospital, describing the Coombe as the 'home of grand multiparity', meaning for him, women bearing seven or more children, of whom 300 or more gave birth in the Coombe every year. According to Feeney, 75 per cent of all women attending the Coombe Lying-in Hospital in 1950 were affected by anaemia but the worst affected were women with grand multiparity, cases which who were often described as 'dangerous' and 'unpredictable'.[142] Feeney then describes the 'social and domestic deficiencies and disadvantages' faced by women in this position: anaemia and malnutrition are commonplace, he tells us,

> as a result of the high cost of essential foodstuffs, faulty diet habits, lack of cooking facilities in tenement rooms, undeveloped sense of thrift, sacrifice of choice pieces to husband and children, unemployment, poverty, defective physical constitution, very hard work within and without the home, nausea and vomiting, dental caries, rapidly succeeding pregnancies, etc.[143]

In this tangle of accurate description and moral judgement (note the charges of 'faulty diet habits' and an 'undeveloped sense of thrift' following on from the observation of the high cost of basic dietary staples), there is no hint that women's lives, health and birth outcomes might be bettered if they had better personal, social and environmental conditions, including fertility control. In relation to post-partum haemorrhage, the women in this situation are exactly those said to be at risk because of multiple pregnancies and anaemia. But obstetrics has seldom considered that part of its remit is a political demand for an alteration in these conditions, and it is sustained in this perspective by the argument that the hospital is a neutral scientific space in which obstetrics must deal with what it finds in the moment with each woman as she comes through the hospital door.

A more recent and more subtle example of this avoidance of the social location of women appears in a comprehensive effort to evaluate the results of all previous controlled-trial studies on the routine use of oxytocics in third-stage labour. The article appears as a chapter in a wide-ranging work based on the premiss that scientific evaluation of obstetric practices, using what are known as randomised controlled trials, can become the gold standard of measurement whereby individual doctors and hospitals can make informed choices about different regimes and approaches to maternity care.[144] In the instance of post-partum haemorrhage, where studies of active management policies with routine prophylactic administration of oxytocic drugs are compared with studies of 'expectant management' policies, the writers conclude that oxytocics have brought about reduced 'odds of this risk of postpartum haemorrhage in the order of 60 per cent' and 'the odds' of requiring therapeutic oxytocic treatment by 70 per cent'.[145] But are we now not back in the territory outlined by Canguilhem where there is a need for a comparative human physiology which will take into account all 'life's intricacy and its kinds and social levels'?[146] In relation to the article of trials on third-stage labour and post-partum haemorrhage, Begley points out that the nine studies reviewed started in 1951 and thus included women at a time when women had far more pregnancies per person.[147] This factor as well as anaemia and poor nutrition were still significant influences on levels of maternal morbidity and mortality, but the reviewers fail to mention this aspect.[148] In Ireland, levels of anaemia amongst pregnant women had dropped dramatically to between 4 and 7 per cent by 1978–87, as had the numbers of children each woman had; the days of the grand multiparous woman in Ireland had drawn to an end.[149] These shifts, reflecting massive social change, form a critical background to the drop in deaths from post-partum haemorrhage, along with the additions of iron supplementation during pregnancy and workable emergency measures like oxytocics and transfusions when haemorrhage did occur. But the social change is acknowledged, if at all, only mutely or as an aside by obstetric science.

The historical demographer, Thomas McKeown, has written that a common problem in reviewing the history of medicine is 'to confuse the activities of the doctor and the outcome for the patient in dealing with the notion of medical progress'.[150] This is especially pertinent to the issue of maternal mortality and the place obstetrics occupies in reducing the incidence of these deaths to the current relatively rare episodes which occur each year in the developed countries of Europe and North America.[151] Feminist historians and demographers have attributed the dramatic fall in maternal mortality in the North Atlantic countries (Europe, Canada and the United States) during this century to the following combined factors: better general health profiles as a result of vastly improved nutrition and better housing; safe and effective control of a woman's fertility through safe contraception and legal abortion facilities; and the control of infectious diseases. Other major factors were the enforcement of an aseptic regime in hospitals and, from the late 1930s, the introduction of antibiotics to control infection, including infection from obstetric operations, and the increased availability and effectiveness of emergency obstetric procedures.[152] They argue that all these developments reduced maternal death rates from puerperal fever or septicaemia and made it possible for obstetrics to argue for the expansion of hospitalised childbirth.

Obstetricians tended to see only what they had accomplished, exclusive of other factors which lay outside their control. Hence they arrived at a position where they attributed the falls in death to increasing levels of hospitalised childbirth. But there are demographers who are quick to observe that this did not make hospitalised care better care, and there is absolutely no evidence to suggest that hospitalised childbirth became *safer* than birth at home *as women became healthier in general.*[153] Marjorie Tew, in her review of the data in the English context, argues that the two factors of increased hospital births and drop in rates of death were assumed to have a direct relationship by obstetric science. But a wider ranging view would have to include the reduction of dangers in obstetric surgery, much of which initially arose through the misdiagnosis and overdiagnosis of complications. The problem of overdiagnosis most commonly arose because of a change in medical perceptions about the utility of possible interventions. Thus in the United States, once Caesarean operations were considered to be safe, there was a sudden upsurge by 1900 in the numbers of women who were reported as having contracted pelves. These women were still at risk of high mortality rates until sepsis was finally controlled in the 1930s.[154] These and similar operations, including forceps deliveries, were gradually rendered less dangerous because the non-compliance with aseptic and antiseptic regimes came to an end and because there was an effective pharmacological response to sepsis from 1936 onwards.[155] Tew cites extensive class differences in the rates of maternal mortality: for the years 1930–32, for example, the records of the Registrar-General in England and Wales indicate that higher rates of maternal death per 1,000 births were experienced by women from social classes I and II, 4.44 per 1,000 births for all causes, than by women from social class V where the rates were 3.89 per 1,000 births. The latter group would have had least contact with doctors and were dying most frequently from induced illegal abortion and post-partum haemorrhage while women in the former group were dying most frequently from sepsis toxaemia and eclampsia, and phlebitis. The highest combined rate of death still came from sepsis at this time, so that the opportune introduction of sulphonamides from the pharmacologists' laboratories in 1936 came as a significant boost to women's well-being.[156]

Marsden Wagner, in his critique of maternal health policies during this century, argues that the phenomenon during the Second World War of a drop in mortality rates to an unprecedented degree, at a point when what he terms the 'birth machine' had ground to a halt because resources were redirected, has never been adequately explained by the medical profession. And he quotes the WHO report which argues that the profession has never been able to prove that hospital birth is a safer place for a woman with an uncomplicated pregnancy to give birth.[157] It is surely valid to query whether the greater proportion of the drop in maternal deaths should be attributed to the development and availability of basic medical resources, like ergometrine to arrest post-partum haemorrhage, emergency Caesarean section, and blood transfusion, or whether they should be attributed to the factors outlined above: better nutrition, better housing, better general health and the increasing ability of women to control their own fertility.

But obstetric science reads this terrain differently and has argued that, in order to prevent possible poor outcomes, the child-bearing population must be hospitalised and their births managed with appropriate obstetric policies. As a body of knowledge, it has been in a strong position socially and politically to argue its case on its own terms and to remain largely unchallenged by those outside the profession, like policy-makers, to change its intensifying tendencies to intervention on the grounds that it must deal with risk. Obstetrics has its spokespersons who favour the risk perspective it adopts, who argue the exact opposite of what critics like Wagner and Tew have set out. Shorter's contention about obstetrics is that it has released women from an historical position of 'victimisation', both the tyranny of biology which subjected women's bodies to pregnancy and childbirth in the first instance and the tyranny of old wives' tales and 'culture of solace' which saw femininity as a basically negative force, responses in themselves which were the result of a traditional male view of women and their bodies as dangerous and polluting.[158] Shorter contends that obstetric science made it possible to change these views and women's responses to them, making possible the alliance between women and doctors which has rescued us from death, disability and shame.[159]

From the perspective of historical demography, Irvine Loudon puts forward his case for obstetrics as a science whose moves towards more knowledgeable and skilled care and reduced maternal mortality. He bases his analysis on statistical profiles compiled in various clinical settings like those described in this chapter as well as the larger sample profiles which became possible later in the nineteenth century as the modern state demanded an ever greater detailed reading of its population, and birth and death certification became practices required by law. Loudon concludes that levels of maternal mortality were determined most importantly by 'poor obstetric care', be it from 'cheap untrained midwives or expensive over-zealous and unskilled doctors'.[160] The key was to develop 'sound obstetric practice' so that even populations which were economically disadvantaged or even geographically disadvantaged because of remoteness from obstetric-care facilities would benefit from a drop in maternal mortality.[161] For Loudon, the progressive overcoming of the 'primitive state of obstetric knowledge' was unproblematic in that as better knowledge was gradually put in place, women's health and lives were better secured.

As with Shorter, there is no sense that obstetric knowledge is a problematic construct in itself; rather the argument is that internally there are problems of knowledge accretion, as with puerperal fever, but these problems are gradually resolved.[162] And even though Loudon outlines problems of both reclassification and non-classification of maternal deaths, reflecting the personal susceptibilities on the parts of doctors in so doing, and also refers to the broad factors of social and economic change, and regional and national differences in the politics of maternity care, all of which impact on statistical enumeration, he returns to the standards of mortality rates as a way of making sense of the causes and determinants of maternal mortality.[163] There is scant sense of doubt or distance about the process whereby numbers are seen as measures of 'positive facts'[164] nor is there any recognition that maternal and perinatal mortality rates of themselves are a kind of artificial creation.[165]

For Loudon, as for Shorter, the problem of examining the risk of death can be dealt with by examining factors which are considered unproblematic categories, such as who attended the birth, the training of the birth attendant, the place of birth and the social class of a woman. There is no dismay that obstetric knowledges are in any way affected by what is 'inherently unmeasurable – attitude or sentiments'[166] or that obstetric science may be far more uncertain and compromised than it presents. There is no suggestion that risk itself is a problematic category, that the statistical schedules on which it relies are themselves flawed by the problem of normality. Finally, there is no suggestion that human biology, the biology of reproduction, is not a series of stable facts but social in nature, as mutable and changeable as the sciences which try to capture it.[167]

Whatever percentage drop in maternal mortality might ultimately be attributed solely to obstetrics, whether it is 20 per cent or 50 per cent, the perspective that it has been the most important contributor to women's health has more frequently than not found favour with the state's policy-makers whose task it is to make provision for the public funding of maternal health care. In 1995, the Irish Department of Health in its discussion document on women's health declared that the decline in maternal and perinatal mortality rates since 1970 was directly attributable to the quality of antenatal and perinatal care provided by Irish hospitals (which increased their coverage of births to almost 100 per cent by that decade, because they and the state progressively withdrew support for alternatives to organising childbirth, including the community-midwife scheme).[168] That there could be another explanation, related to the rapidly falling age-specific fertility rates from the 1970s onwards, as reliable contraception became more possible in the Irish context, and as general health and social conditions improved, compared with the hardship decades of the 1920s through the 1960s, and therefore that there could be different models of maternity care did not surface in the Department of Health document.

In conclusion, it should also be mentioned that as a result of being able to deploy pharmacology, obstetrics' techniques with the third stage of labour, as with the whole of labour, are now far more subtle than they once were; in our contemporary cultural reading of medicine and its technologies, an injection does not have a malign image. It may be worth noting that in Foucault's words, a 'cumbersome form of power was no longer [so] indispensable' and by the 1960s '. . . industrial societies could content themselves with a much looser form of power over the body'.[169] So a blanket policy of active management of the third stage which, at best, appears a bit annoying at the end of a woman's labour is relatively easily tolerated. Within the institution of the hospital, the extension of active management to the entire labour process, possible because of women's tolerance of or acquiescence to the specialist knowledge obstetrics claims, where what the feminist philosopher, Lorraine Code, terms women's 'cognitive authority'[170] is denied, is what I want to explore next.

5

The Production of Norms in Labour: Active Management

Avoidable Foetal Death: The Induction of Labour

The Irish obstetrician, Kieran O'Driscoll, has argued in his influential textbook *Active Management of Labour*, first published in 1986, that 'mothers must . . . be made to face the fact that childbirth is primarily a mother's responsibility, of which she may not wash her hands.'[1]

This assertion may sound strange to those familiar with O'Driscoll's work because he follows in the dominant obstetric tradition of radical intervention which promulgates the danger of childbirth and the consequent necessity of reining in woman as mother. Permitting her any scope to exercise her own judgement is not part of that regime. O'Driscoll, like Ian Craft, the doctor at the centre of the row over the Royal Free Hospital in London discussed in Chapter 1, like Gedis Grudzinskas who suspended Wendy Savage from a London hospital in 1985,[2] reduces pregnant women to 'the mother', to a single object stripped of agency. The process of reduction, which Lorraine Code identifies as part of the positivist-empiricist tradition, also reduces the 'subjectivity and specificity to interchangeable, observable features'.[3] While this may be useful for the operations of a clinical science dealing with the need for a rapid throughput of cases, we shall see in the course of this chapter that the reduction of subject to object, the elimination of agency from the subject and the exclusion of the subject's knowledge carries its own hazards.

The 'dire peril' of maternal death has gradually diminished, for reasons only some of which are attributable to obstetrics. Yet the obstetric imagination is loathe to let go of its use of the risk–death pairing. Edward Shorter has argued that there was a shift in concern from mother to foetus from the 1930s onwards which was made possible by the fall in maternal death rates and which permitted perinatal medicine to establish itself as a significant sub-specialism in obstetrics.[4] It can be seen readily that if obstetrics is unable to employ the starkness of maternal death, that it presents instead the risk of foetal death as the focus of its concerns. And it has expanded this focus to include the social death of the foetus as a result of malformations like severe cerebral palsy which are unassimilable by contemporary society. In placing foetal death in the foreground, the dominant strand of thought in contemporary obstetrics simultaneously offers its solution to avoiding foetal death, known as the active management of labour.

I have argued that from the time of Henrik Deventer's treatise, first published in English in 1716, what is known as a 'natural' or 'normal' birth, that is, a birth which women can accomplish on their own without intervention, assumes the status of a retrospective concept in obstetric discourse. A birth cannot be judged as normal until after it has concluded, when doctors are in a position to say that there has been no pathology present throughout the entire birth process. This is a concept which goes downstream, in Latour's phrase, until in contemporary obstetric practice, women and midwives who have an approach to labour focused on what they view as an ordinary or 'natural', 'normal' process must fight to read each body as an individual entity. They do so against an established body of clinical teaching on risks which states sometimes implicitly but most often explicitly that every birth must be managed as having pathological potential until it is over, at which point it can safely be judged normal.

This retrospective reading of normality and the advancing clinical practices allied to it have not gone uncontested even within the discipline. In the 1930s, Grantly Dick-Read argued that 'misfortunes' rarely happen and the 'fact of unforeseen possibilities should not mar the general expectancy of a successful issue'.[5] In the 1980s, in Britain and France, individual obstetricians like Wendy Savage, Peter Huntingford and Michel Odent, argued in favour of birth as a normal event and against the use of technologies for specific instances of high risk being extended to routine use on women.[6] Huntingford stressed that women should be accorded the acknowledgement that they are highly intelligent and capable of understanding the birth process and therefore obstetricians should allow women the choice on where and how to have their babies.[7] This was a strong strand in the work of Marsden Wagner in the World Health Organisation in the 1980s.[8] It also found its way into the work of Iain Chalmers and his group in the National Perinatal Epidemiology Unit in Oxford who contested the view that the safest place to give birth was in hospital.[9] Chalmers went on to help produce the two-volume *Effective Care in Pregnancy and Childcare* which sought to provide evidence for ending the current system of consultant-led maternal care. Evaluating practices on the basis of being beneficial, ineffective and harmful, the authors concluded that there was overwhelming evidence for turning away from large consultant-led hospitals and returning to locally based midwife-centred care.[10] But these remain minority voices (especially in Ireland) because the issue of risk, now tied to the foetus, dominates obstetric discussions, disputes and practices. As Wagner has pointed out, the obstetric approach to risk results in an 'intense focus' on the foetus to the detriment of the woman. Not only are the contributions of other actors to women giving birth diminished, including those of the midwife, the woman herself is frequently viewed as 'selfish and irresponsible' by obstetricians who have now recast themselves as the advocate for the foetus.[11] Splitting the foetus from the woman and denying to her the role of most interested party creates the context for O'Driscoll's comment that medical staff must confront mothers with their responsibilities, as defined by the obstetricians.

In her research-based text on midwifery, Louise Silverton notes that risk classification has become an intrinsic part of obstetric practice with its effects stretching back into antenatal care. Efforts to utilise risk factors have been either on the basis of scoring systems, where specific signs or symptoms are given a weighting and added up to produce a risk score, or risk for the individual woman is predicated on the basis of previous medical history.[12] With both versions, they can, at best, indicate that the individual has a higher *risk* of facing a certain outcome and with very few exceptions, these risk-scoring efforts are not predictive or diagnostic of outcome.[13] In relation to risk-scoring systems, this is because the data on which the scores themselves are based are drawn from large populations of women and then applied to each pregnant woman, a technique which can have many more weaknesses than strengths.[14] The outstanding problem remains that women identified as low risk will have problems and even serious complications and that many women identified as high risk will have none. This becomes more complicated still during labour where there is now a reliance on electronic foetal-heart monitors which, although they produce continuous information tracings, are notoriously open to different interpretations, while the machinery itself is open to mechanical and technical failure.[15] This should teach obstetricians that they urgently require an alternative method of appraising women's bodies, a method grounded in reflexivity and an understanding of ordinariness and individual variation. But this has not happened, most especially where a strongly interventionist school of thought has influenced obstetric practice.

Silverton notes further that the controversy over labour management can be viewed through the major differences between a medical and midwifery definition of normal labour.[16] In the strict medical classification, normal is retrospective whereas the midwifery classification is a looser, more reflexive, one. The latter states that a

> labour is deemed normal if, following spontaneous onset after 37 completed weeks of pregnancy, the condition of mother and foetus shows no abnormality and the progress of labour is in acceptable limits.[17]

By contrast, the medical definition states that

> if, following spontaneous onset after 37 completed weeks of pregnancy, it ends in the delivery of a live infant (presented by the vertex) and it is completed in no more than 24 hours in the absence of any complications.[18]

Silverton observes that the criteria for the obstetric definition is a prescriptive one and because it can only be judged retrospectively, it has eased the way to extending technologies devised for high-risk women, like continuous foetal-heart monitoring and routine rupture of membranes, into routine practice for women deemed to be low risk. She argues that the midwifery definition permits the labour to be treated as normal, and only reclassified as abnormal if complications arise. In this latter sense, normal can then take in a wide range of variations and permit an assessment of the individual woman who is there in labour in front of you, one which reflects how that woman's labour evolves, rather than a textbook account of how it ought to evolve.

The issue of pronouncing on 'normal' is a source of deepest controversy between women and contemporary obstetric science. On the basis of their research, Hilary Graham and Ann Oakley have argued that the struggle between women and doctors about birth is a struggle pre-eminently between two contrasting frames of reference, where 'normal' for doctors is about medicalising a body which cannot be relied upon to work, and where a successful pregnancy is measured only in terms of whether a well mother and a live baby emerge at the end of it. Graham and Oakley argue that for women, 'normal' conveys the sense of their individual bodies having the capacity to take on pregnancy and labour, in every sense, physically and emotionally, as a 'process rooted in their bodies . . . not in a medical textbook'.[19] Yet what the medical texts insist is that 'no labour is certainly normal until the third stage is concluded.'[20]

If birth cannot be ruled normal until it is over because it is always potentially pathological, then there is a temptation to get it over with as quickly as possible. Staging labour, controlling it, has long been a concern for the interventionists, with attention being given to the different phases of labour, according to different rationales which themselves would change from practitioner to practitioner. As we have seen, well before a stable pharmacological regime was available, the final part of labour could be manipulated externally by manual dilatation of the cervix. The birth of the baby could be speeded by forceps. Similarly, the beginning of labour could be induced or initiated with mechanical interventions like sweeping the cervix, which Ould favoured, or rupturing the membranes with a fingernail or pointed object. William Smellie, Nihell's protagonist, favoured the artificial rupture of membranes in order to initiate labour. Nihell opposed this practice as did Deventer, who wrote that the membranes bulging with amniotic fluid played a key role in helping the cervix to dilate: 'the Humours much more commodiously open the Mouth of the Womb than the Head of the Infant.'[21]

For Nihell, the deliberate 'premature discharge of the waters' was a 'very blameable practice', one 'that all capable midwives reprove and forbid, as it is robbing the part of the most natural and necessary lubrication for facilitating the launch in due course of the foetus.'[22]

But it was a method which nonetheless became a mainstay of available induction techniques, and continues to be used today. Rupturing the membranes in many ways is limited in usefulness as the action of removing the amniotic fluid does not initiate labour so much as the absence of intact membranes allows the foetal head to fit onto the cervix and stimulate it.[23] Of course, it also deprives the woman of a protective barrier against infection and the foetus of its shock-absorbing qualities in the hydrostatic balancing of pressure on the foetus.[24] Left intact, the membranes do not usually rupture of their own accord until the end of the first stage of labour and for a minority of women may still be intact at delivery.[25] While artificial rupture was popular in nineteenth-century obstetrics because it was so easy to do,[26] it was not the only method tried for induction. In his 1878 clinical report on the Rotunda, Lombe Atthill mentions the use of mechanical interventions like gum catheters or bougies (thin, flexible pieces of India rubber or waxed linen), sponge tents, and pieces of laminaria (seaweed) introduced into the uterus to induce labour.[27] Oakley points out that bougies were still popular in the 1930s, despite foetal and maternal deaths which could be attributed to their use; but by then, doctors had also become keen on the wider use of non-mechanical modes of induction such as ergot, quinine, or castor oil.[28]

The significant breakthrough for labour induction first emerged during the 1930s. The hormone, oxytocin (meaning 'swift birth' from 'oxy' – swift, and 'tocos' – birth),[29] had been isolated from pituitary extract in the early 1900s, its action on the uterus recorded by researchers and the product soon marketed by commercial companies. However, the effects were uncertain and with maternal and foetal deaths occasionally occurring when it was used for accelerating a tedious labour, it had limited appeal.[30] Bethel Solomons, in his 1932 clinical report for the Rotunda, declared that 'the dangers of pituitary extract cannot be too strongly stressed.'[31]

But what is perceived as dangerous can be normalised over time and, like active management of the placenta, oxytocic drugs gradually achieved obstetric approval in the search for control over the uterus. As with ergot, the production of pituitary extract was not standardised until the early 1930s. In its earlier guises, it had been administered by intramuscular injections, by tablets which were sucked, or it was absorbed under the skin, nasally or through the rectum.[32] The uncontrollable aspect via any of these routes was the rate of absorption and its uneven and unpredictable impact on women. The production of the Cardiff Infusion Unit, in 1948, permitted the dosages of oxytocin to be introduced intravenously on a phased basis as a dilute solution and in response to the strength of uterine contractions it was stimulating.[33] This technology effectively opened up a new field of operations. Prolonged labour continued to be an obstetric concern in the 1960s, and by then oxytocin had been joined by a synthetic hormone, Syntocinon, which was marketed from 1954 onwards, as a pharmacological aid to bring labours to an end.[34] However, once the rate of infusion could be adjusted and monitored for each individual patient, the list of indications for induction with oxytocic infusions expanded dramatically. If, as Oakley comments, the perfect means by which to control labour became the lodestone of obstetrics in the twentieth century, titrated administration of oxytocin provided the answer.[35]

Once the principal birth-management problem was no longer viewed simply as one of prolonged labour and what should be done to resolve it in order to reduce maternal mortality, the ambition shifted to the reduction of perinatal mortality rates, as Shorter has indicated.[36] The tool for measuring success became the perinatal mortality rate, which was determined by the number of stillbirths of babies from the twenty-eighth week of pregnancy (later changed to twenty-four weeks) plus the number of babies who die in the first week after birth, divided by the total number of live births and stillbirths. Now, any pregnancy or labour which fell outside the criteria of what obstetric practice was defining as acceptable was drawn into an interventionist net in order to achieve the goal of lowering those rates still further. This agenda coalesced with the technological range made possible by a reliable infusion system for oxytocin-based drugs.

So, from the 1960s, any pregnancy which exceeded the averaged 280 days of the 'typical pregnancy' became a target for induction on the grounds that a foetus would be at risk after that time span. The figure of 280 days was based on the averaged menstrual cycle of twenty-eight days × the average ten months since cessation of a woman's last menstrual period before becoming pregnant, a formula which exists in textbooks but not in women's everyday experiences where cycles have complete variability from one individual to the next. Notwithstanding this variability of calculation, by 1974, 38.9 per cent of all births in England and Wales were induced,[37] while the routine use of partograms and foetal-heart monitors and foetal-scalp blood sampling to measure the progress of labour and its impact on the foetus had become part of routine care.[38] In Ireland, the rates of induction at the beginning of the 1970s were thought to be around 36 per cent.[39] The adverse impact of this trend on women giving birth was central to the work of feminists like Oakley and Ann Cartwright, writing about the problem of women's lack of control over pregnancy and birth.[40] Interestingly, Oakley and Cartwright also pinpointed a problem that emerged in relation to inductions (one which is similar to the current problem over the use of epidurals): many of these inductions were for social reasons, like obstetricians' working schedules and availability of staff, but some of these so-called social inductions reflected women's own personal wishes to have a precise control over their labours (perhaps for reasons of scheduling their lives, perhaps because so much emphasis was placed on the expected date of delivery that women felt pressured to produce the baby). Induction was classed as a beneficial form of intervention; going over the 280-day mark meant that the baby was 'late' according to obstetric criteria and therefore at risk (or so women had been led to believe) and so women themselves demanded induction. The fact that without induction, only 5 per cent of all babies are born on what can only ever be an approximate due date escaped discussion and consideration.[41]

However, women's decisions to seek out such care were already embedded in an approach to childbirth within consultant obstetric units that processed women through a series of standardised procedures and time bands just like an assembly line. The routes to handling labour differently in order to facilitate and support the woman to draw on her physical capacities and resources were simply not available in the hospital setting. From the 1960s to the 1980s, there was also an official policy to have all women deliver in hospital. In England, three official reviews of maternal-health policies, the Cranbrook Committee in 1959, the Peel Committee in 1970 and the Short Committee in 1980, all focused on the necessity of hospital confinement for women, the Peel Report requesting a policy of 100 per cent hospital birth, with an emphasis on the consultant obstetrician-led unit.[42] The Short Report was a specific inquiry into perinatal mortality rates due to

> the mounting public concern that babies were unnecessarily dying or suffering permanent damage during the latter part of pregnancy and the earliest part of infancy.[43]

The same trend was evident in Ireland with the 1968 Fitzgerald Report on General Hospital Services, and especially the 1976 Discussion Document on the Development of Hospital Maternity Services by the Comhairle na n-Ospidéal which recommended not only hospital birth for all women but births in consultant-led hospitals, which led to the closing down of smaller maternity units across the country; the rationale was the same as in Britain, the obstetric belief that a reduction in rates of maternal and perinatal mortality would be best aided by hospital birth.[44]

By 1993, only 5.5 per cent of all hospital births in Ireland (which was virtually all births with only several hundred women giving birth at home of a total of 49,456 births) were outside the net of the obstetric-led maternity units, while in Britain, by the late 1980s almost 99 per cent of women gave birth in hospitals, overwhelmingly dominated by the consultant obstetric unit.[45] This lack of choice and the imposition of induction policies fuelled the growing pressure to challenge maternity services, and maternity policies arose in response to women's poor experiences of induced labour during the 1970s.[46] Midwives and childbirth educators like Caroline Flint, Sheila Kitzinger and Sally Inch were quick to point out that induction led to the so-called 'cascade of intervention'.[47]

Inch employed this term, 'cascade of intervention', to produce a diagrammatic account of possible outcomes, beginning with artificial rupture of membranes, which leads to other routine interventions like oxytocic-induced induction, epidural, episiotomy, and forceps delivery. She built up a picture of how labour goes wrong for women because obstetrics cuts across a woman's labour in order to prevent a possible outcome which may never arise. With a labour induced by oxytocin, for example, there is frequently an increased need for heavy-duty analgesics because of the extreme intensity of oxytocic-induced contractions, which are markedly different in nature to physiologically produced contractions, with two to four times more oxytocin in the system than would normally be physiologically produced. Epidural pain relief is the proffered solution but itself is implicated in increased percentages of forceps deliveries due to a complex of interrelated reasons, including the timing of their administration in relation to how advanced a woman's labour is and the lack of sensation coming from the contracting uterus, reducing a woman's ability to push.[48] In Oakley's *Transition to Motherhood* study, she compiled a technology score based on fifteen different forms of intervention that were accepted obstetric practices and found that an outcome of depression in the women who formed her study group strongly correlated with medium to high technology scores, which included the combination of induction, epidural and forceps delivery.[49]

Induction to Acceleration: Obstetric Systems of Labour Management

Induction with oxytocin did not necessarily find favour throughout the obstetric community. There were medical professionals who queried the benefits of a largely untested and unevaluated routine system.[50] However, it was here in Ireland, in the largest maternity hospital in Britain and

Ireland, that induction with oxytocin was jettisoned as a focus for labour management and was replaced instead by the system known as active management of labour. This change was introduced by Kieran O'Driscoll, who was Master of the National Maternity Hospital in Holles Street from 1963–69. He argued that induction of labour put a woman under great stress because in bringing the pregnancy to an end before its time, it exposed the woman to a longer and more difficult labour, with the accompanying burden of painful contractions as a result of oxytocin. He proposed instead a system which relied on three component clinical practices, radically divorced from any input or decision-making by women themselves: the accurate diagnosis of labour, the artificial rupture of membranes if labour were not proceeding at a satisfactory pace, and most importantly, the acceleration of labour by oxytocin to keep a woman on course. Acceleration of labour was a totally different process, he argued, to induction, even though both availed of the same technology, artificial rupture of membranes (ARM) and oxytocin. In O'Driscoll's reading, acceleration was an augmentation of a labour which had already begun, and far from making labour longer as induction tended to do, acceleration was designed to bring a labour more rapidly to a close. This outcome was seen as the key to lower rates of perinatal mortality.

In 1980, O'Driscoll published the textbook *Active Management of Labour: the Dublin Experience*, in which he characterised the old school of watchful waiting as the 'Passive Management of Labour', a misplaced obstetric system that allowed labour to go on until problems arose in the second stage, whereupon it resorted to interventions to achieve a quick delivery which could prove difficult and dangerous to mother and foetus. By contrast, 'Active Management of Labour' was characterised as a mode of organisation whereby the consultant obstetrician became actively involved in the conduct of labour on an ongoing basis, 'as never before', with the delivery unit of the hospital redesignated as an intensive-care unit. The unit's attention was focused on the exact diagnosis of the onset and progress of labour, with an emphasis on bringing the whole labour to a successful conclusion in twelve hours or less. So if labour were not proceeding satisfactorily, 'augmentation' or acceleration provided the answer to the problem of how to secure a safe labour, with a special focus on the woman giving birth for the first time.[51] The implied sense of precision and hands-on medical management achievable only with a consultant-led unit, struck a chord internationally and active management as an idea was widely adopted in Britain, Australia and the United States, albeit with widely varying interpretations as to what it comprised. No mainstream textbook is now published without reference to the system of active management and the book is currently in its third edition, presenting what it argues are the benefits of a unified management system which has accommodated around 200,000 births between 1963 and 1993.[52]

Like Hamilton some 150 years earlier, O'Driscoll argues against watchful waiting; like Hamilton, O'Driscoll also influenced teaching for twenty-five years and longer in his hospital. There are other points of comparison. Robert Collins wrote of Hamilton that his two-volume work was couched 'in language the most decided, and sometimes even a little dogmatical'.[53] The reader of *Active Management* might well arrive at a similar conclusion about O'Driscoll. Most of the elements in *Active Management*, including the style of argument, are familiar themes, with a history as long as obstetric science, although risk of foetal death replaces risk of maternal death as the worst possible outcome. But female vulnerability and emotional fragility are retained and presented as 'the age-old problem of maternal stress' which requires active management, specifically and especially with women giving birth for the first time.[54] This is no apprenticeship system for the woman; she will not be learning to make decisions about her labour. The focus is on the labour itself, not the woman, and the overall duration of labour is the central problem, increasing stress on the woman and risks for the foetus. Time, obstetric definitions of time rather than the physiological time of the individual woman, are imposed, along with a guarantee of a trained 'nurse' to stay with her throughout labour:

> every expectant mother who attends this hospital for antenatal care is given two firm assurances . . . that labour will not last longer than 12 hours and that she will never be left alone, without a personal nurse by her side at all times.[55]

In his introduction to *Active Management*, O'Driscoll argues, again in a vein reminiscent of Hamilton, that the 'well-tried doctrine of watchful expectancy' does not serve the best interests of mother and child, not least because it comes to an end at the point of full dilatation, after which 'almost any procedure aimed at vaginal delivery becomes acceptable'.[56] Active management improves on this scenario because it returns the 'person ultimately responsible' for labour to the delivery unit, the obstetrician:

> The consultant, rather than remain off-stage waiting for a summons to perform an emergency operation in a belated attempt to retrieve a situation, now had to seek to prevent such emergencies arising in women who were normal when they first entered hospital in labour. Ironically, it is in [completely] normal women that most of the problems of labour arise.[57]

On this encouraging note, O'Driscoll and his colleagues set out to explain the novelty of active management, which is that Caesarean sections and forceps deliveries, noticeable statistical trends on the rise elsewhere, are held to an absolute minimum under active management, due to the short duration of labour and a trauma-free delivery. They argue that the success of active management is measured by lower perinatal mortality rates and lower rates of cerebral dysfunction, like cerebral palsy, in the case of the foetus, and for women, by low rates of Caesarean section, which they now consider the best measure of good obstetric care, given that maternal mortality is no longer a significant problem.[58] In the first and second editions of the book, its authors claim a Caesarean-section rate of less than 5 per cent per annum of all deliveries in the National Maternity hospital, during a period when those rates are topping 20 per cent and more in the United States.[59] O'Driscoll argues that the indications for Caesarean section have expanded to include 'abnormal' or 'dystocic' labours (which are analogous to the slow, tedious labours noted by Clarke, Collins and Hamilton), which are dealt with far more successfully under active management, without recourse to surgery. Active management prevents unnecessary Caesarean sections because it recognises 'the fundamental truth that efficient uterine action is the key to normal labour', especially for the first-time mother with a foetus presenting in the vertex (head down) position.[60] And it is active management, O'Driscoll contends, which leads to the reduction of outcomes like cerebral palsy, not a policy of Caesarean sections as some proponents of the latter would like to maintain.[61] Indeed, O'Driscoll asserts that 'permanent brain damage that could have been avoided may well be regarded as the ultimate failure in obstetric practice',[62] and compiles cumulative statistics on cerebral dysfunction as a further measure of the success of his system.[63] To O'Driscoll's eye, the 'explosive growth in Caesarean sections' presented the 'most striking change in the practice of obstetrics over the past 20 years' and was a move to be resisted.[64]

The issue of Caesarean-section rates was used astutely by O'Driscoll in an obstetric climate where practitioners were growing ever more sensitive, on the one hand, to the possibilities of litigation if anything 'went wrong' during birth, but on the other hand, were perhaps reluctant to face into the reliance on major abdominal surgery as a commonplace obstetric practice, for reasons of complications to the mother and cost alone, reasons which O'Driscoll is quick to point out.[65] They were perhaps also aware of the growing resistance to rising rates of Caesarean section, coming from maternity-care pressure groups in Ireland who were equally aware of trends elsewhere and who, small as their numbers were, frequently occupied newspaper and magazine space, in addition to their own publications, in order to emphasise the need for women to have good birth experiences.[66]

To the obstetric audience, active management presented the seductive combination of monitoring labour with the partogram, pharmacological control and a personal nurse for every woman undergoing labour. It also enjoyed wide appeal within the international obstetric community on this basis. The notion of providing support for a woman, albeit support from someone who was part of the hospital staff, fitted into an ongoing agenda about women's emotional lability during and after childbirth which was linked to women's inherent instability (in other words, the strong emotions aroused by birth were distrusted). Ongoing support also fitted in well with mother–infant bonding (a scientific thesis which itself was suspect in terms of its reading of women as valuable only in their private domestic role of child-rearers and carers).[67] In a recent article, the American paediatricians, Klaus and Kinnell, who produced the 'theory' of maternal bonding, report on O'Driscoll's system as one where 'gentle caring, encouragement, warmth and displays of real affection' predominate as part of the solution to prolonged labour.[68] The 'thoughtfully orchestrated' approach to labour that O'Driscoll has promoted

> allows her [the woman] to feel attended at all times – allows her to feel that she will be able to handle her labor, that she will be safe, that her dignity and experiences matter, and that her body's responses are natural and normal.[69]

Despite these rosy images, emotional support for women, let alone women directly taking control of their own labours, is not the primary agenda of active management; events are only meant to be orchestrated so that women *feel* in control, not that they *are*. The primary objective is efficient uterine action at the individual level and, at the level of the hospital as a whole, a rapid throughput of patients.[70] Handling a woman's emotions so that they do not get in the way of the labouring uterus facilitates that overall goal. The 'efficient uterine action' which O'Driscoll wants to set in place (the notion of efficiency itself amplifying that sense of a factory system with targets of efficient production) 'can be provided with a very high degree of safety, subject to a small number of rules'.[71] So the 'normality' of labour has become an adherence to a set of rules, from which the individual body cannot offer any deviation, and which, for the individual woman, invokes a highly regimented approach to labour. The Foucauldian analysis of prisons, the 'carceral' institutions which produce 'docile bodies',[72] is germane to O'Driscoll's agenda in the way power is exercised in the panopticon: the obstetrician's rules, his system, dominates, not the person. In the sense that Foucault writes, this is making bodies 'operate as one wishes, with the techniques, the speed and the efficiency one determines'.[73] As a system to produce normality, active management carries people, women and staff alike, through their allotted paces. And, in the allotted paces of labour, the outside margin that O'Driscoll is prepared to permit is a duration of twelve hours.

The feminist theorist Sandra Bartky points out that in the disciplinary regimes of modern society, 'the body's time ... is as rigidly controlled as its space.'[74] In Holles Street hospital (the National Maternity Hospital), the adherence to the twelve-hour rule for the duration of labour is inscribed in the graphs or partograms that the staff use to record the progress of labour for each woman:

> Full dilatation is equated with 10 cm [centimetres] because this is the diameter of the baby's head. The maximum time allotted is 10 hours. It follows that the slowest rate of dilatation acceptable is 1 cm per hour.[75]

O'Driscoll was able to base these precise-sounding protocols on work first carried out by an American, E.A. Friedman, and in his *Introduction to Active Management*, O'Driscoll acknowledges Friedman's role in developing the 'graphic representation of cervical dilatation'.[76] And, if active management was made possible in part by the technical development of the titration method of administering oxytocic drugs, the other half of its success relied on the statistical measurement of the average rates of dilatation, known as the Friedman curve, which resulted in the design of the partogram to measure labour progress. Friedman argued that dilatation advances in even stages of one centimetre per hour from a passive to an accelerated phase to a decelerated phase, over a twelve-hour period and that any labour which falls outside that time frame is abnormal. Within each of these three phases, there can also occur abnormal or inefficient patterns of contractions which necessitate action on the part of the obstetrician to correct them. Friedman also argued that the longer a labour lasts outside that time frame, the greater risk the foetus runs of a damaging birth outcome.[77] The partogram, which is the conceptual tool expressing this thinking, is described in O'Driscoll's *Active Management* as 'an identikit with which it is possible to construct an endless variety of profiles in labour, to meet almost any clinical circumstance'.[78]

O'Driscoll and his colleagues go on to explain that 'the design and content of these visual records are matters that have an immediate effect on the conduct of labour' and that

> every detail not immediately relevant to the main issue is rigorously excluded. The graph that portrays progress dominates the picture and no provision is made for labour to last longer than 12 hours.[79]

So what has happened here with the Friedman curve and the partogram is that a set of mathematical averages has been used to create a 'truth' about labour, about what is normal and what is abnormal, normality being uncritically appended to this notion of average in order to interpret what then may be abnormal. As we saw in Chapter 4, this notion of normality presents a difficult if not insurmountable problem; in this instance, each individual woman must match this averaged rate of dilatation, or otherwise her labour will be considered as 'abnormal'. It is in this sense, as O'Driscoll states, that the graph, putting forward the 'truth' of labour determines the conduct of labour under medical supervision, with the strict understanding that none of that process nor the decision-making about labour is within the control of the individual woman; all of it is an obstetric problem to be undertaken and pursued within an obstetric-dominated institution. The authors claim that the 'educational potential' of these records is unbounded for 'doctors, nurses' and 'mothers' also; they recommend that teaching on the partogram and its meanings be included in antenatal education. The sub-text here is that antenatal teaching within the hospital system is there to support the aims and objectives of active management, rather than equipping a woman to pursue her own objectives for her labour and birth.[80] It is in this sense that O'Driscoll describes women as 'better educated' about childbirth once this 'simple logic of procedure' called the partogram is explained to them.[81]

And women require sound education in the principles of labour because the 'average woman' is under such stress during labour that 'the morale of the average woman begins to deteriorate perceptibly after six hours. After 12 hours the deterioration accelerates rapidly.'[82]

Once more, O'Driscoll's thinking has interesting echoes of Hamilton's position on the duty to intervene to prevent the 'sufferings of the woman'. Yet O'Driscoll is reputed to have been quite distant in his relations with women who were actually patients in his hospital.[83] O'Driscoll argues that the memory of a bad labour threatens a woman's emotional well-being and he is keen to convince his readers of the validity of his notion 'that labour, especially first labour, is the most disturbing emotional event in the lifetime of one-half of mankind' (*sic*).[84] In the first edition of *Active Management*, its authors write that this can provoke 'a profound emotional disturbance . . . [which] may last a lifetime'.[85] In the second edition, this is amended to read:

> the birth of a first child is almost surely the most profound experience, for good or ill, in a lifetime . . . a woman who has had an unhappy first experience is likely to be terrified . . . these fears can have serious consequences outside the narrow confines of obstetrics. They can haunt a woman for the rest of her life and affect her attitude to her husband and possibly her child.[86]

This is a clever amendment seemingly bending towards the emphasis of individual women, childbirth campaigners and many midwives on the emotional importance of birth, while in fact the assertion steadily underscores the view of women as too emotional and thus dangerous to themselves and others.

A further serious dimension of a woman's deteriorating morale is the impact it has on medical staff whom O'Driscoll claims are rendered powerless when faced with a disintegration that is shaming in its depth:

> A shared sense of impotence in the face of widespread physical suffering, and even moral degradation, frequently colours the attitude of nurses and doctors from their early student days so control of the duration of labour is almost as important for staff as it is for mother and baby.[87]

Instructing a woman about the 'conduct' of her labour has everything to do with preserving order, from the order of the social domain of the family to the labour ward to the internal ordering of her uterus. The intricate experience of a woman's time in labour finds no part in the thinking about active management and a labour curve which must accomplish its work within strict limits.[88]

There is some confusion around the first phase of labour, the so-called passive phase. For the partogram to work as the determinant measure, hospital staff need to know when to start counting the twelve hours of normal labour, beginning with the passive phase. O'Driscoll tackles the issue of who decides when labour begins by challenging the 'altogether anomalous situation' in which the basic decision that determines all subsequent management 'is surrendered to the patients'. He states that because a woman admits herself to a maternity hospital 'the result [is] that she tends to dictate her own treatment': 'This procedure, which leaves the initiative in the hands of the patients, has no parallel in other branches of medicine'.[89] O'Driscoll asserts that a woman's 'presumptive diagnosis' that she is in labour must be replaced by 'objective' clinical evidence established in the hospital: 'no allowance is made for time spent in labour at home' as it is of 'no relevance to clinical practice.'[90] Instead, he proposes that 'A diagnosis of labour is made when a woman admits herself to this hospital . . . and the cervix is found on pelvic examination, to be completely effaced.'[91]

Thereafter, the ten-centimetre rule takes over. According to O'Driscoll's text, if the membranes have not already ruptured spontaneously, they are ruptured artificially, once labour has been diagnosed, no later than one hour after admission. If dilatation does not then proceed at the 'acceptable' rate, as measured by the partogram and its 'action line', the hospital accelerates labour through an oxytocic infusion.

O'Driscoll argues that a 'clear pattern' of dilatation should emerge within three hours but the evidence to the contrary is substantial. Uterine contractility is affected by factors which are not well documented by the obstetric profession, including maternal and foetal position, but also including women's reactions to place. Those midwives who provide ongoing care and who have been in a position to observe labour outside the parameters of an active-management regime are aware, for example, that contractility slows down, lapses or even goes into reverse in the move from home to hospital and can take some time to reassert itself.[92] Louise Silverton points to patterns of initial slowness of dilatation with a significant acceleration towards the end which is why the linear model of one centimetre is of dubious value, most specially when it is accompanied by a rigid programme of obstetric interventions, to accelerate labour.[93]

O'Driscoll states that the 'manifold pressures' of his 'busy delivery unit' notwithstanding, the hospital can accommodate all women who come in and each will be accommodated with regular pelvic assessments, using rectal examination, all of which make it 'eminently feasible' to predict the time of delivery within the first three hours of admission and to take action against a 'drift into prolonged labour'.[94] O'Driscoll believes fully in the promise that modern science makes, which is that it can eliminate risk, for although anything can be a risk, science can deal with all risks by systematising them. This 'dynamic approach' of active management is offered to clinicians everywhere as 'a consequence of these new-found certainties' about effective uterine action.[95] As a text, *Active Management* invokes the Cartesian tradition of rhetorical certainty. Excluding 'every detail not immediately relevant to the main issue',[96] as O'Driscoll intends, through this schematisation of labour ensures that all errors and doubt can yield to the scientific method and are subject to its logic.

As a system, active management in operation is a fine example of the necessity to rigorously discipline bodies within an institution, the lying-in hospital. The 'identikit' which the partograms 'constitute', with the patient's rate of cervical dilatation being plotted against the 'normal' curve, enables the clinicians, we are told, 'to meet almost any clinical circumstance',[97] easily done when normality to a clinical eye is an averaged central mass, not an individual body. O'Driscoll's definition of normal labour has passed into general obstetric texts and midwifery texts alike as an ontological truth, where the first stage of labour lasts up to but no more than ten hours.[98] The educational potential of the partograms provides 'fertile ground' we are told for clinical research and for teaching seminars, 'which can be conducted like exercises in map-reading where abstract names become real places as soon as they are located in relation to the surrounding terrain'.[99] Another way of phrasing this is that the process of 'reading' each body in labour through the partograms represents what Robert Castel has termed a modern ideology of prevention.[100] Such mechanisms do not work by identifying 'a particular precise danger embodied in a concrete individual' but by deducing a specific situation 'from a general definition of the dangers one wishes to prevent'.[101] In other words, abstractions are made into realities, not least because the process of defining risk itself entails power/knowledge: what obstetrics can do in order to enforce its regimes constitutes a formidable exercise of power.

But active management is also a contradictory account, and this shows up on closer examination. The cumulative statistics over the twenty-five years since the beginning of active-management policies make odd reading. In presenting comparative statistics, O'Driscoll tells his audience that 'as the general principle of this hospital is to achieve, the best results with the least interference', what will be of interest to them are the rates of perinatal mortality, Caesarean section, induction and forceps use. Here the claim is repeated that active-management policies have resulted in better and lower rates of all these measures, and thus make good obstetric practice. Rupturing the membranes artificially and accelerating labour by oxytocic augmentation is left out of the table altogether. The fact that acceleration with oxytocin is as painful as it is with induction and certainly equally invasive does not figure in this account.[102] O'Driscoll also presents a table which he terms obstetrical norms for primigravidae and states that these norms have been 'adopted to ensure that the rising tide of intervention is kept in check'.[103] But a comparison of this table between the second edition of the book in 1986 and the third edition of the book in 1993 shows a 'norm' of acceleration changing from 30 per cent of all women giving birth for the first time to 45 per cent.[104] At the same time, O'Driscoll does mention that the increase in 'general health'; the reduction of grand multiparity and the reduction in maternal age are 'notable changes in the social background of the population served' which have 'contributed more to the improvement [in the perinatal mortality rate] than any advance in medical science'.[105]

Must we assume that as Irish women have established reliable fertility control for themselves, and in general become far healthier, that there is now an increased need for the interventions of active management, an increased requirement to accelerate labours with oxytocin to deal with inefficient uterine action? That more rather than fewer women of a huge population of child-bearing women can be designated as faulty in the task of giving birth? Surely, this is only possible within this system of obstetric rationality where the partogram 'excludes every detail not immediately relevant to the main issue', namely its own version of events.

One final point to note about O'Driscoll's system of active management is the demand that women be accountable for their actions in his hospital, while at the same time medical accountability is only at best implicitly stated and rests on claims to expertise alone. According to O'Driscoll, 'mothers' have a 'duty' to the hospital to 'learn how to behave with dignity and purpose during the most important event in their lives' and 'there should be no hesitation' on the part of medical staff in rebuking a woman to circumvent 'the sometimes outrageous conduct' and 'degrading scenes that occasionally result from the failure of a woman to fulfil her part of the contract'.[106] Furthermore, she may not 'demand specific methods of treatment which do not serve the real interests of her and her child',[107] those true interests defined of course by the hospital. And although he adds that 'straight talking is a necessary feature of any contract in which there is mutual trust',[108] it is not clear how trust can be constructed in a situation which is essentially a coercive one.

In O'Driscoll's terms, responsibility on the part of 'mothers' is about following medical orders, not about a woman assessing her own needs in labour and what might assist her to labour most beneficially. Yet when it comes to the hard issues of who might be held accountable for adverse birth outcomes, doctors melt away behind the institution of the hospital and the woman is left with few, if any, satisfactory answers. At that point, her only redress is through the limited and costly redress of the legal system, given the current hegemonic position of the obstetric profession in our system of maternity care and the extent to which the state has invested in this system.

What O'Driscoll claims is that if women submit their bodies to active management, as long as the woman adheres to this regime, all risks will be dealt with by the system, including what is now seen as the ultimate risk of foetal death.

Active Management and the Dunnes' Case

When the death of a baby occurs or, rarely now, the death of a mother, it exposes the obstetric system at its most vulnerable point, revealing such guarantees about its capacity to deal with risk to be meaningless. Death intrudes painfully on the certainties which are crucial to maintaining the hospital domain, and the obstetric response to death indicates an acute unwillingness to acknowledge the failure of its claim to certainty. This factor certainly emerged in the case which the Dunne family took against the National Maternity Hospital in 1988. In *Active Management*, O'Driscoll consistently asserts that his regime is based on rigorous empiricism, pragmatism, precision, and clearly stated rules, the very essence of scientific method. The reader is left in no doubt that when 'fundamental truths of obstetric practice' are cited,[109] these boys know exactly what they are doing. Twins, for example, are regarded as an

> obstetric abnormality mainly because the second twin is exposed to special hazards during the course of labour. The second twin may suffer the effects of hypoxia [diminished levels of oxygen in body tissues] because, not being so readily accessible, he/she cannot be properly supervised. Not infrequently, he/she may be a victim of chronic placental insufficiency, with retarded growth, resorption of liquor and passage of meconium, none of which is suspected until the membranes rupture after the first twin is born, when it may be too late to take effective action. . . . Slow labour in twins is treated always by caesarean section. Oxytocin is never used.[110]

As for the woman who has already given birth, O'Driscoll says she 'may as well belong to a different biological species'.[111] In setting out his partograms for the 'multigravid labour', O'Driscoll also writes:

> Significantly, the sole difference in content [with primigravid labour] is that the word oxytocin is omitted. Lack of appreciation of the reasons for these distinctions leads to the most enduring of all obstetric errors: the practice of extrapolating from a first to a second birth. This results in much unnecessary intervention and iatrogenic disease . . . The duration and consequent stress bear no comparison with first labour because the parous woman rarely suffers from inefficient uterine action and because her genital tract has been stretched before. In the event of slow progress, therefore, another explanation should be sought, the most likely being that she is not in labour. Failure to advance in a parous woman is often a manifestation of obstruction arising from a fetal cause. This can be easily overlooked with disastrous consequences because the capacity of the pelvis is taken for granted.[112]

The language that O'Driscoll employs to describe the context of twins or the most likely complication that might arise for a woman who has already given birth, like the rest of his text, abundantly illustrates how science strives to prove its increasing rationality, its progression towards definitive truths. However the price for this is the denial of any interruptions and displacements to which it is subject. For science to preserve its hegemonic account, it must deny events which fall outside its definitions.[113] For example, O'Driscoll argues that active management, over a period of twenty-five years, has made the greatest progress of any obstetric system towards eliminating the risk of foetal death and maternal distress. The Dunnes' case was an event which substantively challenged the position of certitude and authority which active management presented.

The problematic and contradictory aspects of active management emerged in 1988 and 1989 in the course of legal action taken by the parents of William Dunne against the National Maternity Hospital and one of its consultant obstetricians. The case had three hearings: a High Court trial, a Supreme Court hearing and a retrial in the High Court. The original action, charging the hospital and the consultant with negligence, stemmed from the circumstances of William's birth in March 1982. His twin brother was stillborn and William was subsequently diagnosed as severely brain-damaged and quadriplegic.

As the case unfolded, the main charges of the plaintiffs were that aspects of a high-risk birth were ignored by hospital staff and that the surviving baby was born 'without the benefit of [an] obstetrician or anyone of similar status'.[114] The pregnancy was a second one for Catherine Dunne, William's mother, after an uncomplicated first pregnancy. For the second pregnancy, she arranged to have combined care, seeing her own GP and a consultant, whom she attended alternately, as a private patient. Like the first, the second pregnancy was trouble free. By the fifth month, however, her GP suggested she might be carrying twins. The consultant did not confirm a twin birth until much later, ordering an ultrasonic scan ten days before she went into labour. The scan indicated that one of the twins was in a breech position. Mrs Dunne was then thirty-six-and-a-half weeks pregnant.

Early on 20 March 1982, Mrs Dunne concluded that labour had begun. She went to her GP in Wicklow town at 9 a.m. He measured the dilatation and confirmed she was in labour, dilatation already being two to three centimetres. The Dunnes rang Dr Jackson, the consultant, to say labour had begun. By 11.15 a.m., she had been booked in to the hospital and examined. Dilatation was measured as being two centimetres. At the time, the hospital was conducting a randomised trial of electronic foetal-heart monitoring. All women who were 'low-risk pregnancies' were included in the study, half being assigned the foetal-heart monitor, which meant having a scalp electrode attached to the baby's head, and half being examined by auscultation, where the foetal heartbeat is picked up through a trumpet placed on the woman's abdomen.[115]

Around noontime, Mrs Dunne was examined by a registrar who found her cervix was three-centimetres dilated. He performed an artificial rupture of the membranes and reported grade one meconium present. But as the first twin was presenting head down, and its foetal heartbeat had already been picked up, she was included in the study as a low-risk pregnancy by the doctor, and assigned to continuing auscultation every fifteen minutes. Hospital policy states that there should be a rectal examination every hour,[116] but there was no such examination at 1.15 p.m. because the midwife assigned to her care had gone to lunch just after 1 p.m.[117] At 1.40 p.m., Mrs Dunne felt a tumultuous kicking which lasted about fifteen minutes. Only her husband was present. Mrs Dunne told her husband that something was wrong and asked him to get a nurse. She asked the nurse to inform Dr Jackson and tell him that she wanted him to come to the hospital.

According to Dr Jackson's testimony, he was contacted around 2 p.m. but was not told that Mrs Dunne had requested his presence nor that she had experienced this tumultuous movement (no nursing staff testified at the first trial). He was told that her labour had slowed down, contractions now coming only every four to seven minutes. Dilatation was still only three centimetres. Dr Jackson told nursing staff to get Mrs Dunne to walk in the hope that ambulatory motion would advance labour. At 3.15 p.m., dilatation remained unchanged. She continued to walk although she reported to the nursing staff that she felt very unwell. She repeatedly asked to see Dr Jackson. By 4 p.m. she said she felt absolutely dreadful, refused to walk any more and demanded to see her obstetrician. Dr Jackson was again contacted by telephone and he ordered an oxytocin drip to be set up. Shortly afterwards, a registrar examined Mrs Dunne and found that the membranes, which had been ruptured at noon, had resealed. Upon puncturing the membranes a second time, the registrar recorded grade two meconium.

In *Active Management*, O'Driscoll states 'meconium is regarded as a clinical sign of great potential significance', although according to its properties, it is then subdivided into grade one, two, and three.[118] At the outset of labour, when artificial rupture of the membranes is done to identify the foetus who might be at risk, women are divided into two groups, those with clear liquor, thought to number some 90 per cent of labours, and 10 per cent of those with some grade or other of meconium, a division, O'Driscoll says, into low-risk and high-risk labours.[119] In the Dunne case, finding grade one meconium at noon did allow the doctor some leeway in diagnosing its significance, according to the rules. However, with grade two meconium, a foetal-blood sample was mandatory. The oxytocin drip was discontinued and an electronic foetal-heart monitor was set up. Fifty minutes later, the first baby was born. Dr Jackson arrived to deliver the second twin, who was the breech baby. He was born dead at 5.30 p.m.

The surviving baby, William, was taken to the intensive-care unit where that night he suffered three episodes of cyanosis, that is, turning blue from lack of oxygen. He had already received a blood transfusion and was being treated for brain-swelling. In the first few days after birth, he suffered convulsions, flailing limbs and rolling eyes, signs which are associated with acute oxygen deprivation at birth, one of the outcomes which active management as a system is designed to prevent. When William came home seven days later, there were further disturbing signs. His breathing was weak, he was cold to the touch, and he soon began to cry incessantly with a high-pitched scream. Many rounds of medical consultations later, the Dunnes' suspicion that William was suffering from cerebral palsy was confirmed. He was eventually diagnosed as quadriplegic. Estimated to have a mental age of a tiny child, with no capacity to walk, feed himself, or control his bowels, William is nevertheless expected to live out a full adult span.

The Dunnes, while dealing with this tragedy, were also attempting to find out from Holles Street medical staff what had happened. How had the twins, seemingly perfectly healthy throughout the pregnancy, come to face such a disastrous end? In their interviews with hospital doctors, the term maceration, or the rate at which a body decomposes, kept recurring. The importance of the term appeared to be that the second twin had died *in utero* before Mrs Dunne entered the confines of the hospital. The Master of Holles Street said that there would be an internal inquiry but that the Dunnes could not be present and would not be informed of its outcome.

It took the Dunnes two years to get a copy of the autopsy report, despite the fact that O'Driscoll states that the hospital has 'expert post-mortem examination'.[120] Finally, after the Dunnes had approached the Minister for Health to request a public inquiry and been turned down, they resorted to a court case. They were warned from the outset that, given the international pre-eminence of the hospital, they stood little chance of bringing about successful legal action.

The Dunnes' case contained all these elements: female fragility expressed as unreliability; the hospital regime of active management in all its order to protect women and foetuses from the risks of birth; the objective evidences about the body in labour which are independent of the woman's account; the use of auscultation to establish foetal well-being independent of the woman's account; clinical pathology and what dissection can say about the body in death.

This was not a case of the intuitive mother vs. the science of childbirth. From the outset, both plaintiffs and defendants were anxious to present their arguments as strict scientific accounts. The National Maternity Hospital argued that what had occurred was a twin-to-twin transfusion in the uterus which had killed one twin and severely handicapped the second; in de la Motte's resonant phrase from the seventeenth century, a 'melancholic accident'. The crucial part of their defence turned on the nature and timing of this posited event. For the hospital to be in the clear, they had to argue that it took place after the ultrasound scan, done ten days prior to the birth, at which point heartbeats of both twins were detected, but before Mrs Dunne entered hospital to give birth. Their evidence to support this view was drawn from the interpretation of a number of cases in medical literature where twin-to-twin transfusion appeared to have ended in a similar manner. They also relied heavily on the autopsy report which stated that the body of the dead twin showed signs of an excess of blood and was subject to a degree of maceration indicating that death had occurred before labour began. On this basis, and the fact that there were no untoward factors at the outset of labour, the hospital and Dr Jackson contended that management of the labour was consistent with hospital practice for 'normal labours'. In their eyes, there had been no evidence that a Caesarean section was necessary.

The Dunnes' case contested both elements of this argument and also strongly criticised hospital management. Their medical experts rested their evidence on relevant cases of twin births in current medical literature. They argued that death and damage were the result of acute oxygen deprivation attributable to an unnamed 'accident', that term again, during labour. They contended that staff should have taken account of certain warning signs: the grade one meconium, the tumultuous kicking, the obvious slowness of dilatation, especially within the criteria about both dilatation and twin births laid down by Holles Street. A Caesarean section could have been performed, if not in time to save the twin who died, at least in time to rescue William from brain damage as a result of asphyxia. The autopsy notes, they argued, were unclear about maceration, about how long the second twin had been dead, and about the degree of blood present. Further objections were raised about the procedures for dissection, whether some organs should have been weighed to measure degeneration, and the temperature at which the body had been stored, all of which could contribute to a different conclusion on when death had occurred, later being the plaintiffs' contention rather than earlier. Above all, they argued that both foetal hearts should have been monitored electronically whereas Holles Street staff said, in accordance with its policy in *Active Management*, that only one foetal heart could be monitored, as proper supervision for the second twin was difficult.

The High Court judgment delivered in July 1988, held that William Dunne suffered brain damage as a result of oxygen deprivation during labour and that hospital and obstetrician were equally negligent. The consultant should have ensured that both foetal hearts were identified and monitored. Damages, awarded on the basis of William's need for lifelong care, were just over one million pounds. The hospital and the consultant appealed the case to the Supreme Court in February 1989 seeking a retrial or, if this could not be obtained, a reduction in the damages awarded. Their appeal focused on how the jury had been instructed by the High Court judge and the fact that the jury was composed of lay people who would find if difficult to follow complex medical issues. In April 1989, the Supreme Court ordered the retrial and its judgment expressed particular doubts about the instructions to the jury in the High Court in relation to medical negligence. The Dunne family was ordered to pay costs for the hospital's appeal action.

The retrial in October 1989 was controversial, with a number of anomalies about hospital records and practice emerging. The Dunne family had found ten women who had given birth to twins in Holles Street around the same period Mrs Dunne had given birth who could testify that both foetal hearts were monitored throughout labour even though the hospital had consistently denied that this was part of its practice. On the heels of this evidence, the trial ended abruptly when the hospital made an offer of an out-of-court settlement of £400,000 to the Dunnes, without admission of liability. A former master of the hospital, Dermot MacDonald, was to say some years later in a televised interview, that given the international stature of the hospital, the Dunnes' case 'ended in an appropriate way' and added that morale in the hospital had dropped during the litigation with all the attendant publicity to an all-time low; the hospital had been 'naïve' and 'totally unprepared' for legal action.[121]

Jeopardising Obstetric Knowledge

The Chief Justice concluded the Supreme Court appeal in April 1989 with a striking comment:

> The development of medical science and the supreme importance of that development to humanity made it particularly undesirable and inconsistent with the common good that doctors should be obliged to carry out their professional duties under frequent threat of unsustainable legal claims.[122]

It indicates unquestioning acceptance of the totalising account that obstetrics deploys which excludes all other perspectives, when it declares it can and must move towards ever greater progress. If one accepts the goal of a perfect science which progressively eliminates doubt, then it follows that the fundamental seriousness of its endeavour must not be impeded or questioned. This view is evident throughout all three court hearings in which even the legal process was subordinated to the claims of scientificity and a knowledge that presumes itself so specialist that facts had

> to be proved by inferences drawn, analysis made and diagnostic signs recorded during and after the birth. Such inferences and analyses could not be drawn or made by a layman except by accepting expert medical evidence.[123]

A lay person could intrude only with the greatest difficulty into what might be differences of opinion between acknowledged medical experts and therefore not negligence at all. The obstetric claim to primacy because it is epistemic knowledge has precisely this effect of subordinating all other knowledges to it.[124] This meant that despite anomalies in the presentation of both side's arguments, the court proceedings as a whole were exclusively determined by obstetric categories, in particular, the notion of risk to the foetus. Both plaintiffs and defendants relied on the interpretation of case histories to prove patterns of probabilities and frequencies which have become the hallmark of medical positivism. Catherine Dunne's testimony had a minor part despite the fact that it was she who attempted to alert the medical staff to the fact that something was seriously wrong.

Inevitably, it was around the categories of risk and death that the arguments were sharpest. With different interpretations as to when these elements were present and what their effects were, both sides were nonetheless compelled to use the obstetric frame of reference which meant returning to the argument of norms. It was not possible, for instance, to argue the case for the Dunnes on the grounds that Catherine Dunne's requests for help were a part of the contractual relationship between her and the consultant and then to argue that the contract had been breached because they were ignored. In court, her voice counted least of all, mirroring the role women are allotted within obstetrics. As the 'mother', she was in the terms that Holles Street employs, 'disorganised', 'frightened', in need of 'straight talking', in other words, emotionally incompetent. There was no route whereby Catherine Dunne could claim an authority of knowing, an 'epistemic authority' similar to that of obstetric science, for she was not recognised as in any sense expert about her own pregnant body.[125] Obstetric science thus predetermined the role that she was left to assume.

Obstetric science also to a considerable extent determined the ground rules for debate in court. Ironically, the hospital's assertion that even normal births must be treated as having the potential to become high risk and therefore require the presence of the specialist had great impact on how the Dunne family's counsel proceeded (while the National Maternity Hospital ducked away from its own rhetoric). This accounts for the Dunnes' counsel's contention that William, in being delivered by a pupil midwife, had been put at risk because he had not had the 'benefit' of an obstetrician. And in fact, the trial evidence never grapples effectively with the question of how active management fails as a system in its identification of normality and abnormality; the plaintiffs' arguments called instead for an intensification of high technology in labour and birth, demanding electronic foetal monitoring as well as Caesarean section. The High Court judgment in the first trial favoured this view and the out-of-court settlement in the retrial also gave credence to the obstetric argument that birth is always a high-risk event until it is concluded so there is considerable congruence between the Dunnes' defence and the tenets of active management.

More puzzling is the congruence achieved on the issue of being able to eliminate risk for clearly the Dunnes' defence believed this was possible while the ethos of active management declares precisely the same. Yet as the anthropologist Mary Douglas rightly reminds us, risk is a basic condition of human knowledge and being, and it is only as part of the conditions of modernity that we have sought to quantify risk around the economic relations of probability and loss.[126]

Active management is the most detailed systematisation of labour to date, categorising every birth in terms of its potential to go wrong. Its belief in and reliance on clinical signs to forestall risk; the attention to the basic rules of procedure and uniformity of care to eliminate prolonged labour; the careful assessment of the rate of dilatation; all are the basis for asserting an impeccable scientificity. What this system cannot deal with is death as the Dunnes' case inadvertently revealed. When the outcome is death, the obstetric system is as jeopardised as the women it has mandated itself to protect, if not more so. This de-centring of its power by the realities of death and a consequent confusion as to how to respond has to account for the contradictory use the hospital immediately made of its physical boundary. If death has occurred outside that boundary, the hospital and its obstetricians make an extraordinary bid for non-involvement, turning their own rationale about their total responsibility to mother and foetus on its head. Yet within that boundary, their quasi-legal status is such that the persons most immediately affected will be excluded from any review or inquiry into the events and will not receive formal autopsy reports.[127] A final quote illustrates the rigidity of obstetric thought, its concern to deny any disruption which challenges its theories. It comes from O'Driscoll's testimony in the first trial, and is his opinion on the correctness of hospital procedures: 'given the same set of circumstances all over again, he would pursue precisely the same course of action.'[128]

On the surface, O'Driscoll's statement points to his feeling most secure in the conclusion that the preventative work of active management is not 'meddlesome midwifery', to use the nineteenth-century term, but obstetric science at its most vigilant. However, his reaction also reveals the extent to which the relationship between 'truth' and 'error' in obstetric thinking is, as Foucault writes, about

> what effects of power circulate among scientific statements, what constitutes, as it were their internal regime of power, and how and why at certain moments that regime undergoes a global modification.[129]

What the second trial does establish is that within that internal regime, the movements are shifting, fluid. A 'principle' is that the second foetal heart is hard to supervise. The practice is haphazard, sometimes monitoring, sometimes not. Medicine's 'solid scientific armature'[130] rarely lets us hear so much of the intensely social construction of its 'fundamental truths' (although as women we experience them). But when we can listen in, as with the Dunnes' case, it is actually extremely difficult to make sense of what obstetrics means by normal and pathological, by the logic of its risk–death pairing. Are we seeing an irreducible concept, as obstetric science would want, that risk can be identified and death circumvented or at least predicted, or are we rather seeing, as with all science, 'how effects of truth are produced within discourses which in themselves are neither true nor false'.[131]

Perhaps what we must see as the critical problem is 'the political, economic, institutional regime of the production of truth'[132] and where we are located in relation to the production of those truths. Catherine Dunne was told that she could not read her own body; the tumultuous movements she felt at 1.40 p.m., the day her sons were born, were dismissed as not relevant by the institutional regime of the hospital and by a science which argues that it alone can properly read the maternal body. Her position therefore was one of a radical silencing which was imposed upon her by obstetric science.

Avoidable Death: Arguing Obstetrics as Continuous History

Ludwig Fleck states that speculative knowledge does not simply increase, it also changes. Yet obstetrics, like other sciences, wants to work with a totalising history, with a claim that its knowledge production is continuous and progressive, building from strength to strength. Conceptual continuity, its 'continuous history',[133] is one way it proves its case for its ever greater scientific understanding; schedules of statistics proves the success of obstetrics in effecting change and bringing about great improvements in women's lives.

We have already encountered an example of the way obstetrics argues continuous history, in the debate on the management of the third stage of labour. Jellett's paper, establishing the historical continuity of the 'Dublin Method' for delivering the placenta, does so by denying the internal logic of the various strands he attempts to present as an integrated whole, denying also the evidence of danger to women in following through his line of argument.

Statistics is the other great tool of continuous history, whether used in producing the 'identikit' of labour in Holles Street, based on the ten-centimetre rule, or in compiling definitions of measurable obstetric outcomes and aggregate profiles of these outcomes. In the case of Holles Street and their thesis of active management, they make interesting reading. Between 1968 and 1992, some 65,000 women who gave birth for the first time were delivered in the National Maternity Hospital, with 40 per cent of that number receiving oxytocin 'to ensure effective uterine action during labour'.[134] This figure is usefully read in the context of the metaphors of production that surround childbirth management in the modern period with its links to industry and the logic of capital wherein the obstetrician as overall production manager ensures a smooth and continuous turnover.[135] There may be no other way to read a figure which claims that 40 per cent of this particular child-bearing population, with the highest standards of general health ever, have uteruses which are incapable of functioning without artificial stimulus. (The composite figures for first-time mothers for the whole of the country are, if anything, more discouraging, with only 58 per cent of women having spontaneous births while forceps are used in 19 per cent of all cases and Caesarean section in 14 per cent of all cases.)[136] The production metaphor makes more sense still when we recall the several points in *Active Management* where the authors place such emphasis on a 'reasonable timescale' being achieved in respect of each labour in a 'busy delivery unit' with 'manifold pressures' on it.[137] Another curious aspect of the text is that the usefulness of ambulation in the first stage of labour (recalling Jackson's instructions about Catherine Dunne to keep her walking) is not even mentioned. Presumably this is because it is considered subclinical and appears only on the fringe of science, something that midwives can do as part of their care package.[138]

The statistics on the time women are actually in labour catch the eye also. According to the latest edition of *Active Management*, over the last twenty-five years 98 per cent of the 65,000 women giving birth for the first time did so in under twelve hours with 25,000 of them subject to oxytocic infusion.[139] Robert Collins' figures on labour time make an intriguing comparison. Here was a vastly different population, all women giving birth, not just first-time mothers, under vastly different circumstances with what would now in the West be unacceptable rates of infant death, and also at a terrible disadvantage because of their poverty and its impact on their health. Yet under Collins' regime of 'watchful waiting', 96 per cent of his 15,716 women were delivered within twelve hours.

What requires examination is oxytocic infusion as a technology of the body, given that approximately 25,000 women were enabled to achieve O'Driscoll's twelve-hour target with it.[140] Commenting on another scientific domain, that of nuclear-missile guidance systems, Donald MacKenzie makes two points critical to the business of inventing technologies, of setting target goals for them, and of achieving accuracy in relation to those target goals which are invented. Firstly, the conditions of possibility for technology are always social. His case-study of the drive to produce increasing nuclear-missile accuracy indicates that any technology is not simply self-sustaining, nor just a product that once invented ceases to be social, one that then gets used in a socially neutral way.[141] The knowledges that go into the formation of new technologies are always social, organisational, and political in their context. Similarly, the technology of active management cannot exist outside the context of the institution known as the lying-in hospital. It requires that social context to be able to continue to work and to achieve those targets, principally because it is bound up with and dependent on the notion of surveillance. But as MacKenzie also points out, 'no knowledge possesses absolute warrant, whether from logic, experiment or practice.'[142] He adds that not all knowledges are challenged nor are all challenges successful, but those conditions of possibility are also always there.

If for argument's sake, one wished to challenge active management, one could ask how Collins' regime, which depended on a conceptualising of women as passive and prone throughout the labour process comes within two percentage points of O'Driscoll's aggregate figures?[143] Are we seeing here female bodies which have surprising resources to draw on in labour no matter what system captures them?

The endgame has shifted since Collins' time though, and perinatal mortality is the focus of the risk–death pairing. There are hotly contested meanings around perinatal mortality rates just as there were with maternal mortality rates,[144] but with the exception of pre-term infants and ranges of congenital abnormalities, which once would have proved fatal, the drop in perinatal mortality rates is largely about social and economic factors quite outside the domain of obstetrics. In a 1985 study of perinatal practices across the European region of the World Health Organisation, although there was as much as a four-fold variation between countries on the rates of intervention, there was no proven correlation between higher rates and improved pregnancy and birth outcomes.[145]

According to one current obstetric text, maternal mortality rates have fallen so low as to cease to be of any value as an index of obstetric success or failure.[146] On the issue of perinatal mortality, we are told that the three major causes of foetal death, congenital abnormality, low birth-weight, and hypoxia account for 75 per cent of deaths, with the remaining 25 per cent the result of haemolytic disease, birth injuries and infection.

In 1992, the perinatal mortality rate in Ireland fell to 9.3 per 1,000 births, compared with rates of 30 per 1,000 in 1965 and 12.8 per 1,000 in 1985.[147] The lowest rates were in the smallest units on the whole, but large units argue that they handle all the complicated cases, including referred ones, because they have the most extensive intensive-care units with staff neonatologists. The highest mortality rates cluster around the lower birth-weight babies, 2,000 grams being a fairly critical cut-off point, above which the chances of death drop dramatically. The success of sustaining babies born below that weight grows steadily greater with neonatology techniques. But as boundaries of prematurity are pressed ever further back, there is an uncomfortable question around attempts to 'save' babies and what the future may hold for them. It is as yet unclear what percentage of very low birth-weight babies survive, without sustaining any long-term damage as a result of their prematurity and the intensive care they must receive, and there is a need for longitudinal studies throughout childhood and adolescence to try and establish the levels and nature of morbidity and handicap.[148] The issue of successful treatment or not is not just about the question of survival however. A crucial dimension is the space the woman is allowed to occupy by a science in relation to her baby.

The novelist Susan Hill has written of the intense grief she and her family underwent with the premature birth of her daughter who received what she considered as unquestioned excellence of care from the neonatal medical staff before succumbing to death at six weeks of age.[149] Hill's description of the tiny scarred body with collapsed veins as a result of intensive treatment to keep her alive is not our image of a newly born infant, and Hill contends that quite the most painful aspect of her daughter's birth and death was her own exclusion from decision-making around her daughter. From point of birth, it was the medical staff who made the decisions about saving her daughter's life, a situation Hill came to regret, concluding that a peaceful death might have been preferable to the obvious physical suffering her daughter endured over those weeks.

But as with the issue of maternal mortality and morbidity, it is also important here to question obstetrics on its quiescence in relation to the issue of social location and survival rates, especially if neonatal technology precludes other forms of support on the grounds of expense. In Ireland, in line with figures from other developed countries, rates of infant death are sensitive to class issues, logically enough in respect to the impact poverty has on women's health and consequently on foetal health. In Ireland, in 1992, the rates of perinatal death amongst babies whose fathers were listed as unemployed was 3.7 times the rate of perinatal death amongst babies whose fathers were listed as higher professional: 10.2 per 1,000 births compared with 2.7 per 1,000 births.[150] This three- to five-fold difference in the perinatal mortality rate between women from the lowest social classes and highest social classes is paralleled in figures from the United States and England and Wales.[151] In a review of the perinatal mortality figures in England and Wales from the beginning of the twentieth century through six decades, Raymond Illsley commented that this class differential has not been altered at all, even though the overall rate of perinatal mortality rate has dropped dramatically.[152] The British Commons Committee, reporting on the maternity services, in 1992, in a stark reversal of the position of the three previous parliamentary and departmental committees, concluded that improvements in the perinatal mortality rate by social class would be better secured through improved social support rather than the increased use of high technology in the birth process.[153] Their judgement had already been borne out by the above-mentioned 1985 WHO study of perinatal practices across the European region of the World Health Organisation.

Similar evidence has been accumulating slowly to suggest that very low birth-weight, one of the important factors in perinatal death, cannot be dealt with by medical intervention but that contributing factors like stress, anxiety, low social class, lack of social and emotional support, smoking and substance abuse can be taken on board and responded to positively.[154] A recent survey of perinatal survival in Greece is telling. Greece has a low rate of low birth-weight babies compared with more affluent European countries, despite widespread poverty, which suggests that the extensive family system of support for pregnant women appears to have outweighed the negative effect of poverty and secured better birth outcomes for women.[155]

Perinatal mortality rates have been used consistently since the 1940s to justify childbirth management, in the same way maternal mortality rates were once deployed.[156] But as with O'Driscoll's decision to use Caesarean-section rates as the basis for measuring what type of obstetric care is now best for women, the issue is who decides? How are those probabilities weighed up? What sorts of criteria are entailed? The statistician, Marjorie Tew, uses the discourse on statistics to overturn obstetric claims about criteria of risk and safety by examining the Dutch situation. She points out that maternal and child health-care measures in European countries to bring down infant mortality began to take shape in the first decades of the twentieth century but that before these measures could have a real impact, rates of death had already started to fall dramatically; in the last several decades, this trend has continued unabated in The Netherlands, where the proportion of home births remains very high in comparison with its neighbours.[157] In fact, the Dutch statistics indicate that fewer perinatal deaths occur at home with midwife-led care than in hospital. The common argument advanced in obstetrics is that the consultant hospitals get the most complicated cases to deal with: the births identified as high risk before labour begins and the births which turn complicated with the woman being transferred to hospital, and this is why their perinatal mortality statistics are higher than births taking place in other settings. The proportion of births at home in The Netherlands fell from 53 per cent of all births in 1970 to 36 per cent in 1986. In 1953, the perinatal mortality rates in hospital were three times the rates for home births and this trend has also continued. This 'excess mortality', as Tew names it, can be isolated in the Dutch instance because of the nature of their care system where independent midwives can bring women in to deliver in hospital, if they feel it is necessary. The hospital record-keeping on perinatal deaths thus reflects both consultant-led care and midwife-led care. Similarly, figures at home can be broken down into midwife-led delivery and doctor-led delivery. Tew compares the perinatal mortality rates from each separate regime of care to prove that the argument that hospitals deal with the most high-risk cases, resulting in higher perinatal mortality rates because these babies were not saveable, is not plausible.[158] If anything, the hospital figures indicated a gap widening to a six-fold increase in the rate of mortality over the four decades between the 1950s and 1980s. In 1953, the hospital perinatal mortality rate was three times higher than the mortality rate for births at home. In 1986, with much wider hospital coverage, the perinatal mortality rate in hospitals was 13.9 per 1,000 compared with 2.2 per 1,000 at home. The perinatal mortality rates in 1986 break down to 18.9 per 1,000 births for doctors in hospitals; 4.5 for doctors at home; 2.1 for midwives in hospitals; 1.0 for midwives at home; Tew argues that it is not possible arithmetically for very high-risk babies which would be in obstetric care to solely account for this 'excess proportion' of mortality.[159]

What can be made of the risk–death pairing? Is this contest which has caught up our bodies and lives one of statistical outcomes, of normality and regimes? Does agency mean determining one's position in relation to statistics and normality? We have seen ample grounds to question the 'increasing rationality'[160] obstetrics claims. The issues of forceps deliveries, post-partum haemorrhage and active management of labour have enabled us to follow the lines of controversy and so reopen the black boxes obstetrics is continually making for itself and us. Certainly, the interventionist model has set the dominant voice in obstetrics; it uses the risk–death pairing most extensively, supporting that pairing with continuous history, concepts and statistics. This voice is contested, as in the Dunnes' case, but with no clear direction so that interventionism is only forced to somewhat modify itself and its claims and then regroup.[161] The critical problems of knowledge formation and our agency in relation to that process remain.

6

Reading Birth and Death

Maintaining the Discourse on Risk

My principal task in undertaking this book has been to examine the process of theory-building in obstetric science and to see what has happened in the course of that process to perceptions of birth. My concern is the impact of both theory-building and perceptions on the women who must engage with obstetric science in order to give birth. By definition, this is every woman who lives in a setting where obstetric science dominates the experience of childbirth. Arguably, given the power of science in our modern societies and the vital connections between obstetric science and the domains of health care and health planning in a modern state, every woman in a developed country is affected by obstetric thinking. She either accepts it because she believes its arguments to be correct and meaningful or because she doesn't know what else to do, or she rejects it and works in opposition to it in order to emerge with meanings around birth which she wants to have. The numbers of women outside the sphere of the developed world who are affected by its powerful logic are also on the increase.[1] If I were to extract only two words whereby to classify the concerns of contemporary obstetric practice, they would include not birth, but risk and death. These two themes work together to form the system of rationality that underpins contemporary obstetric science, its 'one and only reason'[2] for acting as it does.

Yet neither themes nor practice can point to some pure order of reason, despite claims to the contrary. As can be seen in the obstetric texts which have been considered in the course of this book, obstetrics is an utterly social body of knowledge, that is, a human activity built on strong feelings, intuitions, prejudice, entrenched positions, considerations of institutional power, and high passions, all of which have been an intrinsic part of its reasoning and careful observations as it has slowly lumbered along constructing its theories. This also applies to knowledges it has taken on board, knowledges from other locations within the physical sciences which are equally subject to these same currents. As Evelyn Fox Keller has argued, the difficulty and the difference with these scientific systems of knowledge, compared with traditional or non-scientific thinking, is that they 'work'; they possess extraordinary instrumental effectiveness, despite the 'representational plasticity' of their theories.[3] We can see examples of this instrumental effectiveness in the way obstetrics has dealt with induction or acceleration of labour, for instance, or the avoidance of post-partum haemorrhage. There is no question that the pharmacological regimes they employ are effective in controlling uterine action. What is necessary to question are the theories on which they base these actions and why these theories have sought to bypass the woman as subject altogether. Keller offers us a lead on this. She comments that neither the theories of sciences nor the instrumental outcomes of these theories are without aim or purpose. And the valuable task of feminist scholarship has been to clarify the extent to which the modern scientific culture has been founded on an

> explicit identification of scientific values with the values our particular cultural tradition takes to be masculine, and a collateral and equally explicit exclusion of those values which have been labelled 'feminine'.[4]

If science chooses to move in certain directions, it does so with agendas which foreclose other agendas and the asking of other questions. It is important to recognise the strength and salience of this 'genderisation of science', as Keller terms it, because of the embedded work of authorisation it entails. In brief, the experience of male scientific empiricism counts while women's experiential empiricism is excluded.

An excellent example of this can be found in Freud's account of how he came to theorise that the act of being born is the source of the affect of anxiety. In the *Introductory Lectures*, he tells us that 'speculation' had a small part to play in his discovery. Rather, what he did was to 'borrow from the *naïve* popular mind'. He then relates that when he was a medical student, he was at lunch one day, when a house physician from the midwifery department recounted the 'comic' story of a pupil midwife who was asked what it meant if meconium makes an appearance when the membranes rupture. Her reply 'it means the child is frightened' provoked laughter and she was failed. Freud then writes, 'But silently I took her side and began to suspect that this poor woman from the humbler classes had laid an unerring finger on an important correlation'.[5] Note that the young midwife's knowledge is considered naïve, that is, scientifically unproven and therefore unacceptable and that it is derided by those medics who hear it with the exception of Freud, who at least has the grace to admit from where he takes the observation, which in his hands then becomes authoritative.

The concept passes on into obstetrics also. As we saw in Chapter 5, not only does meconium become an important indicator of 'foetal distress', it gets broken down into categories and grades of viscosity and colour as a fine-grained measure of distress.

In relation to obstetric reasoning, the gendered basis for knowledge acquisition and knowledge creation has been at the very core of its theorising about women and birth. The grounding of the masculinist vision and the excluding of the 'feminine' critically forecloses our subjectivity. Even when women are given nominal 'choices' like epidurals or having their partners by their sides during labour, even when midwives are left to conduct the vast majority of births in a maternity hospital, they work within and are directed by the power/knowledge system of obstetrics. Ceding an appearance of our gaining personal agency through these limited 'choices', obstetrics can easily continue to subvert any move towards agency. The long-time authority and writer on childbirth, Sheila Kitzinger, argues about the growth of obstetrics that:

> The history of obstetrics is a record of men's struggle to construct a system of scientific certainties on which the management of labour can be based, and to eliminate women's inconvenient emotions, their 'old wives' tales', and the passion of birth giving.[6]

In effect, Kitzinger proposes that what obstetrics defines as the inconvenience and presumed irrationality of women can also make strong claims to rationality, when viewed from other stances, and therefore can challenge the 'one and only reason' whereby obstetrics explains its work to itself and to women. While not agreeing with Kitzinger's attribution of feeling and passion only to women, I do think we can frame childbirth differently, based on our own bodily and emotional experiences. I want to return to how we challenge obstetrics later on, but for the moment, I want to pick up again on the problem of risk and death and the part they play for obstetrics.

The historical demographer, Thomas McKeown, has written of infants' survival chances that:

> in technologically advanced countries today, more than 95 per cent survive to adult life. For the first time in history a mother knows that the loss of one of her children before maturity is an unlikely event.[7]

This knowledge is itself problematic. At one level, the outside chance of infant death, rather than death as a fairly commonplace reality, has become part of women's experiences in bearing children in technologically advanced societies. This includes contemporary Ireland where in 1995, for example, of the 48,530 births that year, there were 307 deaths of children before they reached their first birthdays, giving an infant mortality rate of 6.3 per 1,000 babies born (this rate differs from the rate of perinatal mortality discussed in Chapter 5).[8] Thirty-five per cent of these deaths occurred in the first twenty-four hours after birth, while the remainder occurred in the intervals between four weeks of age and one year of age. The biggest cause of death was a range of congenital anomalies, followed by complications of short gestation and low birth-weight. Four deaths were attributed to maternal complications, five to complications of the placenta, three to birth injury and difficult labour, ten to intra-uterine hypoxia and birth asphyxia; twenty-two in total in the circumstances where obstetrics argues that its expertise lies, pregnancy and birth itself.[9] Our latest survey of perinatal statistics by the Department of Health only reaches to 1992, at time of writing, but even here, there are difficult questions posed by the social locations of perinatal deaths that is, total number of stillbirths and early neonatal deaths: in 1992, the rates were 2.7 deaths per 1,000 live births for higher and lower professional groups compared with 10.2 deaths per 1,000 births for babies whose fathers are unemployed.[10] What we might ask, with figures like these, as we saw in Chapter 5, is how much credit obstetric science should take for the drop in perinatal and infant mortality rates, as distinct from how much it does take. Is obstetrics prepared to tackle the social inequalities which lead to such disparate outcomes between social classes?

Before this question has even been addressed by obstetrics, the science has pushed on to issues of morbidity in babies, especially brain damage. The issue of preventing cerebral palsy through a controlled system of birth management was the *raison d'être* for Kieran O'Driscoll. This discourse on morbidity is cut from the same cloth as that on mother and infant death and states that the prevention of brain damage becomes the goal of best-practice obstetrics. And even though there is a dissident minority within obstetrics who would now argue that brain damage is almost never because of what goes on at birth, the range of serious conditions for babies like congenital abnormalities, fits, cerebral palsy, and respiratory problems are fitted into the obstetric agenda to account for their continuing control. But can obstetrics alone resolve these issues? Equally, if explanations emerge that seem to fit better, can this be subsumed into the agenda of science as progressing towards better truths, ignoring the issue of continuing control?

There is a related problem to do with women's perceptions of how far obstetrics underwrites infant survival. I am suggesting that when women become pregnant, the possibility of infant death is much more to the fore than the reality. This skewed picture is maintained by obstetrics in the relations it sets up with each woman, through its discourse on risk. In effect, obstetrics asks women to stick with its guarantees that all will be well as long as women accept the obstetric system. I am also arguing that when women engage with obstetric medicine, they jeopardise their chances to exercise control over their situation because of the demands that the scientific discourse on risk makes. That discourse now centres on risks to the foetus.

It is apparently difficult for medicine in all its branches to relinquish the seemingly close correlation between the drop in total mortality rates and the advances in medical care. Yet the demographic argument, according to Thomas McKeown, about the reductions in mortality rates from infectious diseases during this century is that nutrition, especially the improved nutrition of mothers and children, has been the major determinant in bringing about lower mortality overall, lowering dramatically infection rates and the outcomes of those infected.[11] There is equally no doubt that with non-infectious illness, some medical interventions, like those in the perinatal field dealing with premature babies, have achieved extraordinary survival rates. But the latter is a very limited percentage of total births and the difficulty is the way obstetrics extrapolates from that to include all births. The obstetric thesis that 'no delivery can be regarded as safe until it is over'[12] remains the predominant rationale, even though the majority of infant deaths occur outside the grasp of obstetrical knowledge.

Ann Oakley argues that medicine is quick to 'pre-empt the primacy of non-medical influences by asserting the exclusive right of doctors to improve health'.[13] Arguably, the major non-medical influence of this century on women's health, after the sorts of factors outlined by McKeown, has been the feminist movement itself, which has worked to secure women's rights to deal with unregulated fertility and unwanted pregnancies, both factors that have threatened women's lives and well-being in the past. This necessary and bold public discourse reflects the accumulated experience and struggles of women over many centuries to control their reproduction. In the Irish case, this achievement is a far-reaching, even profound development of the last thirty years, where through a series of complex decisions women have made on their own behalf, there has been a drop in total fertility rates. Yet at the outset of these changes, women were poorly supported by the medical profession, many sections of which were actively hostile to women gaining access to contraception.[14] Now, even the authors of *Active Management* are prepared to admit the importance of individual and social factors in bringing about the general improvement in perinatal mortality rates, albeit in an appendix to the book and without modifying their perspectives on the need for obstetric control to deal with the risk factors in birth, as they see them.[15]

Why then, does obstetric medicine cling to and pursue its commitment to its system as the most critical component in holding off death? Part of the answer has to do with the effectiveness in terms of its organisation, a fine example of patriarchal power which systematically enforces a position of subordination on women. A telling example of the way this subordination works appears in a 1992 article in the *Irish Times* on the 'Rebirthing of Holles Street'. The article presents the human face of Irish obstetrics, complete with a photograph of the Master, in the foreground holding a baby in his arms, 'one of his tiny charges', as the caption under the photograph puts it. The baby's mother is well in the background, which gives a different weighting to the Master's statement in the article that 'the most important person in the hospital is the woman walking in the door.'[16] Bridget McAdam-O'Connell has said of the photograph that it alludes to all the visible conflicts which arise in relation to the negotiation of birth as well as the invisible ones, presenting as it does, both the visible power of the obstetrician to commandeer space within his own institution, and the non-visible power of his legitimated body of knowledge.[17]

And yet this system works exceptionally well, processing almost the whole of the child-bearing population in Ireland and unequivocally affecting the circumstances of all women giving birth, even if they do so outside hospital. In Marie O'Connor's lucid and original study of women who have chosen to give birth at home in Ireland,[18] the women she interviewed were crystal clear that the greatest barrier they had to overcome in deciding in favour of home birth was the obstetric discourse on risk. Each woman had to review these categories of safety and danger, to try and quantify the risk system in relation to her own circumstances and then work out her own position on the safety of home birth. This happened not least because the obstetric establishment had already indicated that the women opting for home birth would have to bear the burden of their decisions. Perhaps this is a better marker than any other that women who give birth in hospital are viewed as having no role in decision-making about birth at all; their responsibility is limited to being compliant patients and to not challenging the system (the corollary of this should be that obstetrics accepts and will take full responsibility for anything that goes wrong in hospital, but its record on this says otherwise). Women who chose to opt out of the hospital system were made to feel that they would be personally culpable if anything happened to their babies. And, even though women developed different rationales to defend their decisions, most often based on what they viewed as a 'normal, natural' undertaking, which did not require medicalisation, the issue of risk to their babies remained the major one which they were forced to address.[19]

The obstetric system offers a complete explanation of pregnancy and birth to the practitioner and participant alike. In a Foucauldian sense, the disciplinary practices of obstetrics that define the female body are so effective in achieving social control because, as Jana Sawicki notes, they succeed in 'creating desires, attaching individuals to specific identities, and establishing norms against which individuals and their behaviours and bodies are judged.'[20] Thus for example, O'Connor's interviewees recount how in previous pregnancies (which were not home births), they took on medical procedures during labour like oxytocic augmentation and epidurals because medical reasoning always appears so correct while the individual woman appears so wayward when compared with medical norms. The tension of this seeming disparity is further heightened by the lack of effective communication with medical and nursing staff during labour. In brief, women are made to feel that they are out of line (which indeed they are if they try to express any individual choice that goes against the obstetric model or impedes the throughput of patients) and are anxious not to incur further disapproval.[21]

A more complicated dimension to this patriarchal power, however, is the role death is still given to play. Obstetrics sets up a strange bifurcation around death which operates one way for itself and another way for women. For obstetrics, death has been endlessly useful, its source of pathological information with which to build knowledge. But for apparatuses like medical knowledge, death has also been, as Foucault argues, 'power's limit, the moment that escapes it'.[22] We have seen the science's doubts and hesitations, its rationalising around that challenge to its power in the past, especially in relation to puerperal fever. Currently, it focuses on the foetus and on the very premature baby, the areas where it now measures its most dramatic gains and losses. Perhaps connected to its 'immortality strategies'[23] and to long-term agendas that concern itself as a science in which women have little share, it incessantly pushes at that moment at a boundary which it appears able to transgress or overcome, only to open up a new boundary, a new challenge.[24] Obstetrics has related to death at this level throughout its history as a heroic science, contesting the foes that beset women in all their frailty. It continues to work this way, protecting its image of women needing the best possible obstetric care because there is an ongoing 'bodily deficiency',[25] a sense of a failed production system.[26]

Their Horror Stories

In contemporary practice, obstetrics operates on the one hand to deny death as a possible though not very likely outcome and, on the other, to treat it as an always pervasive threat, the result of the less-than-perfect body that is female. It sustains this with the discourse on risk that is underpinned by horror stories, by what has gone wrong and by its heroic attempts to then rescue women and their pregnancies. In its horror stories, obstetrics invokes the possibility of death by using the statement 'what if', which increases nameless anxieties in women about all that might go wrong unless they follow the obstetric line of reasoning. Marsden Wagner relates that in conference amongst themselves, obstetricians are currently much given to proposing more equipment and technology on the basis of horror stories, individual cases where they argue that the absence of particular technologies meant that a woman or a baby died, always certain that technology could have averted these deaths.[27] In an interview with representatives of the Home Birth Centre in 1991, the Master of the National Maternity Hospital argued that 'we still lose babies we shouldn't' but apparently with no reference at all to the effect of socio-economic circumstances on perinatal mortality. Instead, he appeared to take the view that technology would help reduce mortality rates still further. Louise McMahon, one of the two women representatives, comments:

> This I believe is the crux of the matter. The medical belief of the late twentieth century is that given the information and technology, we can do anything. It is this belief which drives hospitals to greater and greater lengths to make birth more predictable, more controlled, more assured of outcome. And I believe this is a fallacy.[28]

The sociologists, Stimson and Webb, came up with the term 'atrocity stories' to describe the way patients relate to family and friends their experiences with medical professionals; the story-teller is in the right, a hero, and challenges the doctor about his professional incompetence.[29] Dingwall re-analysed this concept of 'atrocity stories' finding it relevant to how one set of professionals deals with illegitimate actions of others, especially in the context of professional boundary-keeping.[30] Dingwall then extended the concept to argue that accounts like these arise whenever attempts are being made to control aspects of the lives of one group by another group, which the first group sees as illegitimate.

The concept can be extended further still when looking at obstetrics where horror stories, far from coming first and foremost from the arena of wicked-tongued women, in their 'old wives' tales' as obstetrics claims, are created by obstetrics to help legitimate its control (while deriding these 'tales' which just might undermine its authority over women). We have seen the pervasiveness of horror stories in obstetrics' history where what is being accomplished is the task of proving professional worth amongst colleagues. As Dingwall comments, 'by casting occupation members as hero, atrocity stories maintain the intrinsic worth of the teller and, by implication, his colleague audience.'[31] Obstetrics reinforces its control by passing horror stories on to women. This is how 'shroud-waving' works. These stories help reaffirm its status of having profound scientific knowledge compared with the sketchy, inaccurate and non-medical knowledge it presumes women have about pregnancy and birth.

An indirect example of what I mean by horror stories came out during the first trial of the Dunnes' case against Holles Street. Trying to get at the vexed issue of when Catherine Dunne's labour had begun and how far advanced it was when she entered the hospital (the hospital needing to plead that labour had not been strongly established so that its own rules on time, risk and slow labours could not be called into question in relation to how her labour was handled), Dr Jackson was asked by lawyers whether he believed Mrs Dunne was in labour when she saw her GP at the beginning of that day in March 1982. He replied: 'A patient does not visit her GP if she believes she is in strong labour. She would have been too scared.'[32] Jackson's meaning is clear. Women are repeatedly told by the obstetric system that they must report to the hospital 'if anything happens', that they must not ever of their own accord interpret or determine anything about labour and its progress because they might put their baby at risk. Therefore Jackson felt confident in his presumption that Catherine Dunne would go nowhere but to hospital if she had truly begun to labour because she would have accepted completely the tenet that she has no authority whatsoever to assess her own state, that she is completely subordinated to obstetric authority. O'Connor presents accounts from women who reported being unable to do anything in hospital other than what the system demanded, including the classic instance where a woman tried to prevent herself from pushing in second-stage labour, because she had been socialised by the system into accepting that they must tell her when to push.[33] Obstetrics demands compliance and is not prepared to deal with the woman who asserts her own authority as any other than a grossly irresponsible risk-taker, a non-compliant patient, a source of potential disaster.

As we have seen, obstetric texts record many examples of horror stories in which women are held accountable for what goes wrong in pregnancy and birth because they embody unreliability, but also because they act in their own right. In the course of carrying out its work as a science, obstetrics can and does do damage. But when it sees us breaking ranks, taking on what it perceives as an illegitimate exercise of personal agency, it attempts to label us and makes us take the blame for what goes wrong. There is an instance of this in Bethel Solomons' 1932 annual report for the Rotunda in which he recounts the death of a twenty-five-year-old woman in the wake of a Caesarean section that was delayed too long. The reason for the delay is that she was said to have earlier attempted abortion by taking a large quantity of abortifacients. Admitted when continuously vomiting, her condition stabilised somewhat and she was discharged only to be re-admitted three weeks later, very ill. On this occasion, glucose is given internally but jaundice soon appears and hyperglycaemia is diagnosed. Her condition worsens further, despite being given insulin, and finally the decision is made to section her to save her life. She dies within six hours of the operation. In a rare example of honest evaluation amongst colleagues,

Solomons writes: 'This woman might have been saved by an earlier minor section, but her desire for abortion rather cloaked the gravity of her case and probably warped judgment.'[34]

Contemporary horror stories, concentrating on the always unpredictable outcome of death, tend to flow more strongly from the interventionists who back the line of interpretation about the necessity of specialist units for all births; their contention is that if a woman is on site with the most advanced technologies and skilled help, she has reduced the risk of death to her baby as low as possible. This argument appears to run especially strong in Ireland, where successive maternal-health policies have concentrated on the development of high-technology large obstetric hospitals. Amongst other consequences, this has led to the exclusion of a socially based model of maternity care, where a woman's decision-making is considered the main component of successful care alongside her chosen modes of personal and social support during pregnancy and birth.[35] The principal argument in the 1976 Comhairle na n-Ospidéal report on hospital maternity services, that every pregnant woman should have access to care in a consultant-staffed obstetric/neonatal unit, has been fully endorsed by the 1994 *Report of the Maternity and Infant Care Scheme Review* Group.[36] This latter report reduces the problem of the centrality of woman's decision-making and its current absence in the hospital setting to the statement that 'the mother's voice is *sometimes* [italics added] lost in the organised hospital'.[37] In the chapter entitled 'The Mother's Voice', the report states 'in submissions to the Review Group, many women expressed annoyance at the manner in which decisions are taken in hospitals and stated that they felt left out of the decision making process.'[38] The term 'annoyance' does not begin to cover the loss of power about which women speak but the report as a whole remains silent on the substantive issue of relations of power. The review group does recommend, in the same irritating anodyne manner, that women should prepare a birth-plan during antenatal visits, so that preferences may be expressed directly to staff.[39] Evidently, the review group remained completely distanced from contemporary social research which has consistently indicated how difficult it is for women to negotiate in the antenatal clinic, let alone when they are giving birth.[40] And as Marsden Wagner has argued, how real are women's 'choices' when they must be made within a framework of policies not of women's choosing in the first place?[41] The review document is a discouraging development, for even though it states in the preface that documents such as Marie O'Connor's book, the report from the Second Commission on the Status of Women, and the British Winterton Parliamentary Report were available to the group, women's critiques of the hospital system of birth were not adequately contextualised.

In England, both the 1992 Winterton Report and the 1993 government publication, *Changing Childbirth*, marked the beginning of a more explicitly dialogic approach between women and doctors, raising the possibility of reversing the trend towards consultant-led care.[42] The Winterton Committee which held wide-ranging consultations with midwives, childbirth groups, activists and independent experts in addition to input from the obstetric profession, concluded that the medical model of birth should no longer drive maternity services. The official government response to these findings, in *Changing Childbirth*, was to state that choice for women in deciding their preferred maternity care and place of birth would now be policy. There are political and practical problems in realising that potential on the ground, including what remains a tacit acceptance in *Changing Childbirth* that the safety of woman and child in birth must ultimately be decided by doctors. However, despite the two divergent readings which can be given to the report, it does create a discursive space for women to support different more woman-centred models of care.[43]

By contrast, there is still only one official reading here in Ireland. As Patricia Kennedy has argued, Irish maternity-care policies have remained over-determined by the obstetric professionals who are accepted by the state as the principal actors in the birth scenario.[44] The 1994 *Report of the Maternity and Infant Care Scheme Review Group* accepts without demur the obstetric argument that the marked decrease of maternal, perinatal and infant mortality is attributable to delivery in consultant-staffed maternity units.[45] Although by now, this argument has been authoritatively contested elsewhere, discussion about its validity does not even surface in the review and the group goes so far as to reprint the contention that Ireland has the lowest maternal mortality rate in the world at 2 per 100,000 births because of its system of maternity care.[46] The group says it based its opinion on figures printed in the UNICEF *State of the World's Children Report*, seemingly unaware that these Irish figures are somewhat misleading.[47] Nevertheless they have been picked up as an accurate reading by this group and by the obstetric community as well.[48]

The contention that hospital is the only safe place to give birth was put forward by the Master of the Rotunda Hospital during a radio broadcast in 1996 from CKR Community Radio in Carlow on the always troublesome subject of birth at home.[49] At the programme's end, the Master closed the debate with an excellent example of shroud-waving. He was speaking about The Netherlands, where one-third of births still take place at home:

> Maternal mortality, that is the number of women who die, is much higher in Holland than we would accept as reasonable in this country, and this is despite the fact that it is a wealthier country with a better developed health care system. And this loss of mothers is attributable, or is attributed to home delivery.[50]

There is no evidence from the Dutch statistics to suggest that there were more maternal deaths as a result of home births in The Netherlands, compared with totally hospitalised births.[51] In 1994, The Netherlands had a maternal mortality ratio of 6 per 100,000 births; in absolute figures, there were 12 maternal deaths.[52] As it happens, this ratio is lower than the 1994 ratio for Finland, where birth is completely hospitalised, and where the maternal mortality ratio was 10.73 per 100,000 in 1994, with seven women dying as a direct result of childbirth.[53] In Ireland, the provisional figure (the figure was still provisional in 1996) for maternal deaths in 1994 was 2 per 100,000.[54]

What other meanings attach to these figures? They are part of a dense international health-planning discourse, based on attempts to achieve a standardised codification of death and a basis of comparability, over periods of years in any one country and internationally between countries. Yet these statistics can never be assured of the absolute accuracy which they appear to embody because the very processes which have set them in train are social processes, not mathematical laws. As Ian Hacking has pointed out, 'it has long been illegal to die of anything except the causes on the official list'.[55] The classification of death, which is enforced by the World Health Organisation to bring about standardised demographic accounts, must rest in the last analysis on factors like a post-mortem examination and the death certificate which is filed on that basis, uncertain legal routes which may or may not be used to initiate an inquest rather than to rely on the initial post-mortem, the unequally uncertain verdicts from coroners, and the muddy waters of indirect and direct causes of obstetric death.[56] For example, women dying in an emergency or a medical ward from infection or bleeding may well not have the cause of death traced back to an obstetric origin.[57]

In 1987, a young woman gave birth to a baby who was stillborn in a Dublin maternity hospital, after a labour which included the artificial rupture of membranes. Shortly after the birth, the woman was transferred to a general hospital where she subsequently died. Was her death (according to the post-mortem the result of infection followed by septicaemia which led to uncontrollable haemorrhage),[58] an indirect obstetric death, that is a death from a cause not related to her pregnancy and birth, given that she died in a medical ward? The young woman's family, who had difficulty obtaining information from either hospital about their daughter's autopsy, felt this question was never adequately answered.[59] In circumstances like these, can a reluctance to talk with the family be related just to the possible threat of legal action? Is it not also related to the problem of being perceived to fail in defeating death? Why must hospitals pit their word against women's families? Why can death not be discussed more openly by medical authorities who now appear to withhold vital information from families?

The reason that maternal or infant death remains controversial is largely the same as it has been throughout obstetric history: can obstetrics be held to account for deaths which have occurred? Reputations of individuals and hospital systems are riding on this issue and, given the prominence of Irish obstetrics internationally, it is not surprising that there can be a deep sensitivity and a desire to raise the possibility that deaths, when they occur, are the result of situations where women have put themselves at risk by challenging or rejecting the obstetric system. This is why, for instance, obstetricians' comments about maternal mortality in home births are calculated to unsettle, why the women in O'Connor's study reported that they were regularly subjected to hostile and aggressive reactions on the part of medical professionals and health officials once they had taken the decision to give birth at home.[60] They concluded in the main that birth was a 'normal' event, that their pregnancies had been normal and thus that they ran no risk of death, that the outcome would be fine.[61] Even though they very often excluded death as a possibility, in order to emerge with a workable rationale about their decision, these women had become aware of the socially constructed nature of risk. At the very edge of what they could reason for themselves, they accepted that if death did occur, they would take responsibility. In effect, such decisions signify that the notion of risk can be a negotiated response by all participants to a knowledge, in this case obstetric knowledge, which can only ever be partially realised. The dynamic speaks of a strikingly different moral energy around birth, especially compared with the reluctance of obstetrics to accept responsibility within the hospital domain, where there is no possibility of dialogue and negotiation. For the many thousands of women giving birth every year, the possibility of negotiating with obstetrics about the parameters of risk does not enter the picture, not least because it does not enter obstetric consciousness that the notion of risk is part of the territory of probability, one form of rationality and no more than that. Obstetrics could choose to step back from that form and to negotiate birth differently, more openly.

Although obstetrics rarely does, others have stepped back. In the late 1980s, the Innuit women living in Keewatin, in northern Canada, along the western side of the Hudson Bay, entered into dialogue with doctors and health planners who had successively deprived them of resources to give birth in their own communities, instead enforcing a policy of evacuating women south to hospitals several weeks before their babies were due to be born.[62] The isolation this imposed on women, giving birth amongst people whom they did not know, without their families nearby, was not the only loss. Women pointed out that they dealt competently with their harsh and difficult daily environment, a competence they linked directly to their vast base of knowledge about that hazardous environment. They were good judges of risks in their lives. By contrast, the Canadian government's policy on hospital birth had actually deprived them of competencies and knowledges about birth, leaving them powerless and, in that sense, at risk, precisely because they were now dependent on a medicine and a hospital system, and forced to do without the base of knowledge they had once possessed.[63] For these women, the possibility of things going wrong was an acceptable part of their daily lives, nothing from which they had to duck and weave with sophisticated schedules of probabilities. Another way of framing this is to interrogate those schedules of probabilities for, as Sheryl Ruzek argues, is the safety and efficacy of technology on women's reproductive rights knowable?[64]

Following on from that, suppose that the difficulty of obstetrics dealing with what goes wrong, its 'what if' scenario, the substance of its horror stories, is that the cause of death is never quite knowable, despite what science might want to say? With the two maternal deaths which are listed as occurring in the Republic of Ireland in 1990, for example, one from 'abnormality of the forces of labour' and one from 'obstetrical pulmonary embolism',[65] can we really glean from those classifications how those two women died? Beginning with the final listed reason for death tells us very little, if only because the body which obstetric medicine gets is already the end-product of anywhere from twelve to thirty-eight reproductive years, affected by widely varying individual, social and cultural effects. So any attempt to explain how and why disease and death take place is delimited by the ongoing problematic of how we use the central dense mass of bodies in a way which cannot easily absorb difference and divergence. This is why our answers about cause of death are surprisingly general and informative at the crudest levels only.

Because of these unanswered questions and uneasy responses on the part of obstetrics to the problem of death, it is easy to generate new categories for horror stories. The decision in Ireland to progressively wind down community midwifery based on the dispensary, and to close small local hospital units, meant that by 1978, 91 per cent of all births in the Republic were taking place in units with consultant cover.[66] Doctors and health planners unintentionally created a new problem as a result of this policy, of women giving birth at home or on their way to hospital, often completely unattended, because they could not get to the nearest large consultant hospital in time. This category of births has become known in medical terminology as 'BBAs': 'born before arrival' in the obstetric hospital. 'BBAs' can number as many as 150 women every year.[67] In a study on 'BBAs' which has been carried out by the current Master of the Coombe Hospital, the figure is cited of a six-times higher rate of mortality for babies born in these circumstances, because of the higher percentage of such babies who tend to be premature (by as much as three months) and who require neonatal intensive care. The Master also cites the fact that only one in seven of these births are to first-time mothers. The issue is a dual one of both the location of maternity-care facilities and their quality, as perceived by women. Sometimes women may be caught out by the speed of their labours; however women may also have delayed going to the hospital until the last possible minute in order to avoid unnecessary intervention.[68] So obstetric polices continue to create unexpected and untoward problems for women who must deal with the consequences, come what may.

Every year, there are 'BBA' stories in popular women's magazines, where the woman reports giving birth with the help of family and neighbours or gardaí, fire-fighters, and ambulance personnel. A recent offering in *Woman's Way* recounts the story of Catherine, who was delivered by her husband in their home, after her telephone call for the ambulance to come and collect her came too late.[69] Catherine is quoted as saying, 'I had one big contraction and the baby's head came out. It was so natural, I knew then that everything was all right.'[70] Her husband acted with great competence, to turn the baby's head as it emerged to help the shoulders be born more easily, and then cleaned the baby's nose and wrapped him up in anticipation of the ambulance team's arrival to cut the cord and take the mother and baby to hospital. Both Catherine and her baby have flourished with no untoward effects and Catherine reports that she has felt a great sense of achievement and grown in personal confidence, as a result. She compares this second birth favourably with her experience of birth in hospital with her first baby which involved epidural and forceps. Yet at the article's end, the couple say that if they have another child, it will be a hospital birth; a home birth is something they would never plan despite this experience, because they would not want to 'take the risk'.[71] It is in this way that obstetric science manages to get its discourse on risk fitted into our socialisation patterns, without our considering how this state of affairs has been put in place.

Death in birth, for women and for babies, can and does occur. Neither obstetrics, anxious to defend its reputation, nor women anxious to exercise control over their lives, can deny this reality. If there were instead an acknowledgement that death happens, that risk has to be negotiated, that the actions leading to and the limits of death are such as not to be absolutely knowable and quantifiable, there would be no need for the horror stories. But unless and until obstetrics can reconfigure its position on death, it needs these stories and it is out of these unresolved dilemmas about its relationship with death that they flourish.

Our Horror Stories: Dealing with the Contradictions

While obstetric colleagues exchange their catalogue of near-disasters, we have to deal with the concrete effects of their practices and in so doing, we have horror stories of our own whereby we mediate our experiences. There are many sources for these stories. Newsletters of the four voluntary support organisations in the Republic that deal with childbirth issues[72] feature articles and letters to the editor, which regularly appear in newspapers and in women's popular magazines, all reveal how women take on sets of definitions about themselves as reproducers. In reading these first-hand accounts, we can see how women perceive obstetric science doing its work, but how they also seek to overcome the contradictions which confront them.

Many women make sense of and adapt best to obstetric reasoning by accepting the claim that hospital is the safest place to have a baby, without ever interrogating the validity of this contention unless or until a bad birth experience, serious loss or death, take place. They do not see either disadvantage or danger, accepting instead that participating with obstetrics means a controlled and safer body. Agency in this context means that they can choose to explore the very limited scope permissible within hospitals, opting for epidural pain relief, for example, or elective Caesarean section. They can secure the version of self-hood during birth which they want, a version which makes the most sense to them, a self which can be seen to have a workable relationship with the health sciences. However, that relationship is set in a framework which is non-negotiable. Overall, women will not make these choices with any great awareness of what the procedures entail in the way of added discomfort and complications for themselves or their babies. They will not necessarily be aware that the way their bodies are already contained within the hospital system will impact unfavourably on their capacity to labour. What straws in the wind there are, like the recent industrial action by nurses in Louth County Hospital or the announcement of the cancellation of the epidural service in Sligo General Hospital in 1996, are unlikely to be picked up. Louth nurses pointed out that the gross understaffing of the hospital made it virtually impossible to offer the service of epidural on demand, because these require one-to-one nursing which means that there is only one other nurse at night for other patients and for any other woman in labour; the suspension of the epidural service in Sligo was also tied to the lack of sufficient resources to provide the service with regard to the legal implications of not having full back-up resources at that point.[73] The actual and potential range of hazards, which is why epidurals require one-to-one nursing, are not readily going to be perceived by women for what they are, not least because of the malleability of the body in relation to scientific technological medicine. Our bodies appear to 'fit' well with these technologies. In other words, what Foucault refers to as a 'looser form of power over the body' also provides an adequate and comprehensible definition of self.[74]

In other instances, women move towards autonomy in decision-making so as to participate as little as possible in the assumptions of the obstetric model, as with the 138 women who opted to give birth at home whom O'Connor interviewed. They often become activists on the issue of childbirth, their experiences becoming points of resistance to the obstetric definitions of themselves and their bodies, rather than points of congruence. Women in these circumstances are well able to comment in the national press on the meanings of their personal stories and how these reflect unfavourably on the obstetric perspective on birth, the marshalling of their bodies to match the obstetric model of normality. In response to the celebratory article on Holles Street in the *Irish Times* in 1992, one woman protested in a letter about active management of labour and about the Master's comment in the article that 'We do our best for them [the women]':

> In my own case Holles Street's 'best' meant being told not to push for 45 minutes until the midwife arrived at 10 o'clock. The student midwife would not call her before that hour was up. Such inflexibility is not desirable and at the time was downright uncomfortable for this first-time labouring mother.[75]

For this woman, the impulse to organise a maternity hospital in favour of 'unit costs and efficient deployment of nursing staff'[76] had so adversely affected her experience of birth that she chose to have her next two babies at home.

Often there are moves to seek redress through legal action for the perceived failure of obstetric science to deliver on its implicit promise that all will be well. In February 1996, there was a settlement of a High Court action, of £1.67 million for a family with a child who has cerebral palsy and is a spastic quadriplegic. The family's lawyers charged the hospital and one of its doctors with negligence leading to permanent brain damage. The mother's reported story was that she failed to be diagnosed by medical staff as having a baby in a transverse position, a fact which did not emerge until she was given a Caesarean section some twenty hours after entering the hospital; too late, her lawyers argued, to avoid or prevent the brain damage that had already occurred.[77] In August 1996 the *Nationalist* reported the case of a man seeking legal redress in a struggle to determine why his wife had died. She had been in an IVF programme, had become pregnant once before and the pregnancy had been abruptly ended when she required an emergency operation for swollen ovaries. Her husband relates that she had 'absolutely great' care. A second IVF cycle ended in her becoming ill and she died while in hospital. Her death certificate registered cardiac arrest but her husband is dissatisfied with that answer and is determined to take legal action to determine if his wife was properly cared for while in hospital.[78] These accounts make vividly clear the profound falling away of trust in the medical system in the face of death.

—Sometimes there are just bleak unanswered questions as in a letter written to the *Sunday Tribune* in 1983 by a woman who gave birth to a baby in 1981 who died three minutes later from an intercranial haemorrhage. The event had been preceded by 'a long and traumatic delivery which ended in a rather hurried and clumsy high forceps delivery'. The woman makes a plea to prevent similar 'very serious acts of negligence' from happening to other women, but there has been no explanation to this woman as to what caused her long and traumatic labour or her baby's intercranial haemorrhage.[79] Bad birth accounts also come out in the course of local support groups and women's conferences on childbirth, where women give voice to their distress and grief, perhaps raising political awareness a bit more, perhaps contributing to what can feel like an overly long struggle to put women at the centre of childbirth practices.

However, there are also the bad birth stories where women see that technology and medicine have rescued them and their babies. Perhaps the most frequent characteristics these stories exhibit are confusion and despair about our relationship with medicine and it is worth looking in detail at this dimension. In one of the weekly editions of *WOMAN* magazine in 1994, there appeared a story with the title 'There's Your Baby . . . Look How Lively It Is!'[80] It was told by a thirty-four-year-old woman named Sara who was two months pregnant when she reported to her local maternity unit in Cardiff for an ultrasound scan. Ultrasound is the most sophisticated technology to date which obstetrics has employed to carry out surveillance of the foetus inside the uterus. Like all the other technologies that gained support to deal with possible risk and death, ultrasound has become a routine practice, even though there are doubts about its efficacy in doing what it does and doubts about whether it might contribute to growth retardation of the foetus.[81]

It was a second pregnancy for Sara and she had brought her two-year-old daughter to see the ultrasound picture of the expected baby. As she lay on the examining table, the doctor on duty looked at the image on the ultrasound screen, and then told Sara her baby was dead. She said there was no word of comfort, no counselling, no explanation. She was told to go and get booked in for a D and C (dilatation and curettage, the operation where the cervix is opened and the lining of the uterus is scraped off with a curet) and also to book a second scan with the X-ray department. The story then focuses on her shock and grief, how she broke down going through the antenatal area when she saw women with healthy babies. She was told there would be a four-day wait until the D and C could be done:

> Now we had to face the fact that our baby was dead. Even worse we still had to wait for the operation to remove it. Those four days were the worst of my life. We sat around like zombies while I battled with the agony of it all.[82]

But Sara began to have vague doubts about the diagnosis. When she returned for the scan and the D and C, a radiologist was on duty and she did not know the circumstances under which Sara was returning for a scan. Sara did not want to look up at the screen during the scan to see her dead baby. The story continues:

> Slowly passing the scanner over Sara's abdomen, she looked at the screen and cheerfully said: 'There's your baby. Just look how lively it is.'[83]

The foetus was very much alive and Sara went on to have a healthy pregnancy, giving birth to a second daughter seven months after this incident. She then relates that after her daughter's birth, she was 'over-protective because she's extra precious':

> My heart still misses a beat when I think of how easily she might have died. Looking back, it's amazing that all the stress I went through in those four awful days didn't bring on a miscarriage. I still have nightmares thinking about it. What if the same mistake had been made on the second scan? . . . The frightening thing is how quickly it happened. The first doctor pronounced my baby dead and in seconds decided I should have a D and C.[84]

A 'full inquiry' into what happened was promised after the woman complained to the local health authority whose spokesperson said that doctors should seek a second opinion when there is a suspected foetal death. At the article's end, Sara cautions all pregnant women to insist on a second opinion if they have doubts about a doctor's diagnosis.

In this horror story, the woman has undergone a type of politicisation insofar as she is forced into a position of extreme doubt and caution about expert medical opinion. Three aspects stand out about her initial responses: her complete acceptance of the diagnosis at the outset, the extreme grief she endured at the knowledge presented to her, and her acceptance that she must go through a further medical procedure to resolve an early foetal death which, had it been the case, would have resolved itself through a spontaneous abortion, as hormonal production to sustain a pregnancy ceases in the wake of foetal death.

This account highlights the acute problem of the lack of agency when engaging with the obstetric system. The story suggests, for example, the pressures of time factors in a busy antenatal unit, the need for a doctor to make quick production decisions and the fact that his location in that production system is light years removed from her position as expectant mother, anticipating no loss whatsoever until that scan. Her complete dependence on that system and its knowledges means in effect that she must accept their version of events, including an entirely unnecessary obstetric operative procedure. She is not equipped to stand out against the way knowledges are produced and organised in that system and indeed it is sheer luck that the second scan is part of the routine production for a D and C. Her demand for a second medical opinion still locates her firmly within the obstetric system, where the distance between the phantasmal fear of death and the reality of death, when it must be faced, is so great that she is unable to gain any firm footing.

Using the medical system while locating points of resistance, reaching one's decisions on the issue of risk and death and therefore exercising agency is the focus of an article by Shulamith Reinharz.[85] Reinharz's re-analysis of a published account of a woman's experiences of multiple miscarriages and, finally, a successful pregnancy are presented as a series of responses and reactions defining, re-defining and negotiating a particular situation and how this bundle of changing meanings affects a woman's actions. But there are also points of resistance that emerge in this account, by a woman named Chris, who is attempting to get pregnant. The account reveals first of all, issues of temporality in planning a pregnancy, indicating the shared frame of reference we now have with obstetric science about our bodies as production units. Being able to plan successful contraception leads to a feeling of control which is subverted when pregnancy itself does not come so readily. Having planned this pregnancy and become pregnant, Chris suddenly faces a miscarriage. She describes how her doctor reacts when she must ring to report unexpected bleeding that leads to a spontaneous abortion. In the immediate aftermath, which also includes a D and C, Chris is distressed that her body has let her down. She is also shocked by a series of definitional problems. A miscarriage appears to be an event which one can relate to only as an emergency that requires emergency hands-on attention by the doctors. After this first miscarriage, she is 'shocked, frightened, terribly sad'.[86]

She becomes pregnant a second time and reacts to this by taking all sorts of precautions. Within the limits of what she knows, she seeks to actively protect this pregnancy, watching her diet and rest patterns. She again miscarries and again has a D and C. She now believes in her own culpability, believes that her behaviour has somehow jeopardised her body and its fragile hold on pregnancy. However, she also begins to search for a cause. Reinharz suggests that this is because our schematisation of life events leaves us in that cultural relationship to events where we expect to be able to comprehend or discover cause and effect. I would suggest that this is part of our scientific enculturation. Chris pushes for medical intervention and investigation into the reason for miscarriage but her doctor is reluctant. A third pregnancy ends in miscarriage and Chris is now thoroughly ensconced within a medical paradigm. She re-defines previous treatment of her case as insufficiently serious and pushes her obstetrician to order a range of laboratory tests. The turning point comes when there is a suggestion that a t-strain mycoplasma, an infectious disease, has recently been associated with infertility and miscarriage. She tests positive for this and is treated with simple antibiotics. Her joy in being able to reassert control is because there is, after all, a causal explanation for what is going on, namely that hers is a sick body. She enters on yet another pregnancy which is totally medicalised, where she monitors herself in entirely medical terms. It is also a deeply anxious time because her body has failed her so many times in the past and she refrains from announcing her pregnancy until she can no longer fit into any of her ordinary clothing.

These two stories, one in which medicine fails a woman with near dire consequences, one in which the woman forces medicine to respond to her circumstances as a serious problem and eventually gets an answer for her, share the elements of shock and fear on the part of women who confront unexpected outcomes. They also share a subordinate position in relation to obstetric decision-making and power until, in Chris' story, she demands that obstetric medicine fulfil its stated aims of taking women seriously. Ironically, by demanding to be placed at the centre of the medical system, Chris then achieves a kind of resistance to the particular line of response to her by her doctor up to that point, which has been one of dismissing the meanings of early miscarriage as not very important.

Both stories highlight again the profoundly social nature and location of obstetric knowledges. In considering different strategic responses, I am suggesting that assessing and securing agency and then reassessing how to secure a position on the content of obstetric knowledge as a science are necessary steps.

Rewriting the Stories to Secure Agency

Margaret Stacey writes about the problem of risk, that because the obstetric profession has made the assumption that women have placed themselves in the hands of obstetrics, all the risk-taking is done by them on behalf of women.[87] There is no question that we have accepted that reality and that the operation of the risk–death pairing in obstetrics does unbalance us, does create doubt, anxiety and fear. Doubt is central to our discursive engagement with obstetric medicine because, as Martin has argued:

> Medical culture has a powerful system of socialization which exacts conformity as the price of participation. It is also a cultural system whose ideas and practices pervade popular culture and in which, therefore we all participate to some degree.[88]

At no point is our conformity exacted with greater vengeance than over what are presented as life and death decisions. Within that system we have extremely limited purchase on such decisions. In a sense, our fears about death and loss are constructed for us but we are left no way to deal with those fears actively, to exercise agency in relation to them.

Yet think of the many points where women have exercised agency, when death was a central concern for them, a realistic assessment. We have encountered women whose infants have died, but they themselves have recovered after horrendous experiences with impacted labours and puerperal fever; women discharging themselves from the Rotunda before their babies were born; discharging themselves after the birth when they felt they must go (albeit much to the dismay of the hospital); friends of the labouring woman objecting to various forms of treatment, objecting to the use of forceps; refusing permission to have autopsies performed. Frederick Jebb mentions a case in 1772, when he must tell the woman he is called in to attend that she will not live and she calmly proceeds to ask for her papers to be brought to her so she can put them in order.[89] Shorter includes firsthand accounts from Germany and Switzerland from medical doctors who, when they were called in to emergency situations, preparing to carry out operations like forceps or version, were told by the women that they preferred to die undelivered rather than suffer the pain associated with these interventions, a position which would now be untenable.[90] (Indeed, any attempt by women to stave off interventions they do not want can be countermanded by hospitals going to court to overrule women.)[91] This is not to say that women did not fear illness and death. Robert Collins wrote of the problem of women denying they were in any way affected by the symptoms of puerperal fever, hoping they were not, rightly fearful if they were. But all these examples are about what we might now term issues of empowerment, attempts and often successes within a social context around birth to interpose the woman's realities and immediate concerns which were not necessarily the same as those of obstetric science. Women's concerns are utterly material, utterly about the body, even if their fears and anxieties are so frequently a response to what obstetrics has set in train.

In the 1989 British edition of *Our Bodies, Ourselves*, the introduction to the section on child-bearing opens with a statement that child-bearing 'brings with it its own strengths: flexibility, determination, patience, humour, endurance, and if we listen to our own bodies, a wealth of self-knowledge'.[92]

A bit further on, after recounting a story of a woman who stood up to her doctors to get what she wanted, the authors comment:

> Few women have this degree of determination when they are pregnant. It is a time when we need to be supported, not opposed. It takes very little to crush the fragile self-confidence that we need in order to approach labour without fear.[93]

As contradictory as these might sound, strength and endurance on the one hand, and a fragile sense of self and fear on the other, they quite accurately mark out the continuum along which women are situated when trying to make sense of ourselves, our pregnancies and our engagement with obstetric science. It seems to me that the first sentence has to do with aspirations, where we hope to be and also where we often find ourselves when, after birth, we come to reflect on events which typically have seen us caught in a morass where we have ended bewildered, easily shaken and perhaps defeated but also determined not to be caught out again.[94] Fragility and fear, however, are surely far more to do with the confused and phantasmal relationship obstetrics has with death and if we are to transform our relations with the science, we must take hold of that issue firmly and open up a dialogue with obstetrics about it.

I have been struck by Ina May Gaskin's identification of birth as 'life and death tripping', where one must be attentive to the enormity of an event where there can never be any guaranteed outcomes, but an occasion on which every woman can do well because she has the capacity to labour well and to discover 'what a lady can do with her body'.[95] Birth is a time when a woman can discover 'physical transformations of great power, beauty, and great utility'.[96] This is not the enfeebled body or psyche so often attributed to us by obstetrics. An instance of the competence women discover when they are left to do birth on their own terms comes out in a letter published in the *Evening Herald* in 1996 about a home birth and death a year earlier. The woman, Niamh, wrote of how she gave birth to a baby with the fatal condition of Potter's syndrome, in which kidneys are entirely absent. Her son died within minutes of birth:

> If home is the natural place for birth, it is for death too. I have no regrets about having a Home birth, it was a positive empowering experience in which the whole family could share. Phelim's death was gentle and peaceful, in familiar surroundings. However briefly, his brother Ferdia was able to see him alive.[97]

A scan earlier on in the pregnancy had indicated that there was a problem and Niamh had been advised to have the baby in hospital by Caesarean section, which would have made no difference to her baby who would have died no matter where he was born. Niamh makes reference in the letter to the 'bureaucratic wrangling which followed his death, in circumstances where it is known that a baby can't live outside the womb', a statement which hardly begins to convey the hostility, lack of support and absolute incompetence displayed by the medical profession over the next several days as the family endeavoured to deal with the official work of death registration. Their travels included being sent to a maternity hospital where every effort was made to discomfit mother and father about the death of their baby, a death which of course had taken place outside the obstetric domain.[98]

Karina Colgan's account of a stillbirth in hospital, *If It Happens to You*, differs dramatically to this account, not in the grief and the anguish of the parents, but with the extent to which birth and death in hospital is shot through with the belief that women cannot cope.[99] Through ultrasound, Karina also knew in advance that there was something seriously wrong with the foetus and if it did not die beforehand, it would certainly die at birth. The baby did die *in utero* and when this was confirmed by another scan, Karina was told to come back into hospital a few days later to be induced. The attempted induction, by tablets, failed, leaving the woman exhausted and in pain, and it was abandoned after a day. Given more tablets to help the cervix to soften, Karina returned home and went into labour herself just over a week later, returning to the hospital where she gave birth to her dead son. She was immediately given a sedative and later that night sleeping tablets. This could also be read that throughout her ordeal attempts were made to keep her body orderly and her emotions controllable.

Karina writes that the hospital staff responded with great compassion then and later, taking her through the autopsy report in great detail. It is true that there was no issue whatsoever of hospital practices being implicated in the death, as with the second-born Dunne twin nor did the Colgans face the opprobrium that Niamh's family did, because of a birth and death which had occurred at home. Karina's experience points to one way of constructing a sense of self-identity and Niamh's to another; both are being forced to use the issue of death, usually now hidden from public view. But one has the experience mediated entirely by a public institution that demands the modification of behaviour to fit into its way of managing death (written permission sought and baby taken off for post-mortem by doctors as soon as the mother has seen her baby), while death at home, equally shocking and grief-laden, proceeds at a pace determined by the woman until these keeper-institutions of modernity must be involved. And afterwards, the woman who has given birth at home pronounces the immediate experience and place of death as fitting, appropriate, more ordinary, more everyday. So we can manage the worst outcome – death – and if we can manage death it gives us a way of tackling the obstetric schedules of risk on terms where we can negotiate decision-making for ourselves.

One of the more important divergences of opinion during the 1985 WHO Conference on Appropriate Technology for Birth in Fortaleza, Brazil, came when the issue of normal birth was being debated. The obstetricians pursued their usual argument that birth was normal only if there was no pathology which could only be determined after the baby's birth. A midwife argued that birth is a normal life event, no matter what the outcome, including complications, as long as it is seen as normal by the woman involved, something she can relate to in her everyday life, 'if it mirrors her way of living'.[100] Her perspective was backed by colleagues from anthropology, psychology and sociology, all pointing out that the social nature of birth was such that the social context for each woman largely determined what happens, and that birth being treated as normal depends on who has the power to define normality. The obstetricians remained frankly mystified at the midwife's contention, but this is no surprise given that the principal problem in trying to dialogue with obstetric science is its lack of reflexivity, its inability to see connections.[101]

Behind this debate also lie the difficult issues of power relations and whether individuals can achieve a workable expression of agency. Feminists are clear that we cannot talk about agency in the once accepted sense of an autonomous, responsible, unified and rational individual.[102] For women the reality of acting responsibly, most especially around reproduction, is far messier, a context in which our decision-making is utterly social and relational. It is also fragmented because of the ways in which the body has already been fractured: we need to have agency to determine different levels and types of decisions with our bodies at different points in our reproductive lives, and the different selves which are invoked, like the contracepting self, the menstruating self, the pregnant self. That fracturing must be reflected, and along with it, the growing role that technologies play in how our bodies are mediated within a culture which is still deeply patriarchal. Bearing in mind that we will not have complete knowledges from science, we need to negotiate the boundaries around risks in our decision-making but we also need fluid definitions of our bodies and of risk itself, permitting us to take hold of technologies on our own negotiated terms. The urgency of this task comes increasingly to the fore when we view the developments, for example, in foetal medicine.

The mother–foetus dyad in obstetric thinking, once favouring the preservation of a woman and her reproductive capacity, has shifted and the current status of foetal medicine shows an intensifying tendency to split woman from foetus and then to shift meanings around the foetus. In a classic paper, Rosalind Petchesky traces how the technologies of visualisation, most notably ultrasound, have enabled obstetrics to create this new patient, the foetus, with whom they appear to interact directly, because of that image of the foetus floating 'free', without reference to the woman's uterus in which it lives.[103] But science has the capacity to shift the images at will. This can be seen in the differences of language between doctors who practise high-risk uterine surgery, invading the uterus to 'save' a foetus, and the clinical-research use of 'foetal material' gained from abortions; in both instances, the woman fades completely from the scene as a person in her own right.[104] If she requires an abortion, her decision becomes an opportunity for the research scientist quite without her consent. On the other hand, the progressive invasion of the uterus is accomplished not so much by gaining her consent about what may be best for her and her baby as convincing her about what is best for science: the foetus is transformed into a 'baby boy' or 'baby girl' requiring life-saving surgery on vital organs.[105]

The progressive splitting of the mother–foetus dyad and the personification of the foetus make it even more urgent that we respond to the issue of securing agency and developing the flexibility we require to safeguard our individual interests whenever we interact with medicine. It is true that we have already internalised so many of the disciplinary practices of obstetric medicine that we are skilled at responding to and fitting in with the medical regime. Bartky has pointed out that we may lose this sort of skill and a sense of personal competence and personal identity, if we challenge the points where patriarchal power expresses itself in bodily disciplines like medicine.[106]

But in surrendering safe, familiar territory, if we re-work our concepts of the body, we can labour strongly, rather than weakly under patriarchal power. The philosopher Mary O'Brien writes of women having a 'unity of knowing and doing, of consciousness and creative activity, of temporality and continuity' which must include the physicality, the materiality, the corporeal nature of birth.[107] No matter how much obstetrics seeks to manage pregnancy and labour, they are events which push us to edges of self and ultimately expand and change definitions of self. These definitions are available to us to restructure the politics of childbirth.

At present, within obstetrics, there is an acute problem in securing any of what the philosopher Lorraine Code refers to as 'available rhetorical space', a seemingly neutral space into which self-contained knowledge claims are projected but in a restrictive way so that there can be no open debate.[108] Code argues that we must remake or enlarge such spaces into locations of real, everyday context where the issue of who is speaking and why also says something about the nature of knowledge claims, about their legitimacy. At present, women are not heard within obstetric space. We have no authorised knowledge claims. As Code might describe it, our knowledges, often limited because we have conformed to the natural body created by the medical sciences, are not acknowledged. If we are to become our own agents in birth, we must force acknowledgement and legitimation, as well as seeking to create an effective critical engagement with these already established authoritative voices on the female body.[109]

For example, labour has multiple layers of meaning which can contribute to a different sense of self. Elaine Scarry points out that the concept of labour or work has an intensely contradictory location in Western society, in many ways nearly synonymous with pain, yet also synonymous with the created object:

> It has tended to be perceived at once as pain's twin and as its opposite: in its Hebrew and Greek etymological origins, in our spoken myths and unspoken intuitions . . . it has repeatedly been placed by the side of physical suffering yet has at the same time and almost as often, been placed in the company of pleasure, art, imagination, civilisation.[110]

She observes that 'it hurts to work' and yet 'the wholly passive and acute suffering of physical pain becomes the self-regulated and modest suffering of work', 'work in which we create'.[111] It does not take too practised an eye to see that obstetrics excludes labour and birth as being meaningful, in that sense of creation; excludes them, appropriates labour as their work in overseeing women in birth, and then reinterprets women's work in this, tying them to weakness and suffering, and producing a peculiarly disabled version of women and motherhood. This is fertile ground for permitting a technology like the epidural to be viewed as a helpful, if not essential, part of labour. We could be in a position to challenge the conceptualisations which lie behind such technologies, to exercise 'epistemic responsibility' in Code's phrase, to analyse why we have so readily accepted the expertise that goes with the obstetric model, rather than explore our own capacities as 'empiricists' of our own bodies.[112]

Yet even now, even through those perspectives and institutional practices imposed on us, at the time (if we are very fortunate), more often retrospectively, women recognise birth as a 'fateful moment', one that has the potential of being accomplished well. This comes through the interview data in studies on childbirth like Oakley's and O'Connor's, where women state their desire to do birth well, despite its embeddedness, despite their embeddedness, in the medical system. And doing labour well is an agency based on our corporeality.

Hilary Rose warns us that this is a struggle where we must not abandon 'our corporeal identity' and we must also have an interest in the truth claims of science.[113] We must be able to re-work those truth claims. Even when we take on disciplines of the body which are obstetric in origin, we are in and of our bodies, capable of remaking our bodily identities. We do not make sense of our pregnant bodies solely through the terms of reference obstetrics leaves for us, as is abundantly evident from our horror stories, so we require a basis from which to change our embodied sense of self.

Different Models, Different Approaches

We can change and add to our corporeal identity in birth and Evelyn Fox Keller's argument on making science work is suggestive of how this can be done.[114] If, as she contends, particular theories and representations in science lead to particular interventions, the issue becomes how to change direction by changing representations. Over the last two decades, women in the childbirth movement and midwives (and some medical doctors) have worked hard to create those different conditions of possibility. What is fascinating about these alternative readings is that they by no means reject a scientific approach, but they read science differently to mainstream obstetrics. Indeed it is arguable that new knowledges have emerged from the current problematic obstetrics has created, because of its terms of reference, because of the conflicts that it has generated.

Fleck argued about scientific systems, that what is known appears to be systematic, proven, applicable and evaluated to the knower because it has been generated within that framework. On the other hand, an alien or unknown system of knowledge appears unproven, inapplicable, contradictory, even fanciful.[115] I think this expresses very well how obstetric science has seen itself and it also accounts for its lack of reflexivity to what it perceives as challenges coming from outside its ranks. In contrast, the alternative constructs, based on midwifery, have been on the whole more self-conscious, acutely more aware of the challenge to use an inductive approach to understand how women are best supported, in ways that can be evaluated not alone by the 'knower', the creator of a specific knowledge, but also by shifting the definition of the knower to the woman who is labouring.[116] Broadly speaking, these alternatives have focused on the concrete and capable body rather than a version of the body abstracted from the dead science of anatomy. While in some respects they have been reliant on an ideology of naturalism, similar to Nihell's, which celebrates female physiological capacities as a starting point, their conclusions are startling for their rigorous nature. They 'see' the body differently, incorporating a dimension of perception with which formal obstetrics refuses to work (because it then cedes aspects of its control). If obstetrics depends on images alone to confirm or prove what it believes is happening – and nowhere more dramatically than with its routine use of ultrasound – it discards what Scarry describes as a sensorially far more immediate source of proof or substantiation, the literal substantiation of the body, involving the full range of bodily senses;[117] most especially in the instance of pregnancy and birth, touch, touching, and feeling. This degree of being 'sensorially alive' is central to understanding how a woman undergoes pregnancy and birth, to the point that she alone can say truly what that 'feels' like. A more complete definition of sensory perception allows the elements of labour to be re-defined. If, for example, the image of the perineum one has is of a rigid unyielding wall of tissue against which the baby's head will act like a 'pitchfork' in de Lee's memorable phrase (see Chapter 4), one will 'see' the necessity for an episiotomy. If one 'sees' more widely, perceives the fluid, stretchy nature of perineal tissue and what can make it stretchier still, like the position a woman in labour assumes, episiotomy is no longer a necessity. Again, if one sees the perineum tearing during the birth of a baby's head (or buttocks or legs if the baby is still presenting breech) as a birth injury, one comes to see a surgical cut like episiotomy as being somehow cleaner and neater.[118]

But if we define episiotomy more completely, we take into account when it is carried out amidst the usual pressures of a hospital delivery room: often at the beginning of second-stage labour before the perineum is fully stretched, often with scissors that crush the tissue on either side of the immediate cut. The episiotomy becomes an 'artificial production of a wound which requires closing'[119] with sutures which themselves create rigidity and which take far longer to heal, leaving thickened scar tissue, and which are far more painful in the healing than a tear or a nick (which might happen in any given labour but might not happen, especially if the woman can go through the second stage at her own pace and in a position of her own choosing). One can also see that separately as an action in itself which has no other impact or one can see that when the woman is deprived of the movement of the foetal head sliding across the uncut perineum, the woman also loses a subtle endocrinological action, involving the release of oxytocin, a first step to the successful shedding of the placenta.[120]

Yet again if one 'sees' the placenta coming off the uterine wall as an open invitation to haemorrhage, one is going to resort to an 'active management' of the third stage of labour, cutting the cord and seeking to 'deliver' the placenta, rather than seeing a different more inclusive set of connections: how the blood-filled weight, the turgidness of the placenta helps to peel it down off the uterine wall, the blood-filled weight not lost because the cord is not yet cut; how the 'living ligatures' of the uterine muscles wrap round the blood vessels to close them down. (The Irish midwife, Cecily Begley, has pioneered research on this latter approach.)[121] Or take a foetus in the breech position towards the end of pregnancy; this can be perceived as an abnormal presentation, the solution to which is a Caesarean section. Alternatively, one can ask the woman to spend ten minutes a day lying on her back on the floor with her knees flexed and three pillows under her bottom to raise her pelvis, an awkward position which nonetheless results in turning 89 per cent of breeches spontaneously before labour begins. But if a breech delivery is still presenting, one can assure the skilled training of birth attendants to deal with that birth.[122]

A final example where perceptions differ about what one is seeing is the problem of shoulder dystocia in which the anterior shoulder is impacted against the symphysis pubis, preventing the shoulders from descending into the pelvis to be born. Obstetrics classically 'sees' this as an obstruction in which the mother's body must be got out of the way, by putting her feet into a lithotomy position, doing a large episiotomy, as far back as the anus, and getting in with the operator's fingers to get the baby pulled out, often employing excessive traction to do so, often resulting in a fractured shoulder of the infant. At the outside limit, a symphysiotomy may be performed on the woman or a cleidotomy performed on the infant, deliberately fracturing the shoulder, or most controversially, 'returning' the head back into the vagina and performing a Caesarean, the so-called Zavanelli manoeuvre. All of this will be done in the atmosphere of the 'obstetric emergency'.[123]

An alternative way of perceiving this problem, of seeing the planes of the maternal body, has come from Gaskin, who has made a training video of her approach to this. She and other radical midwives encourage the woman to shift into a position on all fours which maximises the woman's physiology insofar as it maximises the pelvic diameters. This either releases the infant's shoulder of its own accord, having created that space in the pelvis, or allows the midwife to insert her hand along the line of the sacrum to deliver the posterior shoulder, thus releasing the anterior shoulder.[124]

Fleck's reminder that there cannot be complete error or complete truth is pertinent here. The irresistible conclusion is that the body works differently according to the ideological frame of reference within which it is thought to be captured and that the problem is one of cognition, which itself is bound up both with the way the production of knowledge is an exercise of power and with the way autonomy and agency are established. Fleck also wrote:

> It is individual experience, which can only be acquired personally, that yields the capacity of active and independent cognition. The inexperienced individual merely learns but does not discern.[125]

How much of obstetric practice has been about learning without discernment? And how does that impact on the training of midwives who have had to pass through the obstetric net in order to qualify?[126] These alternative rationalities can be identified as what Foucault referred to as 'subjugated knowledges', that is knowledges which have been disqualified as being inadequate because they are classified as 'naïve' or low-down on the hierarchy of knowledges, 'beneath the required level of cognition or scientificity' and marginal to the concerns of real science (this is surely the message of Freud's little story).[127] Moving a woman onto all fours to deal with a dystocic shoulder is a perfect example of this seeming lack of scientificity, as is the 'pelvic tilt'. They are both technologies of the body, but technologies in this context can be defined as appropriate birth interventions, which are simple, non-invasive and acceptable to women because they help make them happen.[128]

Both manoeuvres fall outside the scope of heroic practices that obstetrics favours. Both entail the active engagement of the woman and very much restore her personal agency. Both also operate as critiques of formal obstetric knowledge, leading one to reflect about the validity of obstetric claims to a rational and orderly unfolding of hypotheses. If there has been an increasing fragility of institutions and practices since the 1960s, as Foucault contends, that fragility in relation to obstetrics owes much to the production of theory from these lower echelons, amounting to an 'insurrection' in respect of birth practices.[129]

What work like this on birth also points up is the very disorderly movement in the course of knowledge creation over the last 200 years, during which time obstetrics has lost valuable possibilities from within its own domain, like Clarke's advice on delaying the cutting of the umbilical cord until it has ceased to pulsate. The very grounded observations and analyses that have been part of radical midwifery force us to observe how effectively institutional practices operate against the emergence of multiple forms of knowledge.[130] There is a great contrast as well in the way the birth alternatives have dealt with the social relations of why things happen as they do. Recent work on episiotomy gives us an excellent and fitting example, given that Fielding Ould first wrote up the operation for male midwifery in Dublin. It is the most commonly performed obstetric operation in Western countries, one which takes place without a woman's consent and often without her being informed about it. During the 1970s and 1980s, the childbirth movement worked hard to raise consciousness about its unnecessary application and about the harmful consequences for women physiologically and psychologically. When the effects of episiotomy were compared with the effects of tearing, the latter was easier and less painful for women to sustain and they recovered more rapidly.[131] Its postulated benefits as a routine practice (rather than in exceptional circumstances) – reducing perineal trauma, protecting the foetal head and preventing stress incontinence – are not sustainable claims.[132]

So why do 50 to 90 per cent of first-time mothers have this operation? Cecily Begley, in her ground-breaking study on episiotomy in the Coombe Hospital in Dublin,[133] found significant decreases in the use of episiotomy between 1984–8 and 1986–8 from 54 per cent to 34 per cent for first-time mothers. Midwives carry out the vast majority of births in the Coombe, albeit under the direction of medical policy and just one of the strains they experience is whether or not a laceration to the perineum will be frowned upon by doctors as poor delivery practice. But the more episiotomy is used, along with birth positions like the lithotomy position which puts greater strain on the perineum in the first place, the less likely that the skills to shield the perineum will be exercised and tears may well then result. Begley argues convincingly that the rates of episiotomy fell over that period of time because midwives were actively examining their practice and their own rationales and they were engaged in ongoing discussion about the issue of episiotomy with Begley as a midwife who knew their world and their many dilemmas. They had all been taught that episiotomy was essential and only when they were given room to question that practice could they begin to reflect and reorient themselves, rejecting the belief that 'inflicted trauma was acceptable but natural trauma was not'.[134] Begley's is an especially pertinent example of how relations of power work within institutions.

The length of labour is yet another area where midwives have arrived at different conclusions (because no-one knows how long labour can or should be).[135] Advocates of 'active birth' (the phrase is meant to imply a woman's active direction of her own labour as distinct from the 'active management' which characterises mainstream obstetrics) point out that the symphysis pubis can move up to a quarter of an inch to facilitate the passage of the baby through the birth canal and that the female body softens for labour and becomes more flexible.[136] The midwife Caroline Flint argues that a first labour can be expected to last at least twenty-four hours, with no detriment to the woman, provided she has good physical and psychological support, including freedom of movement. If a long, slow first stage ensues (especially common with posterior labours, the increasing numbers of which among first-time mothers Flint connects to the work that requires so much sitting in our culture), she, like others, points to the beneficial effects of physiologically produced oxytocin.[137] Breast stimulation, orgasm and semen are known in many cultures to have an oxytocic effect and Flint adds that the penis pressing against the cervix releases prostaglandin for the woman, further softening the cervix and contributing to dilatation. These techniques are modes of response which are viewed as 'fanciful', as simply not serious by mainstream obstetrics. Yet these approaches (or techniques like the *manteo* used by Andean women), and approaches like ambulatory movement and warm baths (which reduce pain and increase the rate of dilatation during the first stage),[138] can create a very different support structure for the woman in labour. Because of the way in which knowledge equates with power, obstetrics is almost forced to react as it does to these obvious challenges. It is no surprise that it has come to value the images of the ultrasound over the extensive work of palpation that midwives did by the many thousands in the course of their training, and to value also the regularities of the Friedman curve and the protocols on active management of the third stage. Its deployment of its technologies congruent with its version of science, contributes to an appreciable level of de-skilling within the key group of practitioners who can contest its rationalities at the point of their application to a woman – the midwives.

Nevertheless, practitioners who occupy potential sites of resistance are becoming increasingly confident in the critical voice they are developing. Midwives are actively seeking birth technologies which reflect an experiential base of the body and which do not seek to exclude women as subjects, or to foreclose on their subjectivity. They are eager to read the individual body in labour and they do so using the language of science, often now subverting the discourse from within by using the language of evaluation and research studies. The project being proposed by British midwives to evaluate the effectiveness of the 'thin red line', a faint tracing which appears to track the rate of dilatation, extending first from just below the coccyx until it reaches the anus by the end of labour in a line approximately ten centimetres long, is one such technology, a non-invasive way to determine how far a woman is dilated.

There are many problems with the social model of birth based on midwifery care, not least the problem of how independent it can be as a system of childbirth management.[139] Inside hospitals, it is extremely difficult to allow its constructs to work in the face of obstetric norms, while outside hospitals, the possibility of something 'going wrong', of which death is the worst scenario, operates as a threat against the midwife herself by putting her professional status, her livelihood and her self-esteem on the line.[140]

Chris Shilling makes the point that the classificatory schemes we use to make sense of the experiences we have are not disembodied but arise from the way we see, experience and imagine our and others' bodies.[141] In obstetrics we can see how the male imaginative capacity carries our bodies one way and shapes those bodies concretely in labour, from whence arises obstetric power. For example, it is very easy to take on the model of birth that allows for an epidural to be defined as a necessary adjunct to labour. Equally, we can see possibilities of reshaping that bodily set of experiences of pregnancy and birth. The idea of men embodying power is part of Western culture. It is the task of feminism, in the broadest sense of that term, to enable the pregnant and labouring woman to be defined as embodying an exceptional form of power, as she undergoes childbirth.

Developing Corporeal Feminisms for Birth

Birth is a fateful moment, a reproductive moment of consequence that is far more than the static physicality to which obstetrics has reduced it. We have seen that obstetrics' definitions enable us to make sense of that fateful moment insofar as it gives us a certain kind of identity. However, we can push out the boundaries of that self-definition rather than let it remain in the hands of obstetrics. Jana Sawicki has said that women can account for their position as both victims and agents within male-dominated systems because of the self-definition we can achieve.[142] That is the take-off point for resistance, once we can reflect on the way 'power grips us', as Foucault would have it, at the very point where our desires converge with the possibilities for self-definition.[143]

We can see the potential of this convergence at the end of the first trial in the Dunnes' case, when Catherine Dunne declared that if she could have undertaken that labour again, she would have sought out her doctor the minute she entered the hospital. At that point, Catherine Dunne saw no other way to respond. She accepted what obstetrics says of birth, of her, and of itself, and concluded that her obstetrician's presence would have made a signal difference to preventing the nightmare which unfolded around her. However, a different way of defining herself and her relationship with obstetrics would have been to insist from her point of entry that her account of her physical situation be taken as the critical point of reference in determining her care needs. This is the framework we need to negotiate with obstetrics. If the 'melancholic accident' that occurred early in the afternoon of her sons' births, when she experienced the tumultuous uterine movement, had been accepted by staff not as a patient complaining of discomfort and pain but as a sign of crisis, then perhaps the outcome might not have been as it was. But even if the outcome had been the same, her voice would have counted, her bodily experience would have counted; she would have been able to exercise agency. Both then and during the first trial however, her voice in that moment was dismissed as being of no scientific consequence.

If obstetrics seeks to omit the active voice of the woman or to hear only what it wishes to hear, what then can this closed and unreflexive science know of the experiential difference between the contractions of labour and a wholly unusual and untoward physical commotion? In reading the Dunnes' case, we face the painful contradictions for women there are around birth. Emily Martin's work and that of Robbie Davis-Floyd make us realise that there is no unity in women's ideas about obstetric science.[144]

Yet women demand answers of that science when there are untoward outcomes, regardless of how we conceptualise our relationship to it. Catherine Dunne underwent the experience of birth where its proximity to death was exchanged for the certain death of one of her twins, and the effective death in a social sense of another. Seemingly, the only way to obtain answers was through the legal system. However, obstetric rationality was not subverted by the subsequent trials. If anything, its remit to pursue its version of progress was ratified by the arguments of the prosecution, the defence and the judges, and the fundamental problem of there being no guaranteed outcomes was not interrogated at all. The possibility that there was no chance to rescue William and his brother is not one which fits in with the strategies of our planned society. This reality of no guaranteed outcomes is one that we as women are deeply ambivalent about confronting in ourselves, let alone confronting obstetrics about it. If we attempt to confront obstetrics, its response is that it has not learned enough. Let it pursue its work, it says, and it will yet conquer death and throw light on all the eventualities it has not solved; its inexactitude will become ever more precise and focused, given time. It is silent, however, about the nature of the power relations which are entailed in pursuing this ever-receding horizon where knowledge never quite catches up with the untoward.

What I have tried to show in this chapter is that women going through birth are seeking ways to open out this closed discourse of knowledge creation. When women seek answers for unexpected birth outcomes, they go through a process of politicisation about this discourse; when women take on risk themselves by moving outside the hospital system, they become politicised; when midwives change the nature of the representation of birth, using different models of the body, they also begin to subvert this closed discourse.

If we re-position ourselves on the issue of no guaranteed outcomes, if we accept that there cannot be complete scientific knowledge but that we are valuable contributors to multiple knowledges, we can break up the power relations which maintain this closed discourse on risk and death. Women who have been injured by the practices stemming from the 'cloud of hard words' which is obstetric thinking; who have chosen to re-conceptualise their relationship with risk and who have accepted a less than certain outcome, have taken on board Nihell's injunction to ensure that by 'virtue of such your own fair examination, the decision will no longer be dangerously and precariously that of others for you'.[145] They are, alongside research midwives, physiotherapists, childbirth educators, dissident medical voices, sociologists, psychologists, and birth activists, enabling us to 'establish a historical knowledge of struggles',[146] allowing us to tie together and retrieve disqualified forms of knowing, ways of knowing which have been either upstreamed, abandoned, or left unexplored.

This process of disqualification has been carried out by obstetrics in the name of advancing scientific understanding which, rejecting all knowledges outside its models and its control, has also sought to minimise the violent impact of its own historical practices, rejecting them as 'errors' which have been eliminated. Obstetrics' principal claim is about overcoming death once and for all. To pursue this unattainable objective, it has used inappropriate practices in the past which have done profound violence to women; it continues to do violence, even though its technologies have been greatly refined. Obstetrics must no longer be permitted to categorise its strategies as part of its ongoing struggle to overcome death for women and babies, as if it alone can pronounce on that, as if it alone has the remit to produce authoritative knowledge. It must not be permitted to deny its continuing repetition of violence, by denying women's agency, simply because death is its identified foe.[147]

This is a site of open contest where from multiple points of engagement with the obstetric system, as users and as practitioners, we can overturn obstetrics' claims and status. I am proposing that obstetrics can no longer be permitted to set the context and the limits of practice around childbirth; they can no longer set out the rules of negotiation. It is not up to obstetrics to say what its limits are or whether it has exceeded those limits – that must be negotiated by women giving birth, women in the north, women from the south, in hospitals and at home, midwives, feminists, men sensitive to women's needs and others. We must displace the hegemonic grasp of obstetrics with models of practice of childbirth based on our multiple realities as subjects, producing reflexive knowledges which speak about childbirth in all its social diversity. As women and mothers, we need to push obstetric science to be open about its power strategies around birth. The challenge set by the ambitions of obstetric science remains a substantive one for contemporary feminism.

Notes and References

NOTES TO INTRODUCTION

1. Quechua is one of the three official languages of Bolivia (Spanish and Aymara are the other two) but is perceived as an ethnic language almost exclusively associated with the largest indigenous Indian grouping. In the rural areas where we worked, Quechua is the everyday language. Thus, where possible, I have inserted the local Quechua terms and then an English translation, and I want to thank Jacinta Andrade, Sucre, Bolivia and Tristan Platt of the Institute of Amerindian Studies, St Andrew's University, Scotland, for these translations.
2. See B. Arancibia, P. Nina, and T. Platt, *Informe sobre la Encuesta Cuantitativa de Madres Campesinas (supplementado con información de las entrevistas con los medicos y auxiliares de los Hospitales y Postas Sanitarias)*, (Sucre, Bolivia: Institute of Amerindian Studies, St Andrew's University, unpublished, 1995); C. Torrico, *Las tabues y la tecnología del parto en una comunidad de pastores de puna. Informe Qualitativa para Proyecto Para la Reducción en Mortalidad Materna: Prácticas Apropiadas del Parto* (Sucre, Bolivia: TIFAP, unpublished, 1995a) and *Reading Figures* (Sucre: TIFAP, unpublished, 1995b). I also want to thank Balbina Arancibia, Cassandra Torrico and Tristan Platt for their generous assistance in interpreting the data on women's responses to childbirth.
3. See Instituto Nacional de Estadística/Demographic and Health Surveys, *Encuesta Nacional de Demografía y Salud, 1994* (La Paz: Instituto Nacional de Estdística/ Demographic and Health Surveys, 1994). More recent estimates indicate that maternal deaths may be as high as 650 per 100,000 births, with a rate of 887 per 100,000 in the rural *altiplano*. See WHO/UNICEF, *Revised 1990 Estimates of Maternal Mortality: A New Approach by WHO and UNICEF* (WHO: Geneva, 1996), and *MotherCare Matters*, vol. 6, no. 4, October 1997. The large-scale statistical indicators like the maternal mortality ratio (MMR) have been critical to obstetrics' account of itself and of how well it is managing the needs of women during pregnancy and birth. The meanings of this discourse are discussed in full in Chapter 4.
4. See *Plan Vida: Plan Estrategico para la Reducción Acelerada de la Mortalidad Materna y del Menor, 1994–1997, Provincia Chayanta, Causas de mortalidad en la Provincia Chayanta* (Ocuri: Secretaria Nacional de Salud, Secretaria Regional de Salud, Distrito de Salud Ocuri, IIAM-UNICEF-IPTK, 1994).
5. See D. Maine, *Safe Motherhood Programs: Options and Issues* (Prevention of Maternal Mortality Program, Center for Population and Family Health, Columbia University: New York, 1991); B. Kwast (1995), 'Building a community-based maternity program',

International Journal of Gynaecology and Obstetrics, vol. 48 (supplement, *Reproductive Health The MotherCare Experience*), June 1995, pp. S67–S82; UNICEF, *Progress of Nations, 1996* (New York: UNICEF, 1996).

6. See C. Torrico (1995a), op. cit.; D. Arnold and J. Yapita, *Traditional Maternity in Qaqachaka, Oruro: an Outline Summary of the Existing Health Care Facilities, Practices and Beliefs Surrounding Childbirth in One Andean Ayllu* (Preliminary Report to the European Community, La Paz: ILCA, unpublished, 1994); D. Arnold, M. Tito, and J. Yapita, *Vocabulario Aymara del Parto y de la Vida Reproductiva de la Mujer* (La Paz: UNICEF, in press); ILCA, *Maternidad Tradicional en el Altiplano Boliviano: las prácticas del parto en algunas comunidades aymaras. Informe borrador para la comunidad Europea* (La Paz: ILCA, unpublished, 1995).

7. The *sanitarios*, the official state medical officers are most usually trained to the level of auxiliary nurses in conventional Western medicine. There can be doctors as medical officers in the rural *postas* but the work setting is not popular because of the isolation and lack of up-to-date amenities. The relationship between medical staff in the *postas* and the local rural communities is complex. Anthropologists Denise Arnold and Juan de Dios Yapita argue that due to economic and socio-cultural factors, the *postas* are not heavily used. If difficulties arise, the *sanitarios* may be called on during birth but as one more source of help or information, not as the sole source. See D. Arnold and J. Yapita (1994), op. cit., pp. 8–10.

8. See B. Arancibia et al. (1995), op. cit.; D. Arnold and J. Yapita, op. cit; C. Torrico (1995b), op. cit..

9. C. Torrico (1995a), op. cit., pp. 4–5; D. Arnold and J. Yapita, op. cit., pp. 24–5.

10. S. Sherwin, *No Longer Patient: Feminist Ethics and Health Care* (Philadelphia: Temple University Press, 1992).

11. See for example, the latest policy statement from the WHO which speaks of traditional birth attendants as a way of 'bridging the gap' until such time as full-scale biomedical resources can be established. WHO, *Mother-Baby Package: Implementing Safe Motherhood in Countries* (Geneva: WHO, 1994).

12. D. Arnold and J. Yapit, op. cit., pp. 39–40.

13. See for example, C. Torrico (1995a), op. cit.

14. W. Wilde (1849), 'A short account of the superstitions and popular practices relating to midwifery, and some of the diseases of women and children, in Ireland', *The Monthly Journal of Medical Science*, May 1849, no. 35, new series, p. 725.

15. Ibid., p. 723.

16. See for example, F. Cunningham et al., *Williams Obstetrics, 19th Edition* (London: Prentice Hall International, 1993), pp. 615–17, and B. Hibbard, *Principles of Obstetrics* (London: Butterworths, 1988), pp. 676–7.

17. See C. Torrico (1995b), op. cit.

18. C. Lévi-Strauss, *Structural Anthropology* (New York: Basic Books, 1963), chapter X. I am indebted to Gerry Sullivan for bringing this to my attention.

19. This is why the debate on appropriate technologies for birth is frequently such a vexed and angry affair. Obstetrics does not want to cede control to women in this way, which is why it seeks to dismiss and marginalise approaches outside its domain.

20. A. Oakley, 'Wisewoman and medicine man', J. Mitchell and A. Oakley (eds.), *The Rights and Wrongs of Women* (Harmondsworth: Penguin, 1976).

21. M. Foucault, 'Two lectures', C. Gordon (ed.), *Power/Knowledge: Selected Interviews and Other Writings, 1972–77* (Brighton: Harvester Wheatsheaf, 1986), p. 84.

22. W. Wilde (1849), op. cit.

23. See H. Gerth and C. W. Mills, *From Max Weber's Essays in Sociology* (London: Routledge, 1991).
24. See for example, M. Stoppard, *The Breast Book* (London: Dorling Kindersley, 1996).
25. *Guardian Weekly*, 9 June 1996, 'Gene Tests Raise Spectre of DNA Discrimination'. This test is apparently quite complex to carry out and interpret, and because the gene can have several mutations, success in locating it is by no means guaranteed. See *Sunday Times, Style*, 9 June 1996, 'An Extreme Measure'.
26. M. Enkin et al., *A Guide to Effective Care in Pregnancy and Childbirth*, 2nd edition (Oxford: Oxford University Press, 1995), pp. 142–3.
27. M. Wagner, *Pursuing the Birth Machine: The Search for Appropriate Birth Technology* (Sevenoaks, Kent: ACE Graphics, 1994), p. 114.
28. Ireland, Central Statistics Office, *Vital Statistics, 1994*.
29. By 'doctors', I mean here that medical science is deeply rooted in a paradigm that bundles together objectivity and rational practice as male-dominant activities (even if there are now many women doctors), compared with what it considers the deeply female activity of subjective feeling. An account of this gendered dimension of medical science is presented in Chapter 1.

NOTES TO CHAPTER 1

1. The term 'shroud-waving' to describe this tactic has been popularised by Sheila Kitzinger in many of her books, broadcasts and public talks.
2. See P. Wright and A. Treacher, introduction, P. Wright and A. Treacher (eds.), *The Problem of Medical Knowledge: Examining the Social Construction of Medicine* (Edinburgh: Edinburgh University Press, 1982), p. 7.
3. This is quoted in P. Treichler, 'Feminism, medicine and the meaning of childbirth', M. Jacobus et al. (eds.), *Body/Politics: Women and the Discourses of Science* (London: Routledge, 1990), p. 130.
4. *Irish Times*, 12 June 1996, 'Doctor's comments on births at home angers group'; *Irish Independent*, 12 June 1996, 'Doctor under fire'. Here obstetrics speaks with a voice which enforces its own truth claims while reinforcing patriarchal relations in society.
5. See B.E. Adam, *Time and Social Theory* (Cambridge: Polity Press, 1990). The death of a baby at or near birth also disrupts obstetrics' account of its successful productivity.
6. Our expectation is that modernity confers safety from these events and so, when famine and epidemic illness occur in the countries of the South, we argue that this is possible because they are not yet fully evolved modern societies.
7. M. Foucault, *The History of Sexuality, Volume 1: An Introduction* (Harmondsworth: Penguin, 1981), p. 138.
8. E. Martin, *The Woman in the Body: A Cultural Analysis of Reproduction* (Boston: Beacon Press, 1987), p. 194.
9. R. Campbell and A. Macfarlane, *Where to be Born?*, 2nd edition (Oxford: Crown Publications for National Perinatal Epidemiology Unit, 1995).
10. M. Wagner, 'Birth and power', J. Phaff (ed.), *Perinatal Health Services in Europe: Searching for Better Childbirth* (London: Croom Helm, 1986), pp. 199–200.
11. See for example, R. Rapp 'XYLO: a true story', R. Arditti et al. (eds.), *Test-tube Women: What Future for Motherhood?* (London: Pandora Press, 1985); B.K. Rothman, *The Tentative Pregnancy: Amniocentesis and the Sexual Politics of Motherhood*, 2nd edition (London: Pandora Press, 1994).

12. I.M. Gaskin, *Spiritual Midwifery* (Summertown, TN: The Book Publishing Company, 1977), p. 230; L. Hazell, *Commonsense Childbirth* (New York: G.P. Putnam's Sons, 1976).
13. The list of landmark texts in this literature must include the works of Sheila Kitzinger. See P. Treichler (1990), op. cit., pp. 134–5 for an excellent bibliography of writing on childbirth during the 1970s and 1980s.
14. A. Oakley, *Women Confined: Towards a Sociology of Childbirth* (Oxford: Martin Robertson, 1980), p. 272.
15. P. Treichler (1990), op. cit., p. 128.
16. *Guardian*, 6 July 1994, 'BMA presses for ovary donor scheme to help the childless'. The fact that women have no ownership of their 'ovarian material', once 'harvested' or donated, is just one further turn of the screw.
17. C. Weedon, *Feminist Practice and Poststructuralist Theory* (Oxford: Basil Blackwell, 1987), p. 131.
18. P. Wright and A. Treacher (1982), op. cit., p. 9.
19. See for example, A. Oakley and H. Graham, 'Competing ideologies of reproduction: medical and maternal perspectives on pregnancy', H. Roberts (ed.), *Women, Health and Reproduction* (London: Routledge and Kegan Paul, 1981); E. Martin (1987), op. cit.; A. Todd, *Intimate Adversaries: Cultural Conflict Between Doctors and Women Patients* (Philadelphia: University of Pennsylvania Press, 1989); M. O'Connor, *Birthtides: Turning Towards Home Birth* (London: HarperCollins, 1995).
20. E. Martin (1987), op. cit.; L. Jordanova, *Sexual Visions: Images of Gender in Science and Medicine Between the Eighteenth and Twentieth Centuries* (Hemel Hempstead: Harvester Wheatsheaf, 1989); A. Todd (1989), op. cit.
21. *Faulkner's Dublin Journal*, no. 1884 from 23 to 26 March 1745. A lying-in ward was set up within St James' Hospital in London in 1739 by Richard Manningham but Mosse's was the first hospital devoted completely to lying-in women.
22. Quoted in T. Kirkpatrick and H. Jellett, *The Book of the Rotunda Hospital* (London: Adlard and Son, Bartholomew Press, 1913), p. 166.
23. J. Murphy-Lawless, 'Women and childbirth: the institutional experience', S. Deane (ed.), *The Field Day Anthology, Volume IV, Women in Ireland* (Field Day Publications in association with W. W. Norton, forthcoming).
24. E. Boland, *Object Lessons: the Life of the Woman and the Poet in Our Time* (Manchester: Carcanet Press, 1995).
25. F. Jebb, (1772), 'Of an Haemorrhage occasioned by the adhesion of the placenta to the Os Uteri', *Transactions, Medical and Philosophical Memoirs*, vol. 3, 3 December 1772, Dublin.
26. M.L. Londoño (1993), 'Initial document for the study of an ethics from women and for women (Latin American and Caribbean Women's Health Network)', *IN/FIRE Ethics, Newsletter of the International Network of Feminists Interested in Reproductive Health*, vol. 2, issue 3, 1993.
27. But then legal abortion cannot be carried out without medical assistance, so medicine does not lose control.
28. E. Shorter, *A History of Women's Bodies* (London: Allen Lane, 1983).
29. B. Ehrenreich and D. English, *For Her Own Good: 150 Years of the Experts' Advice to Women* (London: Pluto Press, 1979).
30. B.K. Rothman (1986), 'Reflections: on hard work', *Qualitative Sociology*, vol. 9, no. 1, spring 1986; A. Finger, 'Claiming all of our bodies: reproductive rights and disability', R. Arditti et al. (eds.), *Test-tube Women: What Future for Motherhood?* (London: Pandora Press, 1987).

31. S. Reinharz, 'The social psychology of a miscarriage: an application of symbolic interaction theory and method', M.J. Deegan and M. Hill (eds.), *Women and Symbolic Interaction* (London: Allen and Unwin, 1987).
32. L. Silverton, *The Art and Science of Midwifery* (London: Prentice Hall, 1993), pp. 549–52. Isoimmunisation or rhesus disease, where a rhesus-negative woman carries a rhesus-positive baby, is dealt with by testing and injections of anti-D gamma globulin to prevent the growth of antibodies. It does not usually affect a first pregnancy unless the woman has previously received rhesus-positive blood through a blood transfusion but has not received an anti-D injection, in which case the baby's life will be seriously threatened with the development of haemolytic disease.
33. A. Finger (1987), op. cit., p. 287.
34. E. Nihell, *A Treatise on the Art of Midwifery: Setting Forth Various Abuses Therein, Especially as to the Practice of Instruments* (London: Haymarket, 1760), pp. ii–iv. In the English-speaking world, male practitioners commonly called themselves male midwives in the eighteenth century (sometimes they used the French term *accoucheur*). Although the term 'obstetrics' was established as a description of this new branch of medicine by the 1820s, it was much further into the nineteenth century before the term obstetrician, to describe individual practitioners, came into common usage. Orthodox histories of obstetric science, usually written from within the profession, designate it as midwifery. See for example, H. Spencer, *The History of British Midwifery from 1650 to 1800* (London: John Bales, Sons and Danielsson, 1927).
35. The midwife Louise Bourgeois, who was head midwife of the Hôtel-Dieu, where Nihell was to train in the eighteenth century, published her midwifery text, *Observations Diverses* in Paris in 1626. J. Donnison has written a detailed history of men and women midwives from this period: *Midwives and Medical Men. A History of Interprofessional Rivalries and Women's Rights* (London: Heineman, 1977).
36. Women midwives were forbidden by law to use instruments in the delivery of children which meant that in certain difficult circumstances, they called in the barber-surgeon. These men were not physicians, the old academic-based cadre of doctors, but rather men who carried out emergency surgery of amputations and also performed destructive operations with instruments like the crotchet to release a foetus trapped in the womb.
37. The mistress of Louis XIV is thought to have had a man midwife in attendance. For a brief summary, see S. Inch (1989), op. cit., p. 21.
38. E. Nihell (1760), op. cit., pp. 461–2.
39. J. Murphy-Lawless, 'Images of "poor women" in the writings of Irish men midwives', M. MacCurtain and M. O'Dowd (eds.), *Women in Early Modern Ireland* (Edinburgh: Edinburgh University Press, 1991).
40. F. Jebb (1772), op. cit.
41. F. Ould, *A Treatise of Midwifry in Three Parts* (Dublin: Oli. Nelson and Charles Connor, 1742), p. 49.
42. J. Murphy-Lawless (1992), 'Reading birth and death through obstetric practice', *Canadian Journal of Irish Studies*, vol. 18, no. 1, 1992.
43. *Irish Times*, 26 July 1988, 'A court battle won but a childhood lost forever'; *Irish Times*, 26 July 1988, 'Everywoman versus the medical system'.
44. Historians of science, like Canguilhem, ask how this one form of rationality, science, invested or created its objects of attention. See G. Canguilhem (1980), 'What is psychology?', *Ideology and Consciousness*, no. 7, 1980, pp. 37–50. Foucault argues that the related question which needs to be investigated is what the price has been of

investing the human subject as an object of knowledge: 'At what price can subjects speak the truth about themselves?' he asks in 'Critical theory/intellectual history', L. Kritzman (ed.), *Michel Foucault: Politics, Philosophy, Culture. Interviews and Other Writings, 1977–1984* (London: Routledge, 1988). To bring this back to Catherine Dunne, she speaks of herself only as a mother who may be talking nonsense, but who should be listened to whether she is nonsensical or not. Thus she already accepts what obstetrics says of her, that she is essentially unknowledgeable (in their terms) about herself as she goes through pregnancy and birth, but that her possible silliness must be accommodated. There is no sense from her that she is the central actor and that her experience authorises her to speak. The question then is whether your lack of agency is the price you pay in order to be able to define who you are, as a woman and a mother.

45. D.E. Smith, *The Everyday World as Problematic* (Milton Keynes: Open University Press, 1988), p. 18.
46. J. Murphy-Lawless (1988), 'The silencing of women in childbirth or let's hear it from Bartholomew and the boys', *International Women's Studies Forum*, vol. 11, no. 4, 1988.
47. D. Cameron, *Feminism and Linguistic Theory* (London: Macmillan, 1985), pp. 145–6.
48. See B. Easlea, *Science and Sexual Oppression: Patriarchy's Confrontation with Women and Nature* (London: Weidenfeld and Nicolson, 1981); L. Jordanova (1989), op. cit.; E.F. Keller, 'From secrets of life to secrets of death', M. Jacobus et al. (eds.), *Body/Politics: Women and the Discourses of Science* (London: Routledge, 1990).
49. A central element of this process concerns the facts sciences produce as a dominant discourse. Norman Fairclough, Gerhard Nijhof, and Brian Torode all argue that one goal of critical discourse analysis is to 'denaturalise' a dominant discourse, that is, to make visible the constructed nature of what is otherwise presented as a 'natural given'. See G. Nijhof, 'On naturalisation in health care', B. Torode (ed.), *Text and Talk as Social Practice: Discourse Difference and Division in Speech and Writing* (Dordrecht, Holland: Foris Publications, 1989); N. Fairclough (1985), 'Critical and descriptive goals in discourse analysis', *Journal of Pragmatics*, 9 1985; B. Torode, 'Discourse analysis and everyday life', B. Torode (ed.) *Text and Talk as Social Practice: Discourse difference and division in speech and writing* (Dordrecht, Holland: Foris Publications, 1989).
50. See L. Jordanova (1989), op. cit.
51. B. Duden, *The Woman Beneath the Skin: A Doctor's Patients in Eighteenth Century Germany* (Cambridge, MA: Harvard University Press, 1991), pp. 20–2. This argument is also pursued by Nellie Oudshoorn. See N. Oudshoorn, 'A natural order of things? Reproductive sciences and the politics of othering', G. Robertson et al. (eds.), *FutureNatural: Nature/Science/Culture* (London: Routledge, 1996).
52. Boston Women's Health Collective, *Our Bodies, Ourselves* (New York: Simon and Schuster, 1971), p. 1.
53. M. Foucault, *The Birth of the Clinic* (London: Tavistock 1976), pp. ix–x. Foucault quotes Pomme's description of a woman hysteric under his care whose lesions appear after a treatment of baths for ten to twelve hours a day over a period of ten months to cure what is seen as the desiccation of her nervous system, the woman then passing tissue described as being like damp parchment.
54. P. Wright and A. Treacher (1982), op. cit.
55. D. Armstrong, 'Bodies of knowledge: Foucault and the problem of human anatomy', G. Scambler (ed.), *Sociological Theory and Medical Sociology* (London: Tavistock, 1987).
56. Chris Shilling argues that writing about the body has not been 'respectable' in sociology until relatively recently. See C. Shilling (1991), 'Educating the body: physical capital and the production of social inequalities', *Sociology*, vol. 25, no.4, 1991.

57. M. le Doeuff (1981), 'Pierre Roussel's chiasmas: from imaginary knowledge to the learned imagination', *Ideology and Consciousness*, no. 9, 1981-2.
58. L. Schiebinger, *The Mind Has no Sex?: Women in the Origins of Modern Science* (Cambridge, MA: Harvard University Press, 1989).
59. Schiebinger observes that this eighteenth-century movement wiped out possible earlier gains during the Renaissance when men anatomists had argued that women had the same sense organs as men's, even the same mental capacity. This was replaced by the argument that the female body was an abnormal version of the male body, a pale and weak imitation, or that the female body was so entirely Other, belonging to the domain of nature that a separate branch of medicine was required to study that body as an ontologically distinct category. See also O. Moscucci, *The Science of Woman: Gynaecology and Gender in England, 1800–1929* (Cambridge: Cambridge University Press, 1990).
60. J. Gélis, *History of Childbirth: Fertility, Pregnancy and Birth in Early Modern Europe* (Cambridge: Polity Press, 1991), pp. 121–33.
61. Ibid. I am indebted to the anthropologist Cassandra Torrico for pointing out that non-medicalised birth positions are, in physical terms, actively engaged positions. In the Quechua-speaking community of Tomaycurí, in the northern Chayanta province of Bolivia, she has been struck by the fact that the birth positions women use are all 'forceful', positions where physical forcefulness can be easily expressed, and perhaps it is that strength that is recognised in the Quechua word '*wijchuy*', literally 'to throw out' the baby.
62. It is likely that Mauriceau lifted the description of what has become known as the 'dorsal recumbent position for labour' from Aristotle's writings on midwifery which differed from the recommendation of other ancient manuscripts that a woman retain an upright position. See P.M. Dunn (1991), 'François Mauriceau (1637–1709) and maternal posture for parturition', *Archives of Disease in Childhood*, vol. 66, no.1, January 1991. The speed with which a reclining position became accepted practice amongst men midwives in the eighteenth century suggests that the rationale Mauriceau advanced, conserving energy to deal with the pain of labour, fitted in best with the description of women's physiology which highlighted their weakness. The back and left lateral positions and, for instrumental deliveries, the lithotomy position, with feet in stirrups, are still in use in Irish maternity hospitals although the hospitals argue that 'within reason' – theirs of course – there is room for a woman to choose her own position. See Irish Association for Improvement in the Maternity Services, *A Consumer's Guide to the Maternity Units in Ireland* (Dublin: Health Promotion Unit, Department of Health, n.d.).
63. H. Deventer, *The Art of Midwifery Improv'd* (London: E. Curll, J. Pemberton and W. Taylor, 1716), p. 102.
64. F. Ould (1742), op. cit., pp. 32–3.
65. J. Gélis (1991), op. cit., p. 124.
66. The writing of Simone de Beauvoir, Shulamith Firestone and Sherry Ortner are good illustrations of this argument. Although de Beauvoir, for instance, acknowledges in *The Second Sex* that childbirth can be experienced by some women as a source of creative power, she sees childbirth as painful and dangerous and the female reproductive function as a source of slavery from which women should work to be released. This is a controversy that is set to continue, with women's active engagement, because of the success of reproductive technologies, including post-menopausal pregnancy, in relocating the sites of conception and pregnancy. Obstetrics with its increasing

272 *Notes to pp. 38–40*

insistence that it can interact directly with the foetus, for example with intrauterine surgery, creates a climate which accepts that a woman may be bypassed altogether in relation to reproduction. For a discussion of the implications of these moves in how we see the 'natural' order, see S. Kember, 'Feminist figuration and the question of origin', G. Robertson et al. (eds.), *FutureNatural: Nature/Science/Culture* (London: Routledge, 1996).

67. The contemporary naturalist thesis on childbirth in the English-speaking world got its initial inspiration from Grantly Dick-Read, who wrote about 'natural childbirth' and 'childbirth without fear', a form of psychoprophylaxis to prepare women for labour which he argued was far more respectful of women's natural abilities to give birth and of their emotional experiences at this delicate time. See G. Dick-Read, *Childbirth Without Fear: The Principles and Practice of Natural Childbirth*, 5th edition (London: Pan Books, 1969). In England, the National Childbirth Trust (NCT), established in 1956 and the Association for the Improvement in Maternity Services, established in 1961, worked to promote these changes in hospital practices in order to humanise and feminise birth for women. The NCT also encouraged women to continue to think of the possibility of home birth if they were low risk and to demand this against the increasing trend to hospitalisation.

68. S. Arms, *Immaculate Deception* (Boston: Houghton Mifflin, 1977). Women were spurred to hope that birth outside our Western culture was uncontaminated and purely natural and that this could be regained within our culture with the reinstatement of midwives. A much more sophisticated philosophical approach, with a model of the female body as specially gifted, has been put forward by the philosopher Mary O'Brien, in which she argued that women have a special consciousness around the moment of reproduction which is not open to men and, as a result, the latter are alienated from the work of labour and birth. See M. O'Brien, *The Politics of Reproduction* (London: Routledge and Kegan Paul, 1981); and *Reproducing the World* (Boulder, CO: Westview Press, 1989).

69. J. Murphy-Lawless, 'Male texts and female bodies: the colonisation of childbirth by men midwives', B. Torode (ed.), *Text and Talk as Social Practice: Discourse Difference and Division in Speech and Writing* (Dordrecht, Holland: Foris Publications, 1989), pp. 25–7.

70. L. McNay, *Foucault and Feminism* (Cambridge: Polity Press, 1992), p. 21.

71. See S. Romalis, 'Struggle between providers and recipients: the case of birth practices', V. Olesen and E. Lewin (eds.), *Women, Health and Healing: Towards a New Perspective* (Tavistock: London, 1985).

72. The perceived need for anaesthesia cannot be viewed separately from the complex social relations surrounding each woman in labour: what possible alternatives to deal with her labour she has or wants; hospital practices in respect of labour; hospital environment, including staffing schedules and ward routines disruptive to the individual woman; pressure from the woman's partner to make birth less stressful; all come into play.

73. C. Shilling, *The Body and Social Theory* (London: Sage, 1993), p. 69. Shilling discusses the naturalistic body and its emergence in various disciplines from the eighteenth century onwards, save sociology where, as he notes, the body has been 'an absent presence' until quite recently.

74. Ireland, Central Statistics Office. Personal communication. These were the most up-to-date figures available as of January 1998. Although representatives of the Home Birth Association of Ireland feel that the demand for home births is increasing, the tiny number of domiciliary midwives registered to practise limits this option.

75. On the risk-scoring model, see J. Murphy-Lawless, 'Women dying in childbirth: the international context of "safe motherhood"', P. Kennedy and J. Murphy-Lawless (eds.), *Returning Birth to Women: Challenging Policies and Practices* (Dublin: Centre for Women's Studies, TCD/WERRC, 1998); see also M. Akrich and B. Pasveer, 'Technologies of giving birth: Comparing women's bodies and competencies during "normal" birth in France and the Netherlands', paper delivered at the International Workshop, The Mutual Shaping of Gender and Technology, 6–8 October 1995, University of Twente, The Netherlands.
76. The power of the state to pronounce on who must be present at birth is a good example of Foucault's bio-politics, where the intentions of the state to secure the health of the social body leads to the medicalisation of individuals.
77. E. Shorter (1983), op. cit.
78. C. Shilling (1993), op. cit., p. 183. In the case of childbirth, these increasing opportunities are linked to aspects like reliable birth control, etc.
79. P. Kennedy, 'Between the lines: Mother and infant care in Ireland', P. Kennedy and J. Murphy-Lawless (eds.), *Returning Birth to Women: Challenging Policies and Practices* (Dublin: Centre for Women's Studies, TCD/WERRC, 1998).
80. M. Enkin, M. Keirse, M. Renfrew and J. Neilson, *A Guide to Effective Care in Pregnancy and Childbirth*, 2nd edition (Oxford: Oxford University Press, 1995), pp. 257–9. On the problem of pain relief in labour and the specific problems caused by epidurals, see also M. Wagner, *Pursuing the Birth Machine: The Search for Appropriate Birth Technology* (Sevenoaks, Kent: ACE Graphics, 1994), pp. 154–8.
81. See K. O'Driscoll (1972), 'Impact of active management on delivery unit practice', *Proceedings of the Royal Society of Medicine*, vol. 65, August 1972, pp. 697–8.
82. See for example, M. O'Connor (1995), op. cit., pp. 34–6: 16 per cent of her women interviewees experienced direct hostility and/or retaliation on the part of medical staff.
83. M. Poovey, *Uneven Developments: The Ideological Work of Gender in Mid-Victorian England* (Chicago: University of Chicago Press, 1988), pp. 26–7. Poovey refers to Meigs' privileging of the woman's word over the doctor's rationales as a more traditional form or practice of medicine. As ever, there were huge contradictions in the application of this. Women able to deal naturally with pain were also left to deal with the consequences of puerperal fever by Meigs who rejected the theorising around causes which linked puerperal fever to the man midwife.
84. G. Dick-Read (1969), op. cit., p. 29. A very early version of the naturalness of pain came from Frederick Jebb, who became the fourth Master of the Rotunda Lying-in Hospital. See J. Murphy-Lawless (1989), op. cit., pp. 34–5. The panegyric on the natural body is exceptionally rich in possibilities. To the woman it offers an analysis of what she should be feeling, physically and emotionally, a positive association of birth with the immediately assumed capacity to undertake her role as a feeling responsive mother. To the man midwife or obstetrician, it offers a natural body which is endangered by the grip of nature itself. The body can be injured in its transports of pain and joy and therefore must be restrained for its own good.
85. M. Foucault, 'Technologies of the self', L. Martin et al. (eds.), *Technologies of the Self: A Seminar with Michel Foucault* (London: Tavistock, 1988), p. 18. He goes on to explain 'this contact between the technologies of domination of others and those of the self I call "governmentality"', ibid., p. 19. By governmentality he is referring to the 'government of one's self and of others'.
86. E. Scarry, *The Body in Pain: The Making and Unmaking of the World* (New York: Oxford University Press, 1985), p. 117.

87. Ibid.
88. Akrich and Pasveer (1995), op. cit., observe that in the current French context, the pain of labour itself is made part of the pathology of labour. French obstetricians have written at length about the risk to the baby as a result of the production of maternal stress-hormones, hyperventilation and slow-down of dilatation, problems with uterine contractility, increased heartbeat, etc. which are responses to pain. The epidural is seen as a way to counteract these ill-effects of 'natural' but painful labour, which women are said to find so difficult.
89. E. Scarry (1985), op. cit., p. 60. Or, as Foucault has argued, 'nothing is more material, physical, corporeal than the exercise of power'. See 'Body/Power', pp. 57–8, M. Foucault, *Power/Knowledge: Selected Interviews and Other Writings. 1972–77* (Brighton: Harvester Wheatsheaf, 1980).
90. M. Foucault, 'On the genealogy of ethics: An overview of work in progress', H. Dreyfus and P. Rabinow (eds.), *Michel Foucault: Beyond Structuralism and Hermeneutics* (Chicago: University of Chicago Press, 1983), p. 187.
91. L. McNay (1992), op. cit., p. 9.
92. M. Foucault (1976), op. cit., p. 144.
93. D. Coakley, *The Irish School of Medicine: Outstanding Practitioners of the Nineteenth Century* (Dublin: Town House, 1988).
94. P. Ariès, *Western Attitudes Towards Death: From the Middle Ages to the Present* (Baltimore: Johns Hopkins, 1974).
95. C. Shilling (1993), op. cit., p. 7.
96. Z. Bauman, *Mortality, Immortality and Other Life Strategies* (Cambridge: Polity Press, 1992).
97. A. Oakley and H. Graham (1981), op. cit.
98. Z. Bauman (1992), op. cit.
99. This is the position in which Catherine Dunne found herself, for example. Aggregate hospital statistics, compiled in annual clinical reports, support this collective tendency to deny.
100. E. Bronfen (1992), *Over Her Dead Body: Death, Femininity and the Aesthetic* (Manchester: Manchester University Press, 1992), p. 92.
101. L. Jordanova (1989), op. cit., p. 101.
102. E. Bronfen (1992), op. cit., p. 5.
103. Ibid., p. 13.
104. E.F. Keller (1990), op. cit. Keller identifies what she terms a 'perennial motif', inherent in all science, where to seize nature's secrets is to hold the secret of death and thereby forestall death.
105. J. Clarke (1817), 'Abstract of a Registry kept for some years in the Lying-in Hospital in Dublin', *Transactions of the Association of Fellows and Licentiates of the King and Queen's College of Physicians*, vol. 1, 1817, Dublin, p. 373.
106. See A. Oakley, 'Wisewoman and medicine man', J. Mitchell and A. Oakley (eds.), *The Rights and Wrongs of Women* (Harmondsworth: Penguin, 1976), and J. Donnison (1977), op. cit., on England. On the United States, see D. and R. Wertz, *Lying In: A History of Childbirth in America* (New York: Free Press, 1977); J. Donegan, *Women and Men Midwives: Medicine, Morality and Misogyny in Early America* (Westport, CT: Greenwood Press, 1978); and J. Leavitt, *Brought to Bed: Childbearing in America, 1750–1950* (New York: Oxford University Press, 1986). See also, the edited account of the New England midwife, Martha Ballard, who practised from the late eighteenth century into the early nineteenth century, L. Ulrich, *A Midwife's Tale: The Life of Martha Ballard, Based on Her Diary, 1785–1812* (Vintage Books: New York, 1991).

107. There were some women midwives who were licensed by either Church authorities or the Royal College of Physicians. The latter were given power to license midwives in 1692, but between that date and 1742, only two licences were granted to women midwives, a Mrs McCormack in 1696–7 and Mrs Bradford in 1731–2. See I. Ross, 'Midwifery', I. Ross (ed.), *Public Virtue, Public Love, The Early Years of the Dublin Lying-in Hospital* (Dublin: O'Brien Press, 1986), p. 165. But Ireland appears not to have had midwives trained, as Nihell had been, at a hospital like the Hôtel-Dieu.
108. J. Murphy-Lawless (1987), 'Women and childbirth: male medical discourse and the invention of female incompetence' (Ph.D. Thesis. University of Dublin, Trinity College, unpublished, 1987), pp. 143–51.
109. J. Sawicki, *Disciplining Foucault: Feminism, Power and the Body* (London: Routledge, 1991), p. 67.
110. As Starr points out, this was a distinguishing feature of medical professionalisation in general. See P. Starr, *The Social Transformation of American Medicine* (New York: Basic Books, 1982).
111. J. Brown (1986), 'Professional language: words that succeed', *Radical History Review*, 34, 1986, p. 36.
112. F. Ould (1742), op. cit., p. 49.
113. J. Brown (1986), op. cit., p. 48.
114. L. Jordanova (1989), op. cit., p. 20.
115. E. Nihell (1760), op. cit., p. xii.
116. F. Ould (1742), op. cit., p. 74.
117. H. Deventer (1716), op. cit., p. 160.
118. In his preface, Fielding Ould discusses a labour he witnessed in Paris and from which he took his analysis of how the baby's head turns as the baby is being born; he describes 'the Patient' as a woman who was 'strong and robust' and who by her own efforts delivered a baby, after much effort; the final part of labour was slowed, according to Ould, by the umbilical cord which had been wrapped several times around the baby's neck. See F. Ould (1742), op. cit., p. xi. What is so curious is how observations like these did not disrupt the argument about women's weakness in general. For a detailed discussion of how these images of strength and weakness shifted across class lines until all women were included, see J. Murphy-Lawless (1991), op. cit.
119. J. Brown (1986), op. cit., pp. 34–5.
120. These were not their only competitors; the old academic physicians were hostile to the barber-surgeons and chemists from whose ranks male midwifery proceeded to grow.
121. F. Ould (1742), op. cit., p. 2.
122. E. Shorter (1983), op. cit., pp. 37–8.
123. E. Nihell (1760), op. cit., p. 13.
124. J. Clarke (1817), op. cit., p. 377.
125. F. Ould (1742), op. cit., p. 38.
126. W. Wilde (1849), 'A short account of the superstitions and popular practices relating to midwifery, and some of the diseases of women and children in Ireland', *The Monthly Journal of Medical Science*, new series, no. xxxv, May 1849, pp. 724–5.
127. F. Ould (1742), op. cit., pp. 145–6; pp. 57–8.
128. W. Wilde (1849), op. cit., p. 717.
129. It was not just birthing practices which were replicated. Nihell described the Hôtel-Dieu where the training of women midwives was upheld for a long period and where the men had to 'sue' for entry, as the best teaching establishment in Europe. She refers to the fact that the hospital would often admit women fifteen days before their

confinement for teaching purposes. Birth registers were kept there and Nihell described the 'common daily practice of a regular midwife' keeping a register of deliveries for though 'there might not appear so much anatomy in her descriptions, but I am very sure, there would be couched in them much more solid instruction.' See E. Nihell (1760), op. cit., p. 148.
130. J. Brown (1986), op. cit., p. 36.
131. H. Deventer (1716), op. cit., p. 136.
132. See J. Harvie, 'Delivery of the placenta', H. Thoms (ed.), *Classical Contributions to Obstetrics and Gynecology* (Springfield, ILL: Charles C. Thomas, 1935).
133. J. Gélis (1991), op. cit., p. 171. Perhaps there was also the hope that medical control of the placenta would bring an end to the custom known as placentophagy, eating the human placenta either newly expelled or in powdered form. Gélis writes that this was a long-established custom in Europe for dealing with fertility problems, as was using the placenta for treating a range of ailments. See J. Gélis (1991) op. cit., pp. 168–71. In Ireland, Wilde reports the placenta being burned after birth, but also buried, usually under a hedge or some other place where it could not be polluted. See W. Wilde (1849) op. cit., p. 726.
134. E. Nihell (1760), op. cit., p. viii.
135. Ibid., p. 277.
136. Ibid., p. 90.
137. Ibid., p. 162.
138. Ibid., p. 389.
139. Ibid., p. 400.
140. Ibid., p. 441. By reduction, Nihell means she may be dealing with an obstruction or delay like an anterior lip, where the cervix has not completely effaced but the baby's head is pressing down to be born and the midwife will gently lift the remaining rim of the cervix during a contraction to allow passage for the baby's head.
141. Ibid., p. 378.
142. Ibid., p. 362.
143. Ibid., pp. 97–8.
144. The irony of Ould's attacks on women is that his publisher, Charles O'Connor, included a glossary of terms at the rear of Ould's book for the convenience of women midwives 'who live in the country remote from the assistance of skilful Persons'. See F. Ould (1742), op. cit., Explanation of the Terms of the Art.
145. E. Nihell (1760), op. cit., p. 68.
146. Ibid., p. 97.
147. Ibid., p. 88.
148. Ibid., pp. 102–3.
149. Ibid., p. 217.
150. Women in developing countries are also being drawn into the obstetric net and now occupy one or other of these positions. See J. Murphy-Lawless (1998), op. cit.
151. Foucault has stated that part of the problem of the critical history of rationality is that we fall prey to the argument that if rationality is rejected, it is rejected because irrationality has been accepted in its place. But the challenge has been to isolate and present the dominant rationality which seeks to present itself as the one and only rationality, when in fact, it is one of several or even many. See M. Foucault (1988), op. cit., p. 27.
152. See J. Lawson, *A sermon intended to have been preached at the publick opening of the Chapel of the Lying-in Hospital in Great Britain Street, Dublin* (Dublin, 1759).
153. M. Wagner (1986), op. cit., p. 198.

154. G. Bourne, *Pregnancy* (London: Pan, 1975), pp. 7–8.
155. See D. Cooper (1994), 'Productive, relational and ubiquitous: conceptualising power within Foucauldian feminism', *Sociology*, vol. 28, no. 2, May 1994, p. 442; see also J. Sawicki (1991), op. cit.

Notes to Chapter 2

1. F. Ould, *A Treatise of Midwifry in Three Parts* (Dublin: Oli. Nelson and Charles Connor, 1742), pp.145–6. The term itself is attributed to a German doctor, Braun, who in 1857 condemned the operation as unnecessary and potentially harmful.
2. S. Inch, *Birthrights: A Parent's Guide to Modern Childbirth*, 2nd edition (London: Green Print, 1989), pp. 141–2.
3. Many midwives currently argue that supporting the woman, where possible in an upright position, to give birth to the head gently and slowly, permits the perineal tissue to stretch slowly and is the most effective protection against perineal tears. See S. Inch (1989), op. cit., and L. Silverton, *The Art and Science of Midwifery* (London: Prentice Hall, 1993), p. 312.
4. See International Congress of Obstetrics and Gynaecology, *Transactions of the International Congress of Obstetrics and Gynaecology, Rotunda Bicentenary Congress* (Dublin: Parkside Press, 1947), p. 364.
5. H. Deventer, *The Art of Midwifery Improv'd* (London: E. Curll, J. Pemberton and W. Taylor, 1716), p. 16. But can practice be a shadow? Is it not the substance?
6. Ibid.
7. Deventer also recognises that midwifery is an intensely practical business when he states that 'Midwifry is a Work of the Hands, and requires a repeated Practice to make a Midwife ready in that Business', H. Deventer, op. cit., p. 3.
8. See R.A. Erickson, 'The "Books of Generation": some observations on the style of British midwife books, 1671–1764', P. Boucé (ed.), *Sexuality in Eighteenth Century Britain* (Manchester: Manchester University Press, 1982).
9. F. Ould (1742), op. cit., p. viii.
10. Ibid., p. x.
11. F. Jebb (1772), 'Of an haemorrhage occasioned by the adhesion of the placenta to the os uteri', *Transactions, Medical and Philosophical Memoirs*, volume III, 3 December 1772, Dublin, p. 2.
12. L. Fleck, *Genesis and Development of a Scientific Fact* (Chicago: University of Chicago Press, 1979), p. xxvii.
13. Ibid., pp. 27–8.
14. On the construction of female hysteria, see B. Ehrenreich and D. English, *Complaints and Disorders: the Sexual Politics of Sickness* (London: Writers and Readers Publishing Cooperative, 1976), and *For Her Own Good: A Hundred and Fifty Years of the Experts' Advice to Women* (London: Pluto Press, 1979).
15. See M. Foucault (1980), 'The history of sexuality', C. Gordon (ed.) *Power/Knowledge: Selected Interviews and Other Writings 1972–77* (Brighton: Harvester Wheatsheaf, 1988), p. 186.
16. M. Foucault, *The History of Sexuality, Volume 1: An Introduction* (Harmondsworth: Penguin, 1981), pp.120–1, 128–30.
17. L. Fleck (1979), op. cit. p. 30.
18. B. Latour, *Science in the Making: How to Follow Scientists and Engineers Through Society* (Milton Keynes: Open University Press, 1987), p. 21.

19. F. Ould (1742), op. cit., p. ix.
20. Ibid.
21. E. Nihell, *A Treatise on the Art of Midwifery: Setting Forth Various Abuses Therein, Especially as to the Practice of Instruments* (London: Haymarket, 1760), p. v.
22. C. Weedon, *Feminist Practice and Poststructuralist Theory* (Oxford: Basil Blackwell, 1987), p. 78.
23. See L. Jordanova, *Sexual Visions: Images of Gender in Science and Medicine between the Eighteenth and Twentieth Centuries* (Hemel Hempstead: Harvester Wheatsheaf, 1989), pp. 44–50.
24. E. Nihell (1760), op. cit., p. 25.
25. Ibid., p. 250.
26. B. Latour (1987), op. cit., p. 24.
27. There was a lengthy debate in early eighteenth-century texts on the 'obliquity' of the uterus, that is, whether the angle at which it lay relative to the cervical canal rendered labour extremely difficult. Nihell believed in this theory as did Deventer. Ould rejected it. What the theory may have been trying to account for was a uterovaginal prolapse which would have been common enough with high rates of fertility and heavy burdens.
28. H. Deventer (1716), op. cit., p. 91.
29. Ibid.
30. Ibid.
31. Ibid. 'Gossips' here refers to a woman's close friends, presumed to be with her during labour. The word is traced back to the Old English phrase, God sib, meaning sister of God.
32. Ibid., p. 99.
33. Normal labour has become an even more disputed concept in contemporary obstetrics, as we shall see in Chapter 5.
34. E. Nihell (1760), op. cit., p. 257.
35. Ibid.
36. Ibid., p. 258.
37. Ibid.
38. Ibid., p. 152.
39. Jacques Gélis argues that relatively few midwives of this period understood the usefulness of touching in evaluating the progress of a labour. Many midwives had what he terms a 'false' idea of the sexual organs and of the length of gestation. See J. Gélis, *History of Childbirth: Fertility, Pregnancy and Birth in Early Modern Europe* (Cambridge: Polity Press, 1991), pp. 134–5. But this can perhaps also be explained by the traditional body which Barbara Duden describes in her work and which many midwives of the period who were not trained or influenced by the new medicine, as Nihell was, would still have best understood. See B. Duden, *The Woman Beneath the Skin* (London: Harvard University Press, 1991). The dislike of vaginal examinations by midwives practising outside the hospitals survived in England down to the twentieth century, women relying instead on visual and verbal signs. See N. Leap and B. Hunter, *The Midwife's Tale: An Oral History from Handywoman to Professional Midwife* (London: Scarlet Press, 1993), pp. 162–4.
40. H. Deventer (1716), op. cit., pp. 78–9.
41. E. Nihell (1760), op. cit., p. 230.
42. Nihell quotes Smellie approvingly on touching only to point out that as a man he is automatically disqualified from full knowledge of 'those arcana of the female fabric'

because touching violates the bounds of modesty. She goes to great lengths in her treatise to discount men midwives on this point. However, the modesty argument survives as a protest against male midwifery for only a short period of time. Once within the realm of the hospital, the issue of modesty quickly ceases to matter.
43. H. Deventer (1716), op. cit., p. 76.
44. Ibid., p. 77.
45. Gélis comments that traditional midwives continued to use parts of the body to evaluate dilatation, like fingers or the palm of the hand, while men midwives rapidly moved to money coins as a point of comparison, like the size of a silver crown. See J. Gélis (1991), op. cit., p. 135.
46. F. Ould (1742), op. cit., p. viii.
47. Ibid., p. x.
48. Ibid., p. xx.
49. Ibid., pp. 95–6.
50. Ibid., p. xvi.
51. Ibid., p. 28.
52. Gélis argues that many traditional midwives were inclined to favour rapid labours, fearing complications. In contrast, many of the eighteenth-century men midwives saw labour as Nihell saw it, a time to watch and wait. See J. Gélis (1991), op. cit., p. 134.
53. F. Ould (1742), op. cit., p. xix.
54. Ibid., p. xviii.
55. Ibid., p. 46.
56. Ibid., p. xviii.
57. In a series of interviews I carried out some years ago with midwives about their reactions to working under obstetric-led care for women, a senior midwife tutor related seeing this practice employed by a consultant obstetrician. She objected to it and was reprimanded for her audacity in challenging him.
58. J. Gélis (1991), op. cit., pp. 134–5.
59. F. Ould (1742), op. cit., p. 50.
60. E. Nihell (1760), op. cit., p. v.
61. L. Fleck (1979), op. cit., p. 30.
62. W. Dease, *Observations in Midwifery Particularly on the Different Methods of Assisting Women in tedious and difficult Labours* (Dublin: Williams, White, Wilson, Byrne and Cash, 1783), p. 29.
63. Ibid., p. 35.
64. Ibid., pp. 54–6. The term anencephaly to describe this condition was not used until 1836. The list seems to cover obstructed labour, haemorrhage, and eclampsia.
65. Ibid.
66. Ibid., pp. i, 53.
67. F. Ould (1742), op. cit., p. 79.
68. I. Loudon, *Death in Childbirth: an International Study of Maternal Care and Maternal Mortality 1800–1950* (Oxford: Clarendon Press, 1992), pp. 139–40. The problem of contracted pelves was related to rickets, about which Audrey Eccles has argued that it was a disease entity little known before the seventeenth century, when the density of urban living began in earnest with the very poor living in the worst conditions frequently without any sunlight. See A. Eccles, *Obstetrics and Gynaecology in Tudor and Stuart England* (London: Croom Helm, 1982). Shorter argues that rickets was certainly present in traditional society, brought about through excessive swaddling of infants because of a fear of draughts which resulted in inadequate exposure to sunlight. See E. Shorter, *A History of*

Women's Bodies (London: Allen Lane, 1983), p. 23. According to the historical demographer Thomas McKeown, rickets could also have been a consequence of agriculture because as soon as men moved to a diet based largely on cereal, calcium deficiencies brought about by the content of phytate in grain encouraged rickets. At the beginning of the twentieth century, rickets was associated with the inherited burdens of syphilis. See T. McKeown, *The Origins of Human Disease* (Oxford: Basil Blackwell, 1988), p. 46.

69. E. Shorter (1983), op. cit., p. 72.
70. J. Clarke (1817), 'Abstract of a Registry kept for some years in the lying-in hospital in Dublin', *Transactions of the Association of Fellows and Licentiates of the King and Queen's College of Physicians*, vol. 1, 1817, Dublin, pp. 368–9.
71. Ibid., p. 371.
72. Ibid., p. 372.
73. Ibid., p. 372.
74. Clarke's son-in law, Robert Collins, in a biographical sketch of Clarke, later argued that women from 'the upper ranks of life' had a much greater number of premature births than women from the working classes, a phenomenon Collins attributed to 'the greater delicacy of the upper ranks of society, engendered by the mode of life pursued'. See R. Collins (1849), *A Short Sketch of the Life and Writings of the Late Joseph Clarke* (London: Longman, Brown, Green and Longman, 1849), p. 61. On the other hand, Clarke's claims about death from tedious labour were that there had never been a single instance in women from the upper classes whom he attended in contrast with his experience in the Rotunda, where women were exclusively from the poorer classes.
75. J. Clarke (1817), op. cit., pp. 376–7.
76. E. Shorter (1983), op. cit., p. 83.
77. J. Clarke (1817), op. cit., pp. 376–7. The tendency to defend the hospital's statistics and outcomes on the grounds that what has already taken place before a woman enters the hospital is not the hospital's responsibility, grew in importance over time and I will return to this theme in later chapters.
78. Ibid., pp. 373–4.
79. Ibid., p. 375.
80. Ibid.
81. Ibid., pp. 374–5.
82. Ibid., p. 400.
83. B. Latour (1987), op. cit.
84. J. Clarke (1817), op. cit., p. 371.
85. J. Murphy-Lawless, 'Images of "Poor Women" in the writings of Irish men midwives', M. MacCurtain and M. O'Dowd (eds.), *Women in Early Modern Ireland* (Edinburgh: Edinburgh University Press, 1991).
86. E. Nihell (1760), op. cit., pp. 443–4.
87. L. Fleck (1979), op. cit., p. 118.
88. B. Latour (1987), op. cit., p. 40.
89. T.D. O'Donel Browne, *The Rotunda Hospital, 1745–1945* (Edinburgh: E. and S. Livingstone, 1947), pp. 168–70.
90. B. Latour (1987), op. cit., p. 24.
91. R. Collins, *A Practical Treatise on Midwifery containing the Results of Sixteen Thousand Six Hundred and Fifty-Four Births Occurring in the Dublin Lying-in hospital During a Period of Seven Years Commencing November 1826* (London: Longman, Rees, Orme, Browne, Green and Longman, 1836), pp. 7–8.

92. R. Collins (1837), 'Observations on the artificial dilatation of the mouth of the womb during labour, and upon instrumental delivery', *Dublin Quarterly Journal of Medical Science*, vol. xi, p. 43. In his treatise, Collins said that 'strict attention' was paid to a woman in labour 'to keep her cool and her mind easy' including regulating the bladder and bowels and 'diligent and persevering attention at the patient's bedside'. R. Collins (1836), op. cit., p. 16. The regulation of bladder and bowels with clysters was actually a conservative form of induction to stimulate uterine contractions. See S. Inch (1989), op. cit., p. 46.
93. R. Collins (1849), op. cit., p. 59.
94. R. Collins (1837), op. cit., p. 40.
95. R. Collins (1849), op. cit., p. 59. An ongoing issue with this figure concerns how the start of labour is determined and by whom, a point to which I will return in Chapter 5.
96. R. Descartes, *A Discourse on Method* (London: J.M. Dent and Sons, 1912), pp. 23–4.
97. B. Latour (1987), op. cit., appendix 2.
98. H. Deventer (1716), op. cit., p. 140.
99. E. Nihell (1760), op. cit., p. xiii.
100. Ibid., p. 91.
101. R. Collins (1837), op. cit., p. 71.
102. E. Shorter (1983), op. cit., p. 75.
103. J. Hamilton (1838), 'A letter from Professor Hamilton of Edinburgh in reply to the Objections made to his Practical Precepts in Midwifery by Dr Collins', *Dublin Quarterly Journal of Medical Science*, vol. xiii.
104. R. Collins (1837), op. cit.
105. Quoted in J. Hamilton (1838), op. cit., pp. 219–20.
106. E.W. Murphy (1839), 'An examination of Dr Hamilton's Letters in Defence of his Opinions, especially in Reference to the Management of the First Stage of Labour', *Dublin Quarterly Journal of Medical Science*, vol. xiv, January to June 1839, p. 428.
107. Ibid., p. 429.
108. Ibid., p. 441.
109. Ibid., p. 415.
110. L. Fleck (1979), op. cit., p. 42.
111. R. Frankenberg, '"Your Time or Mine": temporal contradictions of biomedical practice', R. Frankenberg (ed.), *Time, Health and Medicine* (London: Sage, 1992).
112. E. Martin, *The Woman in the Body: A Cultural Analysis of Reproduction* (Boston: Beacon Press, 1987).
113. Rotunda Hospital, 'A Copy of His Majesty's Royal Charter for Incorporating the governors and Guardians of the Hospital for the Relief of Poor Lying-in Women in Dublin', 2nd December 1756.
114. This comes from the sermon written by the Reverend Lawson. See J. Lawson, *A sermon intended to have been preached at the publick opening of the Chapel of the Lying-in Hospital in Great Britain Street, Dublin*. The charter specifically says 'that such hospital when established will be a means not only of preserving the lives and miseries of numberless lying-in women but also of preventing that most unnatural (though too frequent), practice of abandoning or perhaps murdering newborn infants', Royal Charter, 1756.
115. F. Ould (1742), op. cit., p. viii.
116. The figures for live births and those for women's deaths covered the period in hospital only to the point of discharge. This would have excluded all infants who died soon

afterwards. It also would have excluded women who died from puerperal infections and complications, some of which would not have shown up in the immediate postpartum period. One Master, Kelly, at the beginning of the nineteenth century, actively discharged women as soon as possible after birth to keep his mortality figures as low as possible. See T. O'D. Browne (1947), op. cit., p. 104. A mid-nineteenth-century midwifery textbook by George Johnston and Edward Sinclair describes the difficulty the Rotunda had in imposing a longer lying-in period on women who were anxious to return to their homes, much to the dismay of the medical staff. See J. Murphy-Lawless, 'Women and childbirth: The institutional experience', S. Deane (ed.), *The Field Day Anthology, Volume IV, Women in Ireland* (Field Day Publications in association with W. W. Norton, forthcoming).
117. E. Shorter (1983), op. cit., p. 165.
118. J. Clarke (1817), op. cit., p. 370.
119. Ibid., p. 369.
120. E. Nihell (1760), op. cit., p. ix.
121. Ibid., p. 133.
122. G. Johnston (1873), 'Clinical Report of the Rotunda Lying-in hospital for the Year ending 5th November, 1872', *Dublin Quarterly Journal of Medical Science*, vol. lv, January and June 1873, p. 192.
123. Ibid., p. 193.
124. G. Johnston (1872), 'Clinical Report of the Rotunda Lying-in hospital for the Year ending 5th November, 1871', *Dublin Quarterly Journal of Medical Science*, vol. liii, January and June 1872, p. 26.
125. F. Churchill, *Researches on Operative Midwifery* (Dublin: Martin Keene and Son, 1851).
126. The child frequently died when internal version was badly employed.
127. The vectis was a variant of the lever, used to free the foetal head from the birth canal.
128. Levret, a French man midwife, gave forceps the curved form and a methodical account of how to apply them.
129. W. Dease (1783), op. cit., p. ii.
130. Ibid., p. 55.
131. Ibid., p. v.
132. F. Ould (1742), op. cit., p. 140.
133. W. Dease (1783), op. cit., p. 45.
134. F. Ould (1742), op. cit., pp. 162–3.
135. L. Jordanova (1989), op. cit., pp. 60–2.
136. F. Ould (1742), op. cit., pp. 163–4.
137. E. Nihell (1760), op. cit., p. 78.
138. In Atthill's clinical report for the Rotunda in 1878, there is an account of a nineteen-year-old woman, 'T. O'N. primipara', who was in labour for two-and-a-half days, at which point, although it was recorded that the membranes had ruptured, the 'os was about the size of a florin, still hard and undilatable'. Chloroform having been administered, forceps were applied 'but so firmly and rigidly did the cervix surround the blade, that it was not thought safe to employ traction and they were accordingly removed'. The woman was then given a warm bath and a douche after which 'matters assumed a more favourable aspect'. Her child 'was shortly afterwards expelled alive by natural efforts'. See L. Atthill (1879), 'Report and Clinical Records of the Rotunda Hospital for the Year Ending 5th November, 1878', *Dublin Quarterly Journal of Medical Science*, vol. lxviii, July to December 1879, p. 339. This case is but one example that begs the question of how many instrumental deliveries were unnecessary, just as Nihell charges.

139. J. Clarke (1817), op. cit., p. 375.
140. Ibid., pp. 392–3.
141. See L. Jordanova (1989), op. cit., pp. 60–1.
142. E. Nihell (1760), op. cit., p. 91.
143. Ibid., p. 444.
144. The Wertzes argue that the wider use of the Caesarean gave the edge to French men midwives throughout the seventeenth century on anatomical knowledge. See D. and R. Wertz, *Lying In: A History of Childbirth in America* (New York: Free Press, 1977).
145. F. Ould (1742), op. cit., p. xxiii.
146. Ibid.
147. Ibid., p. xxiv.
148. Ibid., pp. 196–7.
149. Ibid., p. 197.
150. Stories of surviving the operation did make news. The French man midwife, de la Motte, wrote in his treatise of an account published in *Le journal des Savants*, in July 1693, of a woman having a Caesarean section at Chateau Tierri in 1667. She and her child were said to have survived the operation, the woman dying fourteen years later in the Hôtel-Dieu, as the result of a ventral hernia. See G. de la Motte, *A General Treatise of Midwifery*, 1985 reprint (New York: Garland, 1746), p. 435.
151. W. Dease (1783), op. cit., p. 61.
152. T. Southwell, *Remarks on some Errors both in Anatomy and Practice in a late Treatise of Midwifery by Fielding Ould, Man-midwife* (Dublin, 1742), p. 85.
153. Another instance of an Irish midwife skilled at her work and enthusiastic about it comes from William Carleton's novel, *Fardorougha, The Miser or the Convicts of Lisnamona*, published in 1839. Carleton tells us she was based on the midwife who had delivered him and who was still actively working when he was growing up in Clogher, County Tyrone. See J. Murphy-Lawless (forthcoming), op. cit.
154. W. Dease (1783), op. cit., p. 67.
155. W. Dease (1783), op. cit., p. 71.
156. T.D. O'Donel Browne, *The Rotunda Hospital, 1745–1945* (Edinburgh: E. and S. Livingstone, 1947), p. 184.
157. E.H. Tweedy (1908), 'Clinical reports of the Rotunda Hospital', *Dublin Journal of Medical Science*, vol. cxxxv, July to December 1908, p. 103.
158. F. Churchill (1858), 'Obstetric Mortality', *Dublin Quarterly Journal of Medical Science*, vol. xxvi, August–November 1858, p. 319. In nineteenth-century Germany, the Caesarean was predicted as having a 54 per cent death rate. See T. O'D. Browne (1947), op. cit., p. 183.
159. F. Churchill, *Researches on Operative Midwifery* (Dublin: Martin Keene and Son, 1851), p. 156.
160. A way of pre-empting the threat of obstructed labour carried out by Irish women midwives is recorded by the seventeenth-century man midwife, Percival Willughby: 'the wild Irish women do break the pubic bones of the female infant, so soon as it is born. And I have heard some wandering Irish women affirm the same to be true, and that they have ways to keep these bones from uniting. It is for certain that they be easily, and soon, delivered. And I have observed that many wanderers of that nation have had a waddling and lamish gesture in their going.' See P. Willughby, *Observations in Midwifery* (Reprint. East Ardsley: S. R. Publishers, 1972), p. 16.

161. G. Tierney (1933), 'Maternal Mortality', *Irish Journal of Medical Science*, sixth series, no. 82, October. These were probably underestimated, most especially within the hospital setting.
162. Ibid.
163. T. O'D. Browne (1947), op. cit., p. 206.
164. In a 1969 obstetrics textbook, traces of the old school of 'watchful waiting' are evident in the authors' expression of concern about forceps deliveries. They warn that 'today there are no dangerous obstetric forceps; unfortunately there are still dangerous obstetricians who misuse the instrument.' See D. Llewellyn-Jones, *Fundamentals of Obstetrics and Gynaecology*, vol. 1 (London: Faber and Faber, 1969), p. 338. The high forceps deliveries Dease described are condemned. Llewellyn-Jones is also interesting on the use of the Caesarean for foetal distress: 'the great problem in fetal distress is to be sure that the signs do in fact indicate that the baby is at risk. Fetal distress, real or imagined, undoubtedly accounts for a large proportion of the additional Caesarean sections performed in recent years', ibid., p. 353.
165. J. Clarke (1817), op. cit., p. 373.
166. F. Ould (1742), op. cit., p. xvii.
167. B. Latour (1987), op. cit.
168. Ibid., p. 15.
169. T. de Lauretis, 'The violence of rhetoric: considerations on representation and gender', *Technologies of Gender: Essays on Theory, Film, and Fiction* (Bloomington: Indiana University Press, 1987).
170. These representations continue to have resonance in contemporary culture. The David Cronenberg film, *Dead Ringers*, picks up on the rhetoric of violence when the twin gynaecologist brother, after inflicting grievous bodily harm, declares 'No, no . . . there's nothing the matter with the instrument. It's the body, the woman's body was all wrong.' In other words, give us the tools; we have the radical technology to deal with malfunctioning women's bodies.
171. J. Clarke (1817), op. cit., p. 397.

Notes to Chapter 3

1. N. Hulme, 'On the puerperal fever', F. Churchill (ed.), *Collected Essays on Puerperal Fever* (London: Sydenham Society, 1849), p. 76.
2. G. Johnston (1875), Clinical Report of the Rotunda lying-in hospital for the year ending 5th November, 1874', *Dublin Quarterly Journal of Medical Science*, vol. lix, January and June 1875, p. 142.
3. E. Shorter, *A History of Women's Bodies* (London: Allen Lane, 1983); J. Gélis, *History of Childbirth: Fertility, Pregnancy and Birth in Early Modern Europe* (Cambridge: Polity Press, 1991).
4. F. Churchill, 'Epidemics of puerperal fever', F. Churchill (ed.), *Collected Essays on Puerperal Fever* (London: Sydenham Society, 1849), p. 5.
5. J. Gélis (1991), op. cit.; A. Gordon, *A Treatise on the Epidemic Puerperal Fever of Aberdeen* (London: G.G. and J. Robinson, 1795).
6. F. Churchill (1849), op. cit.
7. J. Gélis (1991), op. cit., p. 247.
8. F. Churchill (1849), op. cit., p. 5.
9. F. Churchill (1849), op. cit., p. 31.
10. M. Foucault (1976), *The Birth of the Clinic* (London: Tavistock, 1976), pp. 23–5.

Notes to pp. 109–15 285

11. Irish Office, *Reports of the Commissioners on Certain Charitable Institutions in Dublin, 1830*, appendix no. 6 (London: Irish Office, 1830).
12. L. Fleck, *Genesis and Development of a Scientific Fact* (Chicago: University of Chicago Press, 1979), pp. 30–1.
13. J. Gélis (1991), op. cit., pp. 248–9.
14. L. Silverton, *The Art and Science of Midwifery* (London: Prentice Hall, 1993), pp. 454–5.
15. E. Shorter (1983), op. cit., p. 108.
16. L. Fleck (1979), op. cit., p. 35.
17. M. Foucault, *The Archaeology of Knowledge* (London: Tavistock, 1974), pp. 4–5.
18. Ibid.; see also G. Canguilhem (1980), 'What is psychology?', *Ideology and Consciousness*, no. 7, 1980, pp. 37–50; F. Jacob, *The Logic of Living Systems* (London: Allen Lane, 1974).
19. L. Fleck (1979), op. cit., p. 30. Fleck points out that classical bacteriology was committed to the existence of one causative agent in respect of infectious diseases, and this viewpoint organised its methods of investigation. He traces the theory of infectious disease to as far back as Varro in 116 BC, who held that serious diseases were caused by 'minute animals'. For modern science, accepting the notion that 'very small living agents' somehow entered the body, the task was to search for direct evidence of the causative factors and, if that were not obtainable, then there was a search for indirect evidence to explain the nature of the disease.
20. Ibid., p. 18.
21. C. Herzlich and J. Pierret, *Illness and Self in Society* (Baltimore: Johns Hopkins University Press, 1987), pp. 7–12.
22. J. Clarke, 'Observations on the puerperal fever', F. Churchill (ed.), *Collected Essays on Puerperal Fever* (London: Sydenham Society, 1849), pp. 354–5.
23. Ibid., p. 355.
24. Clarke refers here to Dr Hulme, whose work we have already encountered.
25. Ibid., pp. 355–6.
26. M. Foucault (1976), op. cit., p. 101.
27. A. Gordon (1795), op. cit.
28. R. Collins, *A Practical Treatise on Midwifery containing the Results of Sixteen Thousand Six Hundred and Fifty-Four Births Occurring in the Dublin Lying-in hospital During a Period of Seven Years Commencing November 1826* (London: Longman, Rees, Orme, Browne, Green and Longman, 1836).
29. J. Clarke (1849), op. cit., p. 356. A nomenclature for diseases was laid down by the Frenchman, Alibert, in the eighteenth century with each disease entity designated by the endings, *osis, itis* and *rhoea* meaning general alterations, tissue irritations, and discharges respectively. See M. Foucault (1976), op. cit., p. 133.
30. A. Eccles, *Obstetrics and Gynaecology in Tudor and Stuart England* (London: Croom Helm, 1982).
31. M. Foucault (1976), op. cit., p. 164.
32. J. Gélis (1991), op. cit., p. 246. Shorter sees these fevers as forms of endometritis, of which puerperal fever was a serious complication or extension. See E. Shorter (1983), op. cit., p. 106.
33. J. Gélis (1991), op. cit., p. 246.
34. A. Gordon (1795), op. cit., pp. 42–3. Loudon, in his work on maternal mortality, notes that this observation was widespread in writing of the period. See I. Loudon, *Death in Childbirth: an International Study of Maternal Care and Maternal Mortality 1800–1950* (Oxford: Clarendon Press, 1992), p. 53.
35. See L. Fleck (1979), op. cit., p. 118.

286 *Notes to pp. 115–22*

36. M. Foucault, 'Nietzsche, Genealogy, History', D. Bouchard (ed.), *Language, Counter-Memory, Practice, Selected Essays and Interviews* (Ithaca, NY: Cornell University Press, 1977), p. 142.
37. A. Gordon (1795), op. cit., p. 2.
38. Ibid., p. 30.
39. M. Foucault, *The Birth of the Clinic* (London: Tavistock, 1976), p. 140. There is an account of Broussais' work in *The Birth of the Clinic* and in I. Hacking, *The Taming of Chance* (Cambridge: Cambridge University Press, 1990).
40. A. Gordon (1795), op. cit., pp. 32–3.
41. Ibid.
42. M. Foucault (1976), op. cit.
43. I. Hacking (1990), op. cit., p. 82.
44. A. Gordon (1795), op. cit., pp. 5–7.
45. Ibid. Gordon distinguished between 'severe pain in the lower extremities' due to puerperal fever, which many women reported, and the pain of rheumatism, and the former too frequently being taken for rheumatism was another 'fatal cause of mistake', one that was usually attributed to nurses and midwives. See A. Gordon (1795), op. cit., p. 5. Later accounts of puerperal fever in the hospital context rarely mention the extreme pain that accompanies it.
46. The historical demographer, Thomas McKeown, argues that reaching conclusions on the extent of epidemic infectious disease in general from the seasonal distribution of deaths was a common fallacy historically but may nonetheless have had meaning in respect of nutritional status being jeopardised in winter. See T. McKeown, *The Origins of Human Disease* (Oxford: Basil Blackwell, 1988), p. 10. On the other hand, Irvine Loudon, in his reading of puerperal fever, has argued that there was a marked seasonality, at least in the late nineteenth and early twentieth centuries, where demographic evidence from England indicated that the peak time for death from puerperal fever and erysipelas was the winter. See I. Loudon (1992), op. cit., p. 536.
47. J. Clarke (1849), op. cit., p. 357.
48. M. Foucault (1976), op. cit., pp. 12–13.
49. A. Gordon (1795), op. cit., p. 4.
50. R. Collins (1836), op. cit., p. 384.
51. J. Clarke (1849), op. cit., p. 357.
52. Ibid.
53. A. Gordon (1795), op. cit., p. 36.
54. C. White, 'A Treatise on Pregnant and Lying-in Women', F. Churchill (ed.), *Collected Essays on Puerperal Fever* (London: Sydenham Society, 1849), pp. 205–7.
55. J. Lawson (1759), op. cit.
56. C. White (1849), op. cit., pp. 207–8.
57. J. Gélis (1991), op. cit., p. 248.
58. C. White (1849), op. cit., p. 212.
59. A. Gordon (1795), op. cit., p. 39.
60. F. Churchill (1849), op. cit., p. v.
61. Ibid., p. vi.
62. Ibid.
63. J. Clarke (1849), op. cit., p. 360. The lime would have been effective in destroying aerobic bacteria.
64. Ibid.; T. Kirkpatrick, H. Jellett, *The Book of the Rotunda Hospital* (London: Adlard and Son, Bartholomew Press, 1913), p. 109.

65. T. O'D. Browne (1947), op. cit., p. 102.
66. C. White (1849), op. cit., pp. 215–22.
67. Ibid., pp. 228–9.
68. F. Churchill (1849), op. cit., p. 216.
69. M. Poovey, *Uneven Developments: The Ideological Work of Gender in Mid-Victorian England* (Chicago: University of Chicago Press, 1988).
70. See L. Fleck (1979), op. cit.
71. J. Clarke (1849), op. cit., p. 362.
72. A. Gordon (1795), op. cit., p. 34.
73. Ibid., p. 51.
74. Ibid., p. 15.
75. Ibid., pp. 44–5. Bleeding or bloodletting was a general therapeutic tool of the period, the most common form of surgical operation, and not simply a part of childbirth. See R. Porter, *Cambridge Illustrated History of Medicine* (Cambridge: Cambridge University Press, 1996), pp. 207–8.
76. A. Gordon (1795), op. cit., p. 51.
77. See B. Duden, *The Woman Beneath the Skin: A Doctor's Patients in Eighteenth Century Germany* (Cambridge, MA: Harvard University Press, 1991).
78. Mercury was used from at least as early as the fourteenth century in the West as an embrocation to treat skin diseases and played a role in the ancient tradition of metallotherapy. Mercury also had an antiseptic action: used as a caustic, irritant or purgative, it was highly poisonous to bacteria and to humankind as well. See L. Fleck (1979), op. cit., p. 4.
79. I am indebted to Cecily Begley for these insights.
80. A. Gordon (1795), op. cit.
81. J. Clarke (1849), op. cit., p. 361.
82. J. Gélis (1991), op. cit., p. 250.
83. R. Collins (1836), op. cit., passim.
84. T. Beatty (1835), 'First report of the new lying-in hospital, Dublin for the year 1834', *Dublin Quarterly Journal of Medical Science*, vol. viii.
85. Ibid., p. 79.
86. Ibid., p. 81.
87. Ibid., p. 83.
88. Ibid.
89. A. Gordon (1795), op. cit., p. 25.
90. E. Shorter (1983), op. cit., p. 109.
91. A. Gordon (1795), op. cit., pp. 23–6.
92. M. Foucault (1976), op. cit., p. 56.
93. F. Churchill (1849), op. cit., p. 5.
94. J. Clarke (1817), 'Abstract of a registry kept for some years in the Lying-in Hospital in Dublin', *Transactions of the Association of Fellows and Licentiates of the King and Queen's College of Physicians*, vol. 1, 1817, Dublin, p. 367.
95. A. Gordon (1795), op. cit., p. 16.
96. On this, see Z. Bauman, *Mortality, Immortality and Other Life Strategies* (Cambridge: Polity Press, 1992), p. 159. Registering the cause of death became a required state practice in Ireland in 1864.
97. J. Clarke (1817), op. cit., pp. 367–8.
98. J. Clarke (1849), op. cit., p. 356.
99. See note 29 above on nosology.

288 *Notes to pp. 129–38*

100. A. Gordon (1795), op. cit., pp. 29–30.
101. M. Foucault (1976), op. cit., pp. 61–2.
102. Ibid., p. 144.
103. Ibid., pp. 88–9.
104. A. Gordon (1795), op. cit., p. 9.
105. Ibid., p. 18. Notice the gathering of colleagues for so important an opportunity as a dissection, in line with Bronfen's and Jordanova's analyses of the anatomist as the central actor.
106. Ibid., p. 36.
107. Ibid.
108. Ibid., p. 37.
109. Ibid.
110. Ibid., p. 56.
111. Ibid., p. 42.
112. Ibid., p. 23.
113. Ibid.
114. Ibid., p. 37.
115. Ibid., p. 63.
116. O. Holmes, 'The contagiousness of puerperal fever', H. Thoms (ed.), *Classical Contributions to Obstetrics and Gynecology* (Springfield, ILL: Charles C Thomas, 1935), p. 182.
117. F. Churchill (1849), op. cit., p. 40.
118. F. Churchill (1849), op. cit., pp. 40–1.
119. F. Churchill (1849), op. cit., p. 41.
120. Ibid.
121. Ibid.
122. Ibid.
123. Quoted in T. O'D. Browne (1947), op. cit., p. 133.
124. I.P. Semmelweis (1981), 'Childbed fever. Classics in infectious diseases', *Reviews of Infectious Diseases*, vol. 3, no. 4. July-August 1981, p. 811. Semmelweis' work is useful to read, if only for his observations like those on 'Street-births': 'parturients' who, on their way to the hospital, gave birth in the street but subsequently had a much lower rate of infection and death in the hospital. Semmelweis's conclusions on puerperal fever were confirmed for him by the death of his colleague, Kolletschka, who in the course of carrying out autopsies, was injured in his finger by the knife of one of the students and proceeded to develop symptoms similar to puerperal fever. The incident brings to mind Gordon's incomplete observation on this phenomenon.
125. T. O'D. Browne (1947), op. cit., p. 127.
126. Ibid.
127. E. Murphy (1857), 'Puerperal fever', *Dublin Quarterly Journal of Medical Science*, vol. xxiv, p. 19.
128. L. Fleck (1979), op. cit., pp. 29–30.
129. C. Herzlich and J. Pierret, *Illness and Self in Society* (Baltimore: Johns Hopkins University Press, 1987), p. 13.
130. Ibid.
131. L. Fleck (1979), op. cit., p. 20.
132. R. Collins (1836), op. cit., p. 380.
133. R. Collins (1849), *A Short Sketch of the Life and Writings of the late Joseph Clarke* (London: Longman, Brown, Green and Longman, 1849), p. 37.
134. R. Collins (1836), op. cit., p. 380.

135. A. Gordon (1795), op. cit., p. 2.
136. T. O'D. Browne (1947), p. 107.
137. Deploying a discourse so as to change the focus in this way, shifting to the conditions of poor women, is not dissimilar to the re-focusing of notions of contagion which have been part of the recent discourse on AIDS and the so-called 'AIDS' virus.
138. R. Collins (1836), op. cit., p. 387.
139. Quoted in F. Churchill (1849), 'Epidemics of puerperal fever', op. cit., p. 18. Note the reasons why the women are coming to hospital for food and shelter during childbirth.
140. D. Armstrong (1993), 'Public health spaces and the fabrication of identity', *Sociology*, vol. 27, no. 3, p. 395.
141. Ibid., pp. 396–8.
142. M. Poovey (1988), op. cit., p. 180.
143. Their success in so doing was limited by the marked lack of enthusiasm for physicians to attend lying-in cases as part of their work in the dispensary system. See entries in the Poor Law Commission, *Report of the Poor Law Commissioners on Medical Charities, Ireland Pursuant to the 46th Section of the Act 1 & 2 Victoria, C. 56*. With appendices and an index (Dublin: Alexander Thom, 1841).
144. J. Elliott (1867), 'Description and statistics of the Waterford Lying-In Hospital', *Dublin Quarterly Journal of Medical Science*, vol. xliv, November 1867. According to Elliott, this Waterford charity was an extension of a system of charitable relief and medical assistance in their own homes for poor lying-in women begun by the Society of Friends. A 'committee of ladies' was set up in 1838 to manage the new establishment and provide for its finance through voluntary contributions.
145. J. Elliott (1867), op. cit., p. 310.
146. D. Phelan (1867), 'Comparative Advantages of Attending Women in Lying-in Hospitals and their own Homes', *Dublin Quarterly Journal of Medical Science*, vol. xliii, February and May 1867.
147. Ibid., p. 76.
148. Ibid., pp. 81–2.
149. Ibid., p. 87. Phelan quotes Simon as saying that lying-in hospitals in England and Scotland were, for the most part, small and insignificant institutions and that the only lying-in hospital of real importance in Britain or Ireland was the Rotunda. So figures on the Rotunda about mortality were viewed as having special importance.
150. Shorter comments that women from poorer backgrounds, giving birth at home, died less frequently from sepsis than middle- or upper-class women and argues that this was due to acquired immunity. They were also less subject to the lethal microbes of the hospital environment. See E. Shorter (1983), op. cit., pp. 128–9.
151. M. Foucault (1976), op. cit. See also Chapter 1 above.
152. In many ways, this is how Catherine Dunne was read, as we shall see in detail in Chapter 5.
153. On how women expressed their fear of death from puerperal fever, see J. Gélis (1991), op. cit., p. 246; E. Shorter (1983), op. cit., p. 70; and I. Semmelweis (1981), op. cit., p. 808.
154. A. Gordon (1795), op. cit., pp. 22–3.
155. R. Porter, 'Death and the doctors in Georgian England', R. Houlbrooke (ed.), *Death, Ritual and Bereavement* (London: Routledge, 1989).
156. Ibid., pp. 91–3.
157. See I.P. Semmelweis (1981), op. cit.
158. J. Clarke (1817), op. cit., pp. 390–1.
159. R. Collins (1836), op. cit., p. 392.

160. J. Clarke (1849), op. cit., p. 358.
161. Ibid., p. 359.
162. R. Collins (1836), op. cit., p. 384.
163. Quoted in F. Churchill (1849), 'Epidemics of puerperal fever', op. cit., p. 18.
164. T. Beatty (1835), op. cit., p. 84.
165. D. Phelan (1867), op. cit., pp. 83–4.
166. E. Kennedy (1869), 'Zymotic diseases as more especially illustrated by puerperal fever', *Dublin Quarterly Journal of Medical Science*, vol. xlviii, February and May 1869, p. 271. The term 'zymotic', as used by Kennedy, broadened the definition of puerperal fever to include peritonitis, metritis, pleuritis, phlebitis, arthritis, pyaemia, purpuric or cerebro-spinal metria, traumatic metria, erysipelas, and hospital gangrene. He considered all these variants part of the same 'family' of zymotic disease. So he was also gathering under one classificatory heading most of the ways that puerperal fever manifested itself and attributing all deaths from all these causes to that heading rather than limiting it to peritonitis.
167. Ibid., p. 297.
168. Ibid., p. 288.
169. Ibid., p. 290.
170. Ibid., p. 294.
171. Dublin Obstetrical Society (1869), 'Proceedings: discussion on Dr Evory Kennedy's proposal', *Dublin Quarterly Journal of Medical Science*, vol. xlviii, August and November 1869.
172. Ibid., p. 294.
173. G. Johnston (1870), 'Clinical report of the Rotunda lying-in hospital for the year ending 5th November, 1869', *Dublin Quarterly Journal of Medical Science*, vol. xliv, February and May 1870, p. 108.
174. G. Johnston (1873), 'Clinical report of the Rotunda lying-in hospital for the year ending 5th November 1872', *Dublin Quarterly Journal of Medical Science*, vol. lv, January and June 1873, pp.182–3.
175. G. Johnston (1879), 'Clinical Report of 752 Cases of Forceps Delivery in Hospital Practice', *Dublin Quarterly Journal of Medical Science*, vol lxviii, January and June 1879, p. 44.
176. Ibid., p. 53.
177. J. Murphy-Lawless, 'The obstetric view of feminine identity: A case history of the use of forceps on unmarried women in 19th century Ireland', A. Todd and S. Fisher (eds.), *Gender and Discourse: The Power of Talk* (Norwood, NJ: Ablex, 1988), pp. 190–2.
178. G. Johnston (1873), op. cit., p. 207.
179. G. Johnston (1879), op. cit., p. 53. In this paper, delivered in 1878 on the usefulness of forceps, Johnston gave details on a few of the unmarried women who died: one had already attempted suicide before coming in. Another, he tells us, 'commenced drinking whiskey on finding she was pregnant. In this case there was sloughing of the perinaeum' (p. 45), Johnston reporting it as if the sloughing were the consequence of her whiskey drinking.
180. G. Johnston (1875), 'Clinical report of the Rotunda lying-in hospital for the year ending 5th November, 1874', *Dublin Quarterly Journal of Medical Science*, vol. lix, January and June 1875, pp. 157–8.
181. J. Lane (1887), 'Report of the Rotunda hospital for three years ending 3rd November, 1886', *Dublin Quarterly Journal of Medical Science*, vol. lxxxiv, p. 480. Outside the lying-in hospital, medical authorities and other institutions directly related to the state were equally unyielding on this question of mania. See the tragic case of Ellen

Owens, in Larne, County Antrim, in 1891, in J. Murphy-Lawless, 'Women and childbirth: the institutional experience', S. Deane (ed.), *The Field Day Anthology, Volume IV, Women in Ireland* (Field Day Publications in association with W.W. Norton, forthcoming), The issue of insanity in pregnancy and birth has been a long-running one. In 1937, Bethel Solomons and Ninian Falkiner in their seventh edition of *Tweedy's Practical Obstetrics* wrote that 'the insanities' of pregnancy, labour and the puerperium, an 'unfortunately common abnormality' occurred because reproduction was the 'test of a nervous woman' and should she 'be in any way mentally or physically weak, her brain may give way under the trial'. See B. Solomons and N. Falkiner, *Tweedy's Practical Obstetrics*, seventh edition (London: Oxford University Press, 1937), pp. 486–7.
182. D. Armstrong (1993), op. cit., p. 409.
183. Ibid.
184. R. Porter (1996), op. cit., p. 231.
185. Quoted in T. O'D. Browne (1947), op. cit., p. 140.
186. M. Foucault (1974), op. cit.
187. T. O'D. Browne (1947), op. cit., p. 120.
188. O.W. Holmes (1935), op. cit.
189. B. Latour, *The Pasteurisation of France* (Cambridge, MS: Harvard University Press, 1988), p. 28.
190. Ibid., p. 37.
191. Ibid., p. 46.
192. J. Lane (1887), 'Report of the Rotunda hospital for three years ending 3rd November, 1886', *Dublin Quarterly Journal of Medical Science*, vol. lxxxiv, p. 476.
193. Ibid., p. 482.
194. See T. O'D. Browne (1947), op. cit., p. 274.
195. Ibid., p. 145.
196. Ibid., p. 146.
197. E. Shorter (1983), op. cit., pp. 130–1. Marjorie Tew also makes the point about deaths from abortions. See M. Tew, *Safer Childbirth? A Critical History of Maternity Care* (London: Chapman and Hall, 1990), p. 203.
198. E. Shorter (1983), op. cit., pp. 132–3.
199. I. Loudon (1992), op. cit., pp. 82–4.
200. Ibid., pp. 295–360, 540–1. The first antibiotics in the form of Red Prontosil, a sulphonamide, were prescribed in the Rotunda in 1936.
201. J. Gélis (1991), op. cit., p. 250.
202. J.A. Musgrave (1932), 'The Role of the Midwife in the Public Health Service', *Irish Journal of Medical Science*, sixth series, no. 77, 1932, p. 205.
203. B. Solomons (1935), 'A letter on maternal mortality, 11 February, 1935', *British Medical Journal*, p. 10.
204. H. Jellett, *The Causes and Prevention of Maternal Mortality* (London: J. and A. Churchill, 1929), p. 227.
205. Ibid., pp. 228–9.
206. Ibid., p. 235.
207. Ibid.
208. J.A. Musgrave (1932), op. cit., p. 204.

Notes to Chapter 4

1. R. Collins, *A Practical Treatise on Midwifery containing the Results of Sixteen Thousand Six Hundred and Fifty-Four Births Occurring in the Dublin Lying-in hospital During a Period of Seven Years Commencing November 1826* (London: Longman, Rees, Orme, Browne, Green and Longman, 1836), p. 390.
2. I. Hacking, 'How should we do the history of statistics?,' G. Burchell, C. Gordon, and P. Miller (eds.), *The Foucault Effect: Studies in Governmentality* (Hemel Hempstead: Harvester Wheatsheaf, 1991).
3. M. Foucault, *The History of Sexuality, Volume 1: An Introduction* (Harmondsworth: Penguin, 1981), p. 139.
4. E. Kennedy (1869), 'Zymotic Diseases as more especially Illustrated by Puerperal Fever', *Dublin Quarterly Journal of Medical Science*, vol. xlviii, February and May 1869, p. 290.
5. This use of numerical data is explored in I. Hacking (1991), op. cit.
6. See B. Supple, *The Royal Exchange Assurance: A History of British Assurance* (London: Cambridge University Press, 1970); R. Porter, 'Death and the doctors in Georgian England', R. Houlbrooke (ed.), *Death, Ritual and Bereavement* (London: Routledge, 1989); I. Hacking, *The Taming of Chance* (Cambridge: Cambridge University Press, 1990).
7. M. Foucault, 'Neitzsche, genealogy, history', D. Bouchard (ed.), *Language, Counter-Memory, Practice, Selected Essays and Interviews* (Ithaca, NY: Cornell University Press, 1977), p. 97.
8. M. Foucault (1981), op. cit., p. 143.
9. Ibid, p. 15.
10. Quoted in I. Hacking (1990), op. cit., p. 53.
11. Ibid.
12. I. Hacking (1991), op. cit., pp. 182–3.
13. I. Hacking (1990), op. cit., p. 52.
14. I. Hacking (1991), op. cit., p. 181.
15. Ibid.
16. I. Hacking (1990), op. cit., p. 56.
17. T. Kuhn, *The Essential Tension: Selected Essays in Scientific Transition and Change* (Chicago: University of Chicago Press, 1977), p. 219.
18. I. Hacking (1990), op. cit., p. 63.
19. I. Hacking (1991), op. cit., p. 189.
20. E. Sinclair and G. Johnston (1858), *Practical Midwifery: comprising an account of 13,748 deliveries which occurred in the Dublin Lying-in Hospital during the course of seven years commencing November, 1847* (London: J. Churchill, 1858).
21. E. Shorter, *A History of Women's Bodies* (London: Allen Lane, 1983), p. 300; I. Loudon, *Death in Childbirth: an International Study of Maternal Care and Maternal Mortality 1800–1950* (Oxford: Clarendon Press, 1992).
22. H. Jellett, *The Causes and Prevention of Maternal Mortality* (London: J. and A. Churchill, 1929), pp. 228–32.
23. I. Hacking (1991), op. cit., p. 189.
24. G. Johnston (1879), 'Clinical Report of 752 Cases of Forceps Delivery in Hospital Practice', *Dublin Quarterly Journal of Medical Science*, vol. lxviii, January and June 1879, pp. 43–65.
25. Ibid., p. 53.

Notes to p. 165 293

26. This line drawing of Johnston's is remarkable for its complete denial of the actual violence done by forceps to maternal tissue, at such early stages of dilatation. It stands in contrast with the scientific realism/eroticised potential of the work of William Hunter (see note 135 in Chapter 2). Johnston's abstracted concentric circles efface the reality of what Gaskin describes as the 'multifolded skin' of the birth canal, the flaps and folds of the lips of the vagina, all infinitely variable in size and shape (I.M. Gaskin, *Spiritual Midwifery* (Summertown, TN: The Book Publishing Company, 1977), p. 296). It is an example of what Elaine Scarry terms the re-describing of injury to make it invisible. See E. Scarry, *The Body in Pain: The Making and Unmaking of the World* (New York: Oxford University Press, 1985).

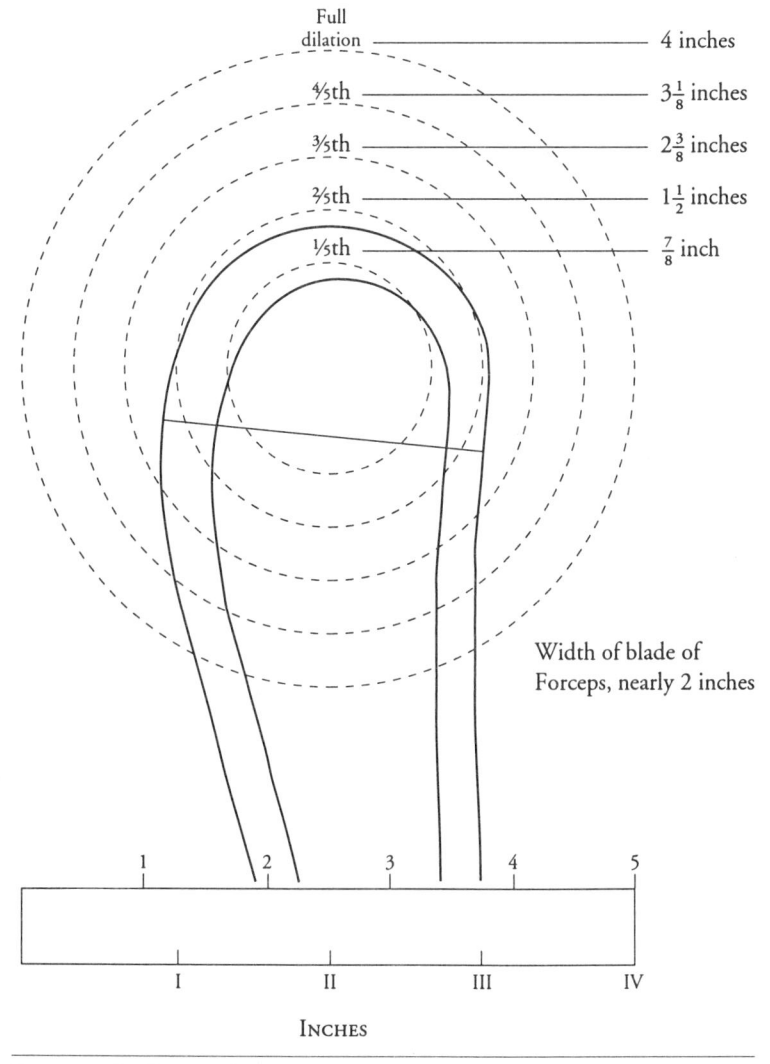

Full dilation — 4 inches
$4/5$th — $3\frac{1}{8}$ inches
$3/5$th — $2\frac{3}{8}$ inches
$2/5$th — $1\frac{1}{2}$ inches
$1/5$th — $\frac{7}{8}$ inch

Width of blade of Forceps, nearly 2 inches

INCHES

Degrees of Dilation of the os uteri

27. J. Clarke, (1817), 'Abstract of a registry kept for some years in the Lying-in Hospital in Dublin', *Transactions of the Association of Fellows and Licentiates of the King and Queen's College of Physicians*, vol. 1, 1817, Dublin, p. 399.
28. G. Johnston (1879), op. cit., p. 63. The comment came from one of Johnston's colleagues in the discussion following the presentation of his paper.
29. E. Scarry (1985), op. cit., p. 119.
30. G. Johnston (1879), op. cit.
31. Ibid., p. 56.
32. Ibid., p. 61.
33. Ibid. Not for the first time, but with damaging consequences, the obstetric concern with constructing a scientific category, in this instance comparability of data, pushes to the rear any analysis of intervention as a preventative practice in itself. And, long after Johnston's scheme of things has been consigned to a backroom of obstetric history, the potential of watchful waiting goes unrecognised by proponents of an interventionist model.
34. Ibid., pp. 58–9.
35. I. Hacking (1991), op. cit., p. 192.
36. G. Johnston (1879), op. cit., p. 64.
37. Quoted in I. Hacking (1991), op. cit., p. 185.
38. I. Hacking (1990), op. cit., p. 61.
39. M. Foucault (1977), op. cit., p. 191.
40. We have already looked at instances when the bodies of soldiers in warfare, torn and infected, exhibited the same symptoms and progression as women with puerperal fever without the connection being made that the same infective, irritating agent was entailed in both. It should also be noted that when men go 'mad' from their war wounds in the aftermath of war, there is some honour attached to it whereas when women go 'mad' after birth it is because of their inherent instability.
41. M. Foucault (1977), op. cit., p. 188.
42. I. Hacking (1990), op. cit., p. 168.
43. Ibid., p. 164.
44. Ibid.
45. Ibid.
46. G. Canguilhem, *The Normal and the Pathological* (New York: Zone Books, 1989), pp. 158–9.
47. Ibid.
48. I. Hacking (1990), op. cit., p. 172.
49. G. Canguilhem (1989), op. cit., p. 159. Canguilhem makes the point that one kind of social and cultural life can produce norms which another does not, so that statistical frequency expresses what he terms vital and social normativity. A human characteristic or trait is therefore not normal because it is frequent, but frequent because it is normal (p.160). He also comments that only a comparative physiology which could take into account the whole of life's intricacy, including social levels and types, could give a precise answer to these queries or hypotheses about average and normality and that such a study remains to be written (p. 163).
50. I. Hacking (1990), op. cit., p. 163.
51. F. Ewald, 'Insurance and risk', G. Burchell, C. Gordon, and P. Miller (eds.), *The Foucault Effect: Studies in Governmentality* (Hemel Hempstead: Harvester Wheatsheaf, 1991), p. 199;
52. M. Foucault, 'The dangerous individual', L. Kritzman (ed.), *Michel Foucault: Politics, Philosophy, Culture. Interviews and Other Writings, 1977–1984* (London: Routledge, 1988),

p. 149; K. Figlio, 'Unconscious aspects of health in the public sphere', B. Richards (ed.), *Crises of the Self: Further Essays on Psychoanalysis and Politics* (London: Free Association Press, 1989), p. 87.
53. F. Ewald (1991), op. cit.
54. Ibid.
55. Ibid., p. 203.
56. Ibid., p. 208.
57. R. Castel, 'From dangerousness to risk', G. Burchell, C. Gordon, and P. Miller (eds.), *The Foucault Effect: Studies in Governmentality* (Hemel Hempstead: Harvester Wheatsheaf, 1991), p. 287.
58. G. Johnston (1879), op. cit.
59. J. de Lee (1920), 'The prophylactic forceps operation', *American Journal of Obstetrics and Gynecology*, 1, pp. 34–44.
60. Ibid., p. 39. De Lee's article has drawings of the damage to the perineum from the foetal head that rival William Hunter's drawings for representational violence.
61. For an account of twilight sleep and its hallucinogenic effects, see J. Mitford, *The American Way of Birth* (London: Victor Gollancz, 1992), pp. 52–5.
62. Ibid., p. 110.
63. G. Johnston (1879), op. cit., p. 53.
64. The problem of what constitutes epidemiological data and how clinicians deal with such data as proof of causation is discussed by M. Wagner, *Pursuing the Birth Machine: The Search for Appropriate Birth Technology* (Sevenoaks, Kent: ACE Graphics, 1994), and D. Maine et al. (1995), 'Risks and rights: The uses of reproductive health data', *Reproductive Health Matters*, no. 6, November 1995.
65. See M. Wagner (1994), op. cit., pp. 97–9.
66. G. Johnston (1879), op. cit., p. 61. Churchill's figures are quoted by Kidd during the debate on Johnston's paper.
67. S. Inch, *Birthrights: A Parent's Guide to Modern Childbirth*, 2nd edition (London: Green Print, 1989).
68. S. Inch (1989), op. cit., pp. 28–31. Every single one of these categories requires close scrutiny. In relation to the measurable uses of medical antenatal check-ups and care to reduce mortality, see A. Oakley, *The Captured Womb: A History of the Medical Care of Pregnant Women* (Oxford: Basil Blackwell, 1984). There is a long-standing problem of women being allocated a socio-economic classification on the basis of her husband's occupation, not her own. On risks to women giving birth over forty, this has been substantively challenged by changing patterns of child-bearing amongst professional middle-class women in the United States. See F. Cunningham et al., *Williams Obstetrics, 19th Edition* (London: Prentice Hall International, 1993). There is an expanding literature on the issue of unnecessary forceps and Caesarean-section deliveries of which an early and influential book is *Silent Knife*; see N. Cohen and L. Estner, *Silent Knife: Cesarian Prevention and Vaginal Birth after Cesarian* (South Hadley, MS: Bergin and Garvey Publishers, 1983).
69. See for example Ireland, Department of Health, *Perinatal Statistics, 1991*, p. 41. Table 18 on perinatal mortality rates indicates that babies born to women from higher professional groups have the best perinatal outcomes.
70. For a critique of antenatal care as an unevaluated system of organisation rather than as a relevant approach to maternal health, see M. Wagner (1994), op. cit. and M. McDonagh (1996), 'Is antenatal care effective in reducing maternal morbidity and mortality?', *Health Policy and Planning*, vol. 11, no. 1, pp. 1–15.

71. The safety of routine ultrasound and its relationship to intra-uterine foetal-growth retardation is being raised in the literature more and more. See M. Wagner (1994), op. cit. for a review of the debate. Two large-scale studies released in 1993, one in Australia and one in the United States, have questioned its usefulness in detecting abnormal babies and in contributing to growth restriction; see *Guardian Weekly*, 26 September 1993, 'Study questions routine use of ultrasound in pregnancy'; *Independent*, 8 October 1993, 'Ultrasound may harm foetuses'.
72. For a discussion on this self-created problem within obstetrics, see M. Enkin, M. Keirse, M. Renfrew and J. Neilson, *A Guide to Effective Care in Pregnancy and Childbirth*, 2nd edition (Oxford: Oxford University Press, 1995), pp. 142–4.
73. D. Maine et al. (1995), op. cit.
74. M. Douglas and A. Wildavsky, *Risk and Culture: An Essay on the Selection of Technological and Environmental Dangers* (Berkeley: University of California Press, 1982).
75. The famous Mrs Delaney, born in England and married to Swift's friend and biographer, Revd Delaney, is credited in the *Oxford English Dictionary* with the first use of the word confinement in relation to childbirth. In terms of modernity's commitment to surveillance, it is no surprise that the use of the word first surfaces in the 1770s.
76. On this, see W. Moore, 'Antenatal care and the choice of place of birth', S. Kitzinger and J. Davis (eds.), *The Place of Birth* (Oxford: Oxford Medical Publications, 1978); M. Richards, 'Place of safety? An examination of the risks of hospital delivery', S. Kitzinger and J. Davis (eds.), op. cit.
77. M. Douglas and A. Wildavsky (1982), op. cit., pp. 5–6.
78. M. Wagner (1994), op. cit., p. 134.
79. I. Hacking (1990), op. cit., p. 20.
80. T.E. Beatty (1842), 'Contributions to midwifery, IV: cases illustrative of the use of forceps', *Dublin Quarterly Journal of Medical Science*, vol. xxi, January to July 1842, p. 343.
81. Note the absence of any mention of the child, common in an era before improved social conditions had been able to make any impression on the rates of infant mortality and before perinatal medicine could begin to build a discipline on the basis of these social improvements. See also T. McKeown, *The Origins of Human Disease* (Oxford: Basil Blackwell, 1988).
82. T.E. Beatty (1842), op. cit., p. 341.
83. I am dealing here only with post-partum haemorrhage relating to the placental site during this final phase of labour, and in the immediate period after expulsion of the placenta. This is the most common type of post-partum haemorrhage and potentially the most serious.
84. J. Gélis, *History of Childbirth: Fertility, Pregnancy and Birth in Early Modern Europe* (Cambridge: Polity Press, 1991), p. 162. Within living memory in inner-city Dublin, women who often gave birth at home in areas like Sheriff Street and Sean McDermott Street with the assistance of a local woman and the help of neighbours, recall that the placenta, once delivered, was wrapped in paper and thrown on the fire to be burned. When it gave out nine cracks from the heat of the flames, it was taken as an indication that the placenta had come out whole and that the woman was therefore safe from haemorrhage. See North Inner City Folklore Project, *Living in the City* (Dublin: Mount Salus Press, 1991), p. 19.
85. See Plato, *Timaeus*, translated by H. Lee (Harmondsworth: Penguin, 1965).
86. J. Gélis (1991), op. cit., p. 163.
87. Ibid., p. 162.

88. Quoted in E. Nihell (1760), *A Treatise on the Art of Midwifery: Setting Forth Various Abuses Therein, Especially as to the Practice of Instruments* (London: Haymarket, 1760), p. 129.
89. G. de la Motte, *A General Treatise of Midwifery*, 1985 reprint (New York: Garland, 1746), pp. 465–6.
90. H. Deventer, *The Art of Midwifery Improv'd* (London: E. Curll, J. Pemberton and W. Taylor, 1716), p. 91.
91. F. Ould, *A Treatise of Midwifry in Three Parts* (Dublin: Oli. Nelson and Charles Connor, 1742), pp. 57–8.
92. T. Southwell (1742), *Remarks on some of the Errors both in Anatomy and Practice in a late Treatise of Midwifery by Fielding Ould, Man-midwife* (Dublin: Thomas Bacon, 1742).
93. E. Nihell (1760), op. cit., pp. 262–5. By 'precautionary bleeding', Nihell is referring to the practice of venesection.
94. Ibid.
95. J. Harvie, 'Delivery of the placenta', H. Thoms (ed.), *Classical Contributions to Obstetrics and Gynecology* (Springfield, ILL: Charles C Thomas, 1935).
96. Ibid., p. 135.
97. Ibid., p. 136.
98. Ibid., p. 137.
99. E. Nihell (1760), op. cit., p. 264.
100. J. Clarke (1817), op. cit., p. 381.
101. Ibid., p. 369.
102. Ibid. Of course it may be that Clarke permitted women to lose more blood than other practitioners before diagnosing a post-partum haemorrhage, which would also have contributed to his low numbers. But if he did so, he moved from a position of cautious and conservative practice which appears to have distinguished his approach to obstetric care in general. It is not mentioned in Clarke's writing whether, during this two-hour waiting period, women were breast-feeding which would have stimulated contractions. The efficacy of feeding-induced contractions would have been part of a more complete model of delivering the placenta.
103. E. Sinclair and G. Johnston (1858), op. cit.
104. Ibid.
105. T.E. Beatty (1834), 'Contributions to midwifery', *Dublin Quarterly Journal of Medical Science*, vol. iv, p. 339.
106. T.E. Beatty (1834), op. cit., p. 334. This last says much about the lack of control over her labour a woman had in the hospital setting and the lack of communication between her and her birth attendants, that a piece of cloth was meant to tell her what point the baby had reached in the delivery process.
107. R. Collins (1836), op. cit.
108. E. Shorter (1983), op. cit., p. 94.
109. Placenta praevia is a condition where the placenta is implanted in the lower part of the uterus, partially or totally covering the entrance to the birth canal. As the uterus stretches in labour, it results in haemorrhage.
110. Churchill did not even refer to 'patients' but always used the term 'females' in his reports. Several sets of Churchill's case notes are on instances of retained placenta and haemorrhage which took place outside and he lavishes blame on both the 'stupidity of the female attendants' and also on the women giving birth themselves, in one instance, giving the second-hand account of a woman who got out of bed after a manual removal at home by one of the hospital men midwives, Mr Speedy, quarrelled

with her lodgers, drank some punch, laid down and died later that night. See F. Churchill (1838), 'Second medical report of the Western lying-in hospital and dispensary, 31 Arran Quay' *Dublin Quarterly Journal of Medical Science*, vol. xiii, p. 245.
111. Quoted in H. Jellet (1900), 'The Dublin Method of Effecting the Delivery of the Placenta', *Dublin Journal of Medical Science*, vol. cix, p. 418.
112. Ibid.
113. Ibid., p. 422.
114. E. Shorter (1983), op. cit. Ergot frequently produced toxic symptoms and, in the Middle Ages, when people could only obtain bread made from infected grain, the resultant epidemics were known as St Anthony's Fire, where the extremities were affected: hands and feet burned and the face reddened due to spasms of the blood vessels, the syndrome leading to gangrene. In another form, the central nervous system could also be affected leading to convulsions.
115. J. Stearns, 'The introduction of ergot', H. Thoms (ed.), *Classical Contributions to Obstetrics and Gynecology* (Springfield, ILL: Charles C. Thomas, 1935), p. 22.
116. L. Atthill (1879), 'Report and clinical records of the Rotunda hospital for the year ending 5th November 1878', *Dublin Quarterly Journal of Medical Science*, vol. lxviii, July to December 1879, pp. 333–7.
117. M. Tew, *Safer Childbirth? A Critical History of Maternity Care* (London: Chapman and Hall, 1990), pp. 210–14.
118. G. Tierney (1933), 'Maternal Mortality', *Irish Journal of Medical Science*, sixth series, no. 82, p. 603.
119. S. Inch (1989), op. cit., p. 147.
120. C. Begley (1990), op. cit., p. 4.
121. E.H. Tweedy (1909), 'Clinical reports of the Rotunda hospital', *Dublin Journal of Medical Science*, vol. cxxviii, p. 27.
122. See D. Llewellyn-Jones, *Fundamentals of Obstetrics and Gynaecology*, vol. 1 (London: Faber and Faber, 1969), p. 303.
123. C. Begley (1990), op. cit.; B. Kwast (1991), 'Postpartum haemorrhage: its contribution to maternal mortality', *Midwifery*, vol. 7, 1991, pp. 64–70. The current international definition for primary post-partum haemorrhage is set at a measurable blood loss of 500 millilitres or over. See WHO, *The Prevention and Management of Post-partum Haemorrhage. Report of a Technical Working Group, Geneva, 3–6 July, 1989* (WHO/MCH/90.7. Geneva, 1990).
124. See B. Kwast (1991), op. cit. and B. Hibbard, *Principles of Obstetrics* (London: Butterworths, 1988).
125. D. Maine et al. (1995), op. cit.; B. Kwast (1991), op. cit. Kwast argues that many of these are not specific enough for purposes of screening. Such predisposing factors are seldom present in more than a third of women who experience post-partum haemorrhage. See B. Hibbard (1988), op. cit., p. 676. Sheila Kitzinger has argued that, for obstetrics, the diagnosis of a pathology, even if it is a provisional diagnosis like the possibility of a post-partum haemorrhage, is preferable to missing a diagnosis which should have been made (S. Kitzinger, 'Why women need midwives', S. Kitzinger (ed.), *The Midwife Challenge* (London: Pandora Press, 1988), p. 15). This line of action perhaps also reveals the inherent lack of belief in its own enterprise for obstetrics, never quite trusting its capacity to respond to the crisis it makes of childbirth.
126. T. Lewis and G. Chamberlain, *Obstetrics by Ten Teachers*, 15th edition (London: Edward Arnold, 1990), pp. 170–1.

127. G.M.L. Gyte (1994), 'Evaluation of the meta-analyses on the effects, on both mother and baby, of the various components of "active" management of the third stage of labour', *Midwifery*, vol. 10, pp. 183–99; B. Hibbard (1988), op. cit., pp. 468–9; F. Cunningham et al. (1993), op. cit., pp. 384–5.
128. B. Hibbard (1988), op. cit., pp. 469, 678; F. Cunningham et al. (1993), op. cit., p. 385.
129. If the cord is not cut, the placenta remains turgid and full, so that it shrinks off the contracting uterus very quickly.
130. S. Inch (1989), op. cit., p. 150.
131. Quoted in S. Inch (1989), op. cit., p. 157.
132. Ibid., pp. 151–3; C. Begley (1990), op. cit., p. 4.
133. F. Cunningham et al. (1993), op. cit., p. 616.
134. C. Begley (1990), op. cit., pp. 4–5, 13–15.
135. S. Inch (1989), op. cit., p. 174.
136. Ibid., pp. 166–9.
137. Ibid., pp. 151–2.
138. Ibid., pp. 164–5; G.M.L. Gyte (1994), op. cit., p. 194.
139. M.C. Botha (1968), 'The management of the umbilical cord in labour', *South African Journal of Obstetrics and Gynecology*, vol. 16, no. 2; M. Enkin, M. Keirse, M. Renfrew and J. Neilson (1995), op. cit., p. 239.
140. S. Inch (1989), op. cit., p. 65. Inch suggests that this may be because the uterine muscle, once exposed to high levels of oxytocin, responds poorly to yet another oxytocic dose in the third stage.
141. M. le Doeuff (1981), 'Pierre Roussel's chiasmas: from imaginary knowledge to the learned imagination', *Ideology and Consciousness*, no. 9. 1981–2.
142. J.A. Feeney (1955), 'The grand multipara: trauma of labour', *Journal of the Irish Medical Association*, January–June 1955.
143. Ibid., p. 12.
144. M. Enkin et al. (1995), op. cit., pp. 3–9.
145. Ibid., pp. 236–7.
146. G. Canguilhem (1989), op. cit., p. 163.
147. C. Begley (1990), op. cit., p. 5.
148. M. Tew (1990), op. cit., p. 213.
149. C. Begley (1990), op. cit., p. 4.
150. T. McKeown (1988), op. cit., p. 78.
151. Whereas 25 per cent of women of reproductive age live in developed countries, only 1 per cent of the world-wide totals of maternal deaths occur in these countries. See D. Maine, *Safe Motherhood Programs: Options and Issues* (Prevention of Maternal Mortality Program, Center for Population and Family Health, Columbia University: New York, 1991), p. 6.
152. See A. Oakley, 'Wisewoman and medicine man', J. Mitchell and A. Oakley (eds.), *The Rights and Wrongs of Women* (Harmondsworth: Penguin, 1976); T. McKeown (1988), op. cit.; M. Tew (1990), op. cit.; N. Dye, 'The history of the relationship between women's health and technology', J. Rodin and A. Collins (eds.), *Women and New Reproductive Technologies: Medical, Psychosocial, Legal and Ethical Dilemmas*. (Hillsdale, NJ: Lawrence Erlbaum Associates, 1991); N. Leap and B. Hunter, *The Midwife's Tale: An Oral History from Handywoman to Professional Midwife* (London: Scarlet Press, 1993).
153. M. Tew (1990), op. cit.; R. Campbell and A. Macfarlane, *Where to be Born?* 2nd edition (Oxford: Crown Publications for National Perinatal Epidemiology Unit, 1995).

154. N. Dye (1991), op. cit., pp. 18–19. Dye comments that as contracted pelves went out of fashion as a reason for using the Caesarean section, the more statistically measurable notion of cephalo-pelvic disproportion came in to use to sustain the Caesarean operation as a mode of intervention, yet another categorisation founded on the ideology of the normal.
155. M. Tew (1990), op. cit., pp. 204–6.
156. Ibid., pp. 209–10.
157. M. Wagner (1994), op. cit., pp. 12–14. See also WHO *Having a Baby in Europe, Public Health in Europe, Number 26* (Copenhagen, 1985).
158. E. Shorter (1983), op. cit.
159. Ibid.
160. I. Loudon (1992), op. cit., p. 517.
161. Ibid.
162. Ibid., pp. 4–5.
163. Ibid.
164. I. Hacking (1991), op. cit., p. 186.
165. David Armstrong (1986), and Peter Wright (1988), have referred to maternal and perinatal mortality rates as artefacts, as an out-of-focus picture of reality, because they are so context-bound and therefore can be so ambiguous. See D. Armstrong (1986), 'The invention of infant mortality', *Sociology of Health and Illness*, vol. 8, no. 3, pp. 211–32; P .Wright, 'Babyhood: the social construction of infant care as a medical problem in the years around 1900', M. Lock and D. Gordon (eds.), *Biomedicine Examined* (Dordrecht, The Netherlands: Kluwer Academic Publishers, 1988). The anthropologists Patricia Kaufert and John O'Neil have referred to such rates in relation to childbirth as statistical conceits (P. Kaufert and J. O'Neil, 'Analysis of a dialogue on risks in childbirth: clinicians, epidemiologists and Inuit women.', S. Lindenbaum and M. Lock (eds.), *Knowledge, Power and Practice: The Anthropology of Medicine and Everyday Life* (Berkeley: University of California Press, 1993), p. 45). Perhaps the major difficulty for all death rates is the impossibility of truly being able to express context and thus to know what is being measured.
166. I. Loudon (1992), op. cit., p. 5.
167. See G. Canguilhem (1989), op. cit. and C. MacCormack, 'Nature, culture and gender: a critique', C. MacCormack and M. Strathern (eds.), *Nature, Culture and Gender* (Cambridge: Cambridge University Press, 1980).
168. Ireland, Department of Health (1995), *Developing a Policy for Women's Health*. For an analysis of the demise of the community midwife see J. Colgan, *The Marginalisation of the Dublin Community Midwife: 1950–1973*, unpublished MA thesis, Women's Studies, UCD, 1992.
169. M. Foucault, 'Body/Power', C. Gordon (ed.), *Power/Knowledge: Selected Interviews and Other Writings 1972–77* (Brighton: Harvester Wheatsheaf, 1980), p. 58.
170. L. Code, *Rhetorical Spaces: Essays on Gendered Locations* (London: Routledge, 1995).

Notes to Chapter 5

1. K. O'Driscoll and D. Meagher, *Active Management of Labour*, second edition (London: Baillière Tindall, 1986), pp. 90–1.
2. See W. Savage, *A Savage Enquiry: Who Controls Childbirth* (London: Virago, 1986). Savage was dismissed from her post as consultant obstetrician at Mile End Hospital in London by Grudzinskas for mismanagement of five cases where she was said to have

put women and their babies at risk in labour by inappropriate management during pregnancy and by allowing labour to proceed without intervention, in circumstances where the clinical protocols would have indicated Caesarean section rather than a trial of labour. She was cleared of all charges and subsequently reinstated.
3. L. Code, *Rhetorical Spaces: Essays on Gendered Locations* (London: Routledge, 1995), p. 44.
4. E. Shorter, *A History of Women's Bodies* (London: Allen Lane, 1983).
5. G. Dick-Read, *Childbirth Without Fear: The Principles and Practice of Natural Childbirth*, 5th edition (London: Pan Books, 1969), p. 185.
6. Their perspectives were not without difficulties, both on the issue of women as a 'natural' entity, which was Odent's model, and on the issue of what constitutes 'normal'. Savage, for example, argued that a breech delivery does not constitute a normal straightforward delivery and should be overseen by a doctor rather than a midwife. See W. Savage (1986), op. cit., p. 37.
7. P. Huntingford (1984), 'Birth Right: The parent's choice', British Broadcasting Corporation. See also Foreword in S. Inch, *Birthrights*, first edition (London: Hutchinson, 1982), pp. 9–11.
8. See WHO, *Having a Baby in Europe, Public Health in Europe*, no. 26, (Copenhagen: WHO Regional Office for Europe, 1985). See also Appendices on the 1980s WHO conferences on appropriate birth technologies in M. Wagner, *Pursuing the Birth Machine: The Search for Appropriate Birth Technology* (Sevenoaks, Kent: ACE Graphics, 1994).
9. R. Campbell and A. Macfarlane, *Where to Be Born?* 2nd edition (Oxford: Crown Publications for National Perinatal Epidemiology Unit, 1995).
10. See I. Chalmers et al., *Effective Care in Pregnancy and Childbirth* (Oxford: Oxford University Press, 1989).
11. M. Wagner (1994), op. cit., p. 98.
12. L. Silverton, *The Art and Science of Midwifery* (London: Prentice Hall, 1993), pp. 253–4.
13. Ibid.
14. M. Wagner (1994), op. cit., p. 99.
15. M. Enkin et al., *A Guide to Effective Care in Pregnancy and Childbirth*, 2nd edition (Oxford: Oxford University Press, 1995), pp. 210–14.
16. L. Silverton (1993), op. cit.
17. Ibid., p. 261.
18. Ibid.
19. A. Oakley and H. Graham, 'Competing ideologies of reproduction: medical and maternal perspectives on pregnancy', H. Roberts (ed.), *Women, Health and Reproduction* (London: Routledge and Kegan Paul, 1981), p. 53.
20. T. Lewis and G. Chamberlain, *Obstetrics by Ten Teachers*, 15th edition (London: Edward Arnold, 1990), p. 162.
21. H. Deventer, *The Art of Midwifery Improv'd* (London: E. Curll, J. Pemberton and W. Taylor, 1716), p. 131.
22. E. Nihell, *A Treatise on the Art of Midwifery: Setting Forth Various Abuses Therein, Especially as to the Practice of Instruments* (London: Haymarket, 1760), p. 322.
23. S. Inch, *Birthrights: A Parent's Guide to Modern Childbirth*, 2nd edition (London: Green Print, 1989), p. 57.
24. Ibid. pp. 82–3.
25. Ibid. An extensive series of studies in Latin America in the 1960s and 1970s concluded that four factors – an upright position in labour, ambulatory labour where the woman was free to walk, the membranes being allowed to rupture in their own time, and a

vertical position for delivery – resulted in less pain for women, less pressure on the foetal head and shorter labours. See R. Caldeyro-Barcia (1960), 'Effect of position changes on the intensity and the frequency of uterine contractions during labour', *American Journal of Obstetrics and Gynecology*, 80; A.G. Diaz et al. (1980), 'Vertical position during the first stage of the course of labour and neonatal outcome', *European Journal of Obstetrics and Gynaecology*, vol. 11, no.1; R. Schwarcz et al. (1976), 'Influence of amniotomy and maternal position on labour', *Proceedings of the VIII World Congress of Gynaecology and Obstetrics* (Amsterdam: Excerpta Medica).

26. This was also known as the 'English method'. See A. Oakley, *The Captured Womb: A History of the Medical Care of Pregnant Women* (Oxford: Basil Blackwell, 1984), p. 196.
27. L. Atthill (1879), 'Report and clinical records of the Rotunda hospital for the year ending 5th November, 1878', *Dublin Quarterly Journal of Medical Science*, vol. lxviii, July to December 1879.
28. A. Oakley (1984), op. cit., p. 197.
29. Ibid., p. 189.
30. Ibid., pp. 200–1; S. Inch (1989), op. cit., pp. 148–9.
31. B. Solomons (1933), 'Report of the Rotunda Hospital (November 1st 1931 to October 31st 1932)', *Irish Journal of Medical Science*, no. 92, August 1933, p. 174.
32. A. Oakley (1984), op. cit., p. 201; S. Inch (1989), op. cit., p. 148.
33. Ibid.
34. S. Inch (1989), op. cit., p. 148. The language used to set out the causes of prolonged labour in a 1960s' text is instructive, as ever. Doctors are urged to remember the 'four Ps: faults in the powers; faults in the passenger; faults in the passages; and faults in the patient's personality', see D. Llewellyn-Jones, *Fundamentals of Obstetrics and Gynaecology, Volume I* (London: Faber and Faber, 1969), p. 275.
35. A. Oakley (1984), op. cit., p. 207.
36. E. Shorter, *A History of Women's Bodies* (London: Allen Lane, 1983), pp. 164–5.
37. A. Oakley (1984), op. cit., p. 207.
38. A. Oakley, *From Here to Maternity: Becoming a Mother* (Oxford: Martin Robertson, 1979); A. Oakley, *Women Confined: Towards a Sociology of Childbirth* (Oxford: Martin Robertson, 1980); A. Cartwright, *The Dignity of Labour? A Study of Childbearing and Induction* (London: Tavistock, 1979).
39. K. O'Driscoll and D. Meagher (1986), op. cit., p. 181.
40. A. Oakley (1984), op. cit., pp. 206–7; A. Cartwright (1979), op. cit.
41. S. Kitzinger, *The Experience of Childbirth*, third edition (Harmondsworth: Penguin, 1972), pp. 153–4.
42. See M. Tew, *Safer Childbirth? A Critical History of Maternity Care* (London: Chapman and Hall, 1990), pp. 155–8.
43. House of Commons, Social Services Committee, *Second Report from the Social Services Committee, Session 1979–80, Perinatal and Neonatal Mortality*, vol. 1 (London: HMSO, 1980), p. 1.
44. See P. Kennedy, 'Between the lines: mother and infant care in Ireland', P. Kennedy and J. Murphy-Lawless (eds.), *Returning Birth to Women: Challenging Policies and Practices*, (Dublin: Centre for Women's Studies, TCD/WERRC, 1998).
45. House of Commons, Health Committee, *Second Report, Session 1991–2, Maternity Services*, vol. 1, p. ix, 1992.
46. On the growth of maternity-care pressure groups in the English context, see L. Durward and R. Evans, 'Pressure groups and maternity care', J. Garcia et al. (eds.), *The Politics of Maternity Care: Services for Childbearing Women in Twentieth Century*

Britain (Oxford: Oxford University Press, 1990), pp. 256–73. The comparable groups in Ireland date from the late 1970s: AIMS, Cuidú, the Irish Childbirth Trust, and the Home Birth Centre.

47. C. Flint, *Sensitive Midwifery* (London: Heinemann Medical Books, 1986); S. Kitzinger, 'Why women need midwives', S. Kitzinger (ed.), *The Midwife Challenge* (London: Pandora Press, 1988); Inch (1989), op. cit.
48. S. Inch (1989), op. cit., pp. 113–14, 244.
49. A. Oakley (1980), op. cit., pp. 123–4, 146–51, 305.
50. See T. Chard and M. Richards, *Benefits and Hazards of the New Obstetrics* (London: Heinemann, 1977); I. Chalmers, 'Implications of the current debate on obstetric practice', S. Kitzinger and J. Davis (eds.), *The Place of Birth* (Oxford: Oxford University Press, 1978).
51. K. O'Driscoll and D. Meagher (1986), op. cit.
52. See F. Cunningham et al., *Williams Obstetrics, 19th Edition* (London: Prentice Hall International, 1993), pp. 378–9, for a debate on differences in the system as applied elsewhere. There are variations even in the clinical system in the National Maternity Hospital, which is what was indicated in the Dunnes' defence, although from the text of active management, we would be led to believe that the system has been a single coherent whole from 1963 onwards. See also G. Kerrigan, *Nothing But the Truth* (Dublin: Tomar Press, 1990).
53. R. Collins (1837), 'Observations on the artificial dilatation of the mouth of the womb during labour, and upon instrumental delivery', *Dublin Quarterly Journal of Medical Science*, vol. xi, p. 40.
54. K. O'Driscoll and D. Meagher (1986), op. cit., p. 5. This argument is particularly geared to women giving birth for the first time; for the woman who has already given birth, O'Driscoll argues that there is a comparatively short duration of labour. K. O'Driscoll and D. Meagher (1986), op. cit., p. 11.
55. K. O'Driscoll and D. Meagher (1986), op. cit., p. 4. All three editions of the book have referred to midwives as 'nurses' or 'obstetric nurses' and the authors state that 'nurses and midwives are synonymous'. This appears to be a clear endeavour to downgrade midwifery as a professional specialism in its own right and to 'engender' the work of midwives in the most essentialist form possible. In the chapter on the role of the nurse, emphasis is placed on the senior nurse in charge knowing the limits of her authority, while for junior nurses, the emphasis is on how to properly instruct them to maintain personal contact with the woman in labour. The junior nurse's task, in addition to recording all information on the woman's partogram or chart, is to tend to all the emotional work of labour: 'In our experience *young properly motivated girls* [my italics] perform this task with remarkable success.' K. O'Driscoll and D. Meagher (1986), op. cit., p. 56. The authors also argue that, with regard to active management, the nurse/midwife role in it has given a 'boost' to 'the professional status of nurses', ibid., p. 87. But the reality is that midwives are reduced under this system to the equivalent of shop-floor supervisors, with their most important task being the measurement of dilatation.
56. Ibid., pp. 1–2.
57. K. O'Driscoll, D. Meagher and P. Boylan, *Active Management of Labour*, third edition, (Aylesbury, England: Mosby Year Book Europe Ltd, 1993), p. 15. This paragraph in the third edition, written with the addition of Peter Boylan, Master from 1991–1998 to the authors' team, has been written in the present tense rather than the past tense and has added the qualifier 'completely' to the sentence on 'normal' women.

58. K. O'Driscoll and D. Meagher (1986), op. cit., p. 2.
59. One of the principal appeals of active management over induction is O'Driscoll's claim that the rate of Caesarean section can be held below 5 per cent (ibid., p. 2). He argues that Caesarean section rates 'are currently the most realistic objective measurement of the standard of obstetric care afforded to mothers [*sic*], replacing maternal mortality rates', ibid., pp. 2–3. In the second edition, the section rate is quoted as 'below 5 per cent', ibid., p. 108. In the third edition, in 1993, a section rate is not specifically quoted at this point in the text, the phrase being instead 'the incidence of which has shown little change over these [twenty-five] years', K. O'Driscoll, D. Meagher and P. Boylan (1993), op. cit., p. 14. In the third edition, the Caesarean section rate is listed as 8 per cent, ibid., p. 190. However, in an interview with the Association for Improvements in the Maternity Services, in 1992, Boylan admitted the rate was as high as 10 per cent. Letters to the Editor, 'Managing Labour', *Irish Times*, 10 February 1992. The appendix on clinical data includes what it terms 'obstetrical norms in primigravidae', norm here being used in the sense of an ideal to attain. The 'norm' in relation to section rates is 5 per cent. See K. O'Driscoll, D. Meagher and P. Boylan (1993), op. cit., pp. 208–9.
60. K. O'Driscoll and D. Meagher (1986), op. cit., p. 111.
61. Ibid., p. 108.
62. Ibid., p. 191.
63. Ibid., pp.190–1. O'Driscoll's model, including artificial rupture of membranes before moving on to acceleration or augmentation of labour by oxytocin, is an invasive one for women. But so is the model of management based on Caesarean section to resolve the problem of dystocic labour. The models and the debates about this problem provide another example of the hotly contested space surrounding women and the importance given over to securing personal and institutional reputations. See F. Cunningham *et al.* (1993), op. cit. on dystocic labour. The British Institute of Epidemiology and Health Services Research, on the basis of its evaluations, has declared that although continuous professional support is an excellent basis for labour management, the routine use of amniotomy and early oxytocin is not justified in respect of perinatal outcomes. *Guardian Weekly*, 14 August 1994, 'Births study downgrades "artificial" aids'.
64. K. O'Driscoll and D. Meagher (1986), op. cit., p. 108.
65. Ibid., p. 108.
66. All the groups have run newsletters.
67. On this issue, see D. Eyer, *Mother-Infant Bonding: A Scientific Fiction* (Woburn, Massachusetts: Yale University Press, 1992). Whatever the rationale of bonding, an unintended consequence was the removal of an aspect of hospitalised childbirth heavily criticised by childbirth groups, namely that their babies were taken to a central nursery after birth. In the 1940s, women were held to be so dangerous to their babies in the post-partum period that forcible separation was the norm. Eyer makes the point that mother–infant bonding – while returning a woman's baby to her in hospital – has been done within the context of a regime where women have lost control over their labours in any case. Oakley's findings on postnatal depression in the wake of a technological hospital birth confirm what Eyer suggests – that mothers lose control over labour within hospitals but that if they experience depression in the postnatal period as a result, bonding theory increases their sense of guilt that they are failing their baby because of their depression.
68. M.H. Klaus et al. (1994), 'The Dublin experience', *Mothering*, no. 72, fall 1994, p. 68.

69. Ibid.
70. See K. O'Driscoll (1972), 'Impact of active management on delivery unit practice', *Proceedings of the Royal Society of Medicine*, vol. 65, August 1992, pp. 697–8. In the book published to celebrate the hospital's centenary, the author points out that although forty-four more beds had been added to the hospital in 1967, by 1973, the hospital was handling 40 per cent more births than in 1963, the first year of O'Driscoll's mastership, and this was only possible because of the 'techniques of active management'. See T. Farmar, *Holles Street, 1894–1994: The National Maternity Hospital – A Centenary History* (Dublin: A. and A. Farmar, 1994), p. 165.
71. K. O'Driscoll and D. Meagher (1986), op. cit., p. 4.
72. M. Foucault, *Discipline and Punish: the Birth of the Prison*. (Harmondsworth: Penguin, 1979).
73. Ibid., p. 138.
74. S. Bartky, 'Foucault, femininity, and the modernization of patriarchal power', I. Diamond and L. Quinby (eds.), *Feminism and Foucault: Reflections on Resistance* (Boston: Northeastern University Press, 1988), pp. 62–3.
75. K. O'Driscoll and D. Meagher (1986), op. cit., pp. 32–3. In the systematic review of obstetric care known as *Effective care in pregnancy and childbirth*, the authors state that this view can be challenged as a 'cut-off point' between normal and abnormal labour. Because many women have a slower rate of dilatation, but proceed to a 'normal labour', they argue that a rate of .05 cm. per hour is a more realistic lower limit, still a normalising rule, of course. They also argue that there is an urgent need for good controlled trials on a prolonged latent phase of labour. See M. Enkin et al. (1995), op. cit., p. 263.
76. K. O'Driscoll and D. Meagher (1986), op. cit.
77. E.A. Friedman (1973), 'Patterns of labour as indicators of risk', *Clinical Obstetrics and Gynecology*, 120; E.A. Friedman et al. (1977), 'Dysfunctional labor. Long term effects on the infant', *American Journal of Obstetrics and Gynecology*, p. 127. Emily Martin has written that the Friedman curve (which makes the partogram possible), conceptualises the uterus as an either good or malfunctioning machine, with dilatation broken into sub-stages. Whereas the progress of dilatation between 4 and 8 cms is 'a good measure of the overall efficiency of the machine', any deviation from these sub-stages will produce 'disorders' in the labour process. E. Martin, 'The ideology of reproduction: the reproduction of ideology', F. Ginsburg and A.L. Tsing (eds.), *Uncertain Terms: Negotiating Gender in American Culture* (Boston: Beacon Press, 1990), p. 302. In practice, clinicians argue that a distinction between the so-called acceleration and deceleration phases are not easily discernible unless frequent vaginal examinations are used. See B. Hibbard, *Principles of Obstetrics* (London: Butterworths, 1988), p. 452. Therefore, applying the whole of this system to a woman is outstandingly invasive.
78. K. O'Driscoll and D. Meagher (1986), op. cit., p. 5.
79. Ibid., p. 6.
80. Margaret Mason points to this precise problem and concludes from the current literature on childbirth teaching that hospital-based antenatal educators are quite limited in their capacity to give unbiased information to their clients because their task is primarily that of enabling women to fit into hospital systems. See M. Mason, 'Childbirth education: empowerment or indoctrination?', P. Kennedy and J. Murphy-Lawless (eds.), *Returning Birth to Women: Challenging Policies and Practices* (Dublin: Centre for Women's Studies, TCD/WERRC, 1998).

81. K. O'Driscoll and D. Meagher (1986), op. cit., pp. 6–7. The third edition omits this particular part of its mission statement although the paragraph on abstract map-reading remains. See K. O'Driscoll, D. Meagher and P. Boylan (1993), op. cit., p. 18.
82. K. O'Driscoll and D. Meagher (1986), op. cit., p. 21.
83. See J. Hamilton quoted in R. Collins (1837), 'Observations on the artificial dilatation of the mouth of the womb during labour, and upon instrumental delivery', *Dublin Quarterly Journal of Medical Science*, vol. xi, p. 40; see also T. Farmar (1994), op. cit., p. 156, on O'Driscoll's reputation for speaking with women about their symptoms but never addressing them by name.
84. K. O'Driscoll and D. Meagher (1986), op. cit., p. 1. In the third edition this use of 'mankind' is finally changed to 'one-half of humankind'. See K. O'Driscoll, D. Meagher and P. Boylan (1993), op. cit., p. 13, employing the phrase that Nihell used in 1760 – see Chapter 1.
85. K. O'Driscoll and D. Meagher (1986), op. cit., p. 11.
86. Ibid.
87. Ibid., p. 22.
88. The sociologist Barbara Adam writes about the overcoming of what she terms 'natural time' by the calendar or clock time of modernity. This shift claims to produce a plane of time that is predictable and efficient. But quantitative time is so limited because it does not include all the 'complex times of our being' including, crucially, variation. Invariable and predictable time is an 'abstract' commodity. See B.E. Adam, 'Time and health implicated: a conceptual critique', R. Frankenburg (ed.), *Time, Health and Medicine* (London: Sage, 1992), p. 160.
89. K. O'Driscoll and D. Meagher (1986), op. cit., p. 24.
90. Ibid., p. 21.
91. Ibid., p. 27.
92. M. Enkin et al. (1995), op. cit., p. 224.
93. Ibid. See also L. Silverton (1993), op. cit., p. 263.
94. K. O'Driscoll and D. Meagher (1986), op. cit., pp. 34–5.
95. Ibid., p. 4.
96. K. O'Driscoll and D. Meagher (1986), op. cit., pp. 5–6.
97. Ibid.
98. T. Lewis and G. Chamberlain, *Obstetrics by Ten Teachers*, 15th edition (London: Edward Arnold, 1990), p. 163.
99. K. O'Driscoll and D. Meagher (1986), op. cit., p. 6.
100. R. Castel, 'From dangerousness to risk', G. Burchell, C. Gordon, and P. Miller (eds.), *The Foucault Effect: Studies in Governmentality* (Hemel Hempstead: Harvester Wheatsheaf, 1991).
101. Ibid., pp. 287–8.
102. K. O'Driscoll and D. Meagher (1986), op. cit., pp. 180–1. O'Driscoll admits that oxytocic-driven contractions are painful, which is why he says he is opposed to induction of labour. But he argues that for the purposes of accelerating labour, oxytocin use is acceptable because the woman is assured that labour will soon be concluded, ibid., pp. 15–16.
103. Ibid., p. 199.
104. See K. O'Driscoll and D. Meagher (1986), op. cit., pp. 198–9; K. O'Driscoll, D. Meagher and P. Boylan (1993), op. cit., pp. 208–9.
105. K. O'Driscoll and D. Meagher (1986), op. cit., p. 183.
106. Ibid., pp. 90–1.

107. Ibid. It is interesting that this rhetoric lasts until the third edition of the book, although one of the authors of the third edition has worked at retrieving the image of the National Maternity Hospital as being more woman-centred.
108. K. O'Driscoll and D. Meagher (1986), op. cit., p. 91.
109. Ibid.
110. Ibid., p. 116.
111. Ibid., p. 18.
112. Ibid., p. 176.
113. As Foucault has argued, in order to sustain its position as the bearer of progress, science must construct a totalising history which denies the epistemological breaks and disruptions which occur.
114. *Irish Times*, 6 July 1988. Sources for details of the Dunnes' case are ongoing news reports of court evidence in the *Irish Times* and *Irish Independent*, an article in the *Sunday Tribune*, 31 July 1988 and G. Kerrigan (1990), op. cit.
115. The practice of auscultation and the use of the stethoscope to determine pregnancy in the 1820s, were initially seen as a breakthrough because they freed the practitioner of any reliance on the woman patient's word in determining pregnancy. See J. Murphy-Lawless (1992), 'Reading birth and death through obstetric practice', *Canadian Journal of Irish Studies*, vol. 18, no. 1, 1992.
116. In the second edition of *Active Management*, O'Driscoll argues that rectal examination is preferred over vaginal examination because there is less chance of infection; also, the infection control procedures required for vaginal examination slow down the rate of examination. He concedes, however, that rectal examination 'is not always reliable even in expert hands' and also reports that as a recent study in the hospital 'revealed to our surprise' that women prefer vaginal examination', 'the choice' is likely to 'remain a matter of local custom'. K. O'Driscoll and D. Meagher (1986), op. cit., p. 34. Whose custom, women's or medical staff, is not clear. The authors of *Effective Care in Pregnancy and Childbirth* have concluded that rectal examination has no place in the measurement of cervical dilatation. See M. Enkin et al. (1995), op. cit., p. 202.
117. The sociologist, Franca Pizzini, has argued that women's bodies are unable to conform to exact regularities in obstetric units. She has observed clock time being used to measure strictly defined versions of normality, at the end of which an intervention like forceps, Caesarean section or acceleration of labour is employed. She has also observed the differences in staff responses to these invariable rules, often in relation to the shift being worked, the number of staff available relative to the women in labour and so on. See F. Pizzini, 'Women's time, institutional time', R. Frankenburg (ed.), *Time, Health and Medicine* (London: Sage, 1992).
118. K. O'Driscoll and D. Meagher (1986), op. cit., p. 92.
119. Ibid.
120. K. O'Driscoll and D. Meagher (1986), op. cit., p. 2.
121. Quoted in the programme, *Birth of a Nation*, broadcast on RTÉ, 29 December 1994.
122. *Irish Times*, 15 April 1989.
123. Ibid.
124. M. Foucault, 'Two lectures', C. Gordon (ed.), *Power/Knowledge: Selected Interviews and Other Writings 1972–77* (Brighton: Harvester Wheatsheaf, 1980), pp. 78–92.
125. Ibid. pp. 41–2. For a discussion of epistemic authority, see L. Code (1995), *Rhetorical Spaces: Essays on Gendered Locations* (London: Routledge, 1995).
126. M. Douglas, *Risk Acceptability According to the Social Sciences* (London: Routledge and Kegan Paul, 1986).

127. This quasi-legal status, where the hospital can insist on its own autonomy within its own space, seems related to the work of medicine in general in extending bio-politics. Foucault argues this as part of the multiple sites which emerge in the social body that are concerned with the global implications of health and illness. See M. Foucault, 'The politics of health in the eighteenth century', C. Gordon (ed.), (1980), op. cit., p. 167.
128. *Irish Times*, 26 July 1988, 'Everywoman versus the medical system'; *Irish Times*, 26 July 1988, 'A court battle won but a childhood lost forever'.
129. M. Foucault, 'Truth and power', C. Gordon (ed.), (1980), op. cit., pp. 112–13.
130. Ibid.
131. M. Foucault, 'Two lectures', C. Gordon (ed.)(1980), op. cit., p. 118.
132. Ibid., p. 133.
133. M. Foucault (1974), *The Archaeology of Knowledge* (London: Tavistock, 1974), p. 12.
134. K. O'Driscoll, D. Meagher and P. Boylan (1993), op. cit., p. 196.
135. See E. Martin, *The Woman in the Body: A Cultural Analysis of Reproduction* (Boston: Beacon Press, 1987); P. Treichler, 'Feminism, medicine and the meaning of childbirth', M. Jacobus et al. (eds.), *Body/Politics: Women and the Discourses of Science* (London: Routledge, 1990), pp. 120–1.
136. Department of Health, *Perinatal Statistics, 1992* (Dublin: Stationery Office, 1996), p. 83.
137. K. O'Driscoll (1972), 'Impact of Active Management on Delivery Unit Practice', *Proceedings of the Royal Society of Medicine*, vol. 65, August 1992, pp. 697–8.
138. There is excellent ongoing evidence to suggest that the upright position and ambulation reduces contractions while increasing the effectiveness of each contraction, increasing also women's physical comfort and ability to deal well with labour. See S. Inch (1989), op. cit., and R. Schwarcz et al. (1977), op. cit.
139. K. O'Driscoll, D. Meagher and P. Boylan (1993), op. cit., p. 205.
140. Ibid., p. 196.
141. D. MacKenzie, *Inventing Accuracy: A Historical Sociology of Nuclear Missile Guidance* (Cambridge, Mass.: MIT Press, 1990), p. 4.
142. Ibid., p. 10.
143. It must be pointed out that active management does not have an ideological anchoring that emphasises women's physical and mental strengths. Delivery with a woman semi-lying on her back and her feet in stirrups was still in evidence at the time of the showing of the television documentary about the National Maternity Hospital, *Birth of a Nation*, RTÉ, 29 December 1994.
144. R. Campbell and A. Macfarlane, *Where to Be Born?*, second edition (Oxford: Crown Publications for National Perinatal Epidemiology Unit, 1995); M. Tew, *Safer Childbirth? A Critical History of Maternity Care* (London: Chapman and Hall, 1990).
145. M. Wagner (1994), op. cit., p. 49. See also WHO, *Having a Baby in Europe*, Public Health in Europe, no. 26 (Copenhagen: WHO Regional Office for Europe, 1985).
146. T. Lewis, and G. Chamberlain (1990), op. cit., p. 340.
147. Department of Health, *Vital Statistics, Fourth Quarter and Yearly Summary, 1995* (Dublin: Stationery Office, 1996a), pp. 17–18.
148. A. Oakley (1984), op. cit., p. 233.
149. S. Hill, *Family* (Michael Joseph: London, 1989).
150. Department of Health (1996), op. cit., p. 35. An article in the *Irish Times*, 6 October 1994, reported on a study presented to the Irish Perinatal Society in which sixteen years of perinatal mortality rates were reviewed for the three largest maternity hospitals. The study indicated that the Rotunda had the lowest rate of perinatal mortality

compared with the Coombe and the National Maternity Hospital, excluding in the instances of all three apparently babies under 2,500 grams and also premature births. Although one co-author regarded the figures as 'not significant', the difference between the Rotunda and the National Maternity hospital being 998 women going home with live babies as compared with 996 women, the second co-author regarded the figures as 'highly significant' because it showed that the Dublin hospital with the lowest rate of medical intervention, the National Maternity Hospital, had the highest rate of mortality. In response, the first co-author stated that high rates of intervention might enable one to save one or two babies per thousand but it would require sectioning hundreds more women to do so. The way these arguments are constructed, concentrating on aggregate outcomes and profiles of each institution, raises precisely the issue of who controls this decision-making.

151. In the United States, maternal and infant health profiles for low-income women of colour have worsened dramatically since the beginning of the 1980s, with rising rates of perinatal mortality and of maternal mortality. See Children's Defence Fund, *A Call for Action to Make Our Nation Safe for Children: A Briefing Book on the Status of American Children in 1988* (Washington, DC: Children's Defence Fund, 1988), pp. 3, 20–1.
152. R. Illsley, ' The sociological study of reproduction and its outcome', S. Richardson and A. Guttmacher (eds.), *Childbearing – Its Social and Psychological Aspects* (Baltimore: Willams and Wilkins, 1967).
153. House of Commons, Health Committee (1992), op. cit., p. lxv.
154. M. Wagner (1994), op. cit., p. 33.
155. Ibid.
156. M. Stacey, *The Sociology of Health and Healing* (London: Unwin Hyman, 1988), p. 162.
157. M. Tew (1990), op. cit., pp. 266–7.
158. Ibid.
159. Ibid.
160. M. Foucault (1974), op. cit.
161. This is by now a long-established strategy in forms of argument in obstetric discourse.

NOTES TO CHAPTER 6

1. Marsden Wagner has cited the conflict about appropriate birth practices as one of the most 'serious challenges facing established healthcare systems worldwide'. M. Wagner, *Pursuing the Birth Machine: The Search for Appropriate Birth Technology* (Sevenoaks, Kent: ACE Graphics, 1994), p. 6. The problem of the uncritical absorption of the Western obstetric package by health authorities in countries from the South is discussed in J. Murphy-Lawless, 'Women dying in childbirth: "safe motherhood" in the international context', P. Kennedy and J. Murphy-Lawless (eds.), *Returning Birth to Women: Challenging Policies and Practices* (Dublin: Centre for Women's Studies, TCD/WERRC, 1998). A recently issued book on obstetrics in Bolivia illustrates how difficult it is for a counter-discourse on conventional obstetric practice to be built up. See A. Gálvez Murillo et al., *Obstetricia Práctica* (La Paz: Medicon, 1997). The chapter on episiotomy as a routine birth practice, for example, reinforces rationales from mainstream obstetrics which have been firmly rejected by counter-arguments, even within obstetrics (by the dissident voices of Iain Chalmers' Oxford group), as being harmful. On the latter, see M. Enkin et al., *A Guide to Effective Care in Pregnancy and Childbirth*, 2nd edition (Oxford: Oxford University Press, 1995), pp. 231–3. It is a

matter of deepest urgency to tackle the circulation of these mainstream practices which are authorised uncritically by international health planners.
2. M. Foucault (1988), 'Critical theory/intellectual history', L. Kritzman (ed.), *Michel Foucault: Politics, Philosophy, Culture. Interviews and Other Writings, 1977–1984* (London: Routledge, 1988), p. 27.
3. E. Fox Keller (1992), *Secrets of Life, Secrets of Death: Essays on Language, Gender and Science* (London: Routledge, 1992), p. 74.
4. Ibid., p. 75.
5. S. Freud, *Introductory Lectures on Psychoanalysis*, vol. 1 (Harmondsworth: Penguin, 1991), p. 445.
6. S. Kitzinger, 'Why women need midwives', S. Kitzinger (ed.), *The Midwife Challenge* (London: Pandora Press, 1988), p. 15.
7. T. McKeown, *The Origins of Human Disease* (Oxford: Basil Blackwell, 1988), pp. 74–5.
8. Perinatal mortality rates include all stillbirths and early neonatal deaths up to the first week of life whereas infant mortality includes all deaths in the first year of life.
9. Department of Health, *Vital Statistics, Fourth Quarter and Yearly Summary, 1995* (Dublin: Stationery Office, 1996a), Table 7, Deaths of Infants under 1 year, classified by cause, sex, and age group.
10. Department of Health, *Perinatal Statistics, 1992* (Dublin: Stationery Office, 1996b), p. 35.
11. T. McKeown (1988), op. cit., pp. 84–5.
12. Council for Science and Society, quoted in M. Stacey, *The Sociology of Health and Healing* (London: Unwin Hyman, 1988), p. 240.
13. A. Oakley, *Women Confined: Towards a Sociology of Childbirth* (Oxford: Martin Robertson, 1980), p. 24.
14. J. Murphy-Lawless (1993), 'Fertility, bodies and politics: the Irish case', *Reproductive Health Matters*, no. 2, November 1993.
15. See K. O'Driscoll and D. Meagher, *Active Management of Labour*, second edition (London: Baillière Tindall, 1986).
16. *Irish Times*, 27 January 1992, 'The rebirthing of Holles Street', p. 9.
17. B. McAdam-O'Connell, 'Risk, responsibility and choice: the medical model of birth and alternatives', P. Kennedy and J. Murphy-Lawless (eds.), *Returning Birth to Women: Challenging Policies and Practices* (Dublin: Centre for Women's Studies, TCD/WERRC, 1998).
18. M. O'Connor, *Birthtides: Turning Towards Home Birth* (London: HarperCollins, 1995).
19. Ibid. pp. 102–6. When they interviewed the Master of the National Maternity Hospital, representatives from the Home Birth Centre were told that his priority was the baby and the effect of the various procedures on the woman were considered more or less incidental. See 'Meeting with Peter Boylan, Master of Holles St.', 9 July 1991, *Home Birth Newsletter*, July 1991–January 1992. The extent to which these interventions also impact on the baby is the issue that obstetrics has been trying to avoid, as technological intervention has intensified in the last four decades. See S. Inch, *Birthrights: A Parent's Guide to Modern Childbirth*, 2nd edition (London: Green Print, 1989).
20. J. Sawicki, *Disciplining Foucault: Feminism, Power and the Body* (London: Routledge, 1991), pp. 67–8.
21. Oakley's interview accounts of births vibrate with this tension. See 'The Agony and the Ecstasy', chapter 5 in A. Oakley, *From Here to Maternity: Becoming a Mother* (Oxford: Martin Robertson, 1979). The women O'Connor interviewed report similar tensions and fears and in chapter 2, accurately entitled 'A Sense of Ice', the stories of the scale of unpleasant behaviour towards the women, ranging from hostility to the inflicting of

outright physical and mental trauma are bitingly clear. See M. O'Connor (1995), op. cit.
22. M. Foucault, *The History of Sexuality, Volume 1: An Introduction* (Harmondsworth: Penguin, 1981), p. 138.
23. Z. Bauman, *Mortality, Immortality and Other Life Strategies* (Cambridge: Polity Press, 1992).
24. I say 'appears' rather than is because the picture is far from consistent across Western countries. The strong and consistent association between social class and perinatal death and the lack of any significant reduction between class-based rates raises the question as to whether the issues of the consequences of poverty and ill-health for women must be made the focus of attention instead.
25. S. Bartky, 'Foucault, femininity, and the modernization of patriarchal power', I. Diamond and L. Quinby (eds.), *Feminism and Foucault: Reflections on Resistance* (Boston: Northeastern University Press, 1988).
26. E. Martin, *The Woman in the Body: A Cultural Analysis of Reproduction* (Boston: Beacon Press, 1987).
27. M. Wagner (1994), op. cit., pp. 18–19.
28. *Home Birth Newsletter* (1991–92), op. cit.
29. G. Stimson and B. Webb, *Going to See the Doctor* (London: Routledge and Kegan Paul, 1975).
30. R. Dingwall (1977), '"Atrocity stories" and professional relationships', *Sociology of Work and Occupations*, vol. 4, no. 4, November 1977.
31. Ibid., p. 376.
32. *Irish Times*, 26 July 1988.
33. M. O'Connor (1995), op. cit., p. 44.
34. B. Solomons (1933), 'Report of the Rotunda Hospital (November 1st 1931 to October 31st 1932)', *Irish Journal of Medical Science*, no. 92, p. 335. A recent version of this kind of horror story emerged in the course of an inquest on the death of a woman after a legal abortion, held in England in west Yorkshire, in March 1994. The twenty-nine-year-old woman died of cardiac arrest after a massive inter-abdominal haemorrhage, the result of a perforated uterus which, the inquest heard, had most likely been caused by a dilator used during the operation (*Independent*, 5 March 1994). During the inquest, it emerged that Mrs Lall, already having three young children between the ages of five and eight, all girls, had sought an amniocentesis test in Manchester which had revealed that the fourth pregnancy was a female foetus. Mrs Lall then sought a termination through the Marie Stopes Pregnancy Advisory Service in Leeds on the grounds that she could not cope with another child as the family was already under pressure, financially and emotionally. The coroner's judgment was that Mrs Lall had died as a result of misadventure, that there had been nothing wrong with her medical treatment, but that she had been 'devious and dishonest' in seeking an abortion:

> I have not throughout the inquiry exposed any evidence of any lack of care on the part of any involved agencies. I have exposed evidence of deviousness and dishonesty in seeking to achieve ends by devious and dishonest means. (David Hinchcliffe, Coroner, quoted in *Independent*, 5 March 1994)

35. Although the precepts of active management of labour appear to have the tantalising possibility of continuous social support for the woman in labour, this support is almost always given by a pupil midwife, as we have seen in Chapter 5. A truly social model of birth would have three interrelated elements in it: an emphasis on birth as an ordinary

life event, a social event; one in which the woman giving birth has her decision-making honoured about what is the most appropriate form of care and attention; and finally an emphasis on the importance of midwives as the primary caretakers of normal birth, who seek to facilitate birth, as distinct from controlling it, with obstetrics playing a back-up role only.
36. Department of Health, Comhairle na n-Ospidéal, *Development of Hospital Maternity Services, a Discussion Document* (Dublin: Stationery Office, 1976), pp. 11–12; Ireland, Department of Health, *Report of the Maternity and Infant Care Scheme Review Group, April, 1994* (unpublished), p. 28.
37. Ibid.
38. Ibid.
39. Ibid.
40. See P. Kennedy, 'Between the lines: mother and infant care in Ireland', P. Kennedy and J. Murphy-Lawless (eds.), *Returning Birth to Women: Challenging Policies and Practices* (Dublin: Centre for Women's Studies, TCD/WERRC, 1998); M. O'Connor (1995), op. cit.
41. See M. Wagner (1994), op. cit.
42. See England, House of Commons, Social Services Committee, *Second Report from the Social Services Committee, Session 1979–80, Perinatal and Neonatal Mortality*, vol. 1. p. 1 (London: HMSO, 1980), and Department of Health, *Changing Childbirth* (London: HMSO, 1993).
43. This is not an easy task. Women and midwives alike are still caught up in the medical paradigm, even when opting for home birth. See J. Murphy-Lawless (1991), 'Piggy in the middle: The midwife's role in achieving woman-controlled childbirth', *Irish Journal of Psychology*, vol. 12, no. 2, p. 199. See also note 119 below.
44. See P. Kennedy (1998), op. cit.
45. Ireland, Department of Health (1994), op. cit., p. 18.
46. Ibid.
47. Over the last fifteen years, maternal mortality from direct obstetric causes has declined to single figures.
48. The same error was made in the United Nations Human Development Report, 1995 which gave prominence to women's issues and listed the average MMR for the period 1980–92 for Ireland as 2 per 100,000. The rate is incorrect: in 1983 alone there were eight direct obstetric deaths in a virtually blanket hospitalised population. See Department of Health, *Vital Statistics, 1983* (Dublin: Stationery Office, 1984).
49. The discussion programme on home births was broadcast on 13 June 1996 from CKR Radio.
50. A tape of the programme was kindly made available to me by Máire O'Regan, of AIMS, who was one of the participants in the discussion.
51. M. Tew, *Safer Childbirth? A Critical History of Maternity Care* (London: Chapman and Hall, 1990).
52. Central Statistics Office, Ireland kindly furnished me with Dutch figures.
53. Finland, Ministry of Social Affairs and Health (1996), *Äitiyskuolleisuus, 1960–1994*, p. 1.
54. Personal communication, Central Statistics Office, Ireland. The reason the figure was provisional is due to a time lag between the ruling on deaths at inquests, their official recording, and their incorporation into our national vital statistics kept by the Central Statistics Office. Unlike other European countries, Ireland still does not have a system of confidential enquiry by an independent board into maternal deaths.

55. I. Hacking, 'How should we do the history of statistics?', G. Burchell, C. Gordon, and P. Miller (eds.), *The Foucault Effect: Studies in Governmentality* (Hemel Hempstead: Harvester Wheatsheaf, 1991), p. 183.
56. Demographic literature refers to ongoing problems of under-reporting and misclassification of maternal deaths, in both developed and developing countries. See J. Murphy-Lawless (1998), op. cit.
57. D. Maine et al. (1996), op. cit., p. 22.
58. *Irish Times*, 25 July 1988, 'Whatever happened to Antoinette?'.
59. Ibid.
60. M. O'Connor (1995), op. cit., pp. 79–80.
61. Ibid., p. 102.
62. P. Kaufert and J. O'Neil, 'Analysis of a dialogue on risks in childbirth: clinicians, epidemiologists and Inuit women', S. Lindenbaum and M. Lock (eds.), *Knowledge, Power and Practice: The Anthropology of Medicine and Everyday Life* (Berkeley: University of California Press, 1993).
63. Ibid., p. 49.
64. S. Ruzek, 'Women's reproductive rights: the impact of technology', J. Rodin and A. Collins (eds.), *Women and New Reproductive Technologies: Medical, Psychosocial, Legal and Ethical Dilemmas* (Hillsdale, NJ: Lawrence Erlbaum Associates, 1991).
65. Department of Health, *Vital Statistics, 1990* (Dublin: Stationery Office, 1991).
66. M. O'Connor, *Women and Birth: A National Study of Intentional Home Births in Ireland* (Dublin: Coombe Hospital and the Department of Health, 1992), p. 7.
67. *Irish Times*, 20 May 1996, 'Born out of the blue', p. 6.
68. Ibid.
69. *Woman's Way*, 20 December 1996, 'I delivered my own son', pp. 12–13.
70. Ibid.
71. Ibid. In August 1994, a petition was handed in comprising some 30,000 signatures protesting about a threat to close the maternity unit at Louth County Hospital. It was pointed out that women from Omeath might have to travel as far as forty-four miles to reach the next nearest hospital with an obstetric unit, in Drogheda, a long journey when one is already in labour. However, a medical source speaking to the *Irish Times* argued that the unit in Louth county hospital was too small to be 'viable' and that in any case, women would prefer to travel to Drogheda where 'the full range of maternity services' would be available. *Irish Times*, '30,000 sign petition to save maternity unit', 31 August 1994.
72. See S. Inch (1989), op. cit., for a discussion of the impact of Caesarean sections and epidurals on women. See also M. Wagner (1994), op. cit.
73. *Irish Times*, 'Nurses step up action in Dundalk hospital', 3 December 1996; *Sligo Champion*, 'No Cause for Alarm', 28 August 1996.
74. M. Foucault, 'Body/Power', C. Gordon (ed.), *Power/Knowledge: Selected Interviews and Other Writings 1972–77* (Brighton: Harvester Wheatsheaf, 1980), p. 58.
75. *Irish Times*, Letters to the Editor, 'Managing Labour', 10 February 1992.
76. K. O'Driscoll (1972), 'Impact of active management on delivery unit practice' *Proceedings of the Royal Society of Medicine*, vol. 65, August 1992, pp. 697–8.
77. *Irish Times*, 22 February 1996, 'Court is told of "missed" chances for baby'; *Irish Independent*, 24 February 1996, 'Family who sued Holles St settle for £1.67m'.
78. *Carlow Nationalist*, 'Man fights to clarify cause of wife's death', 23 August 1996.
79. *Sunday Tribune*, 4 September 1983, 'No change at Holles Street'.
80. *WOMAN*, 21 March 1994, 'There's Your Baby . . . Look How Lively It Is.'

81. One of the most interesting aspects of ultrasound is that its measurement of each foetus is then placed against an averaged-out version of what growth rate each foetus should attain by each week of gestation. In 1987, AIMS reported that in Kings College Hospital, London, as part of a project on neonatal defects, an ultrasound project was under way in which mothers with 'high risk' pregnancies were screened intensively with ultrasound for up to two hours at a time to 'prove' that a foetus was breathing and therefore that the woman did not 'require' an abortion. The doctor leading this project claimed that ultrasound could 'save' up to 2,000 babies each year from unnecessary abortion. AIMS made the obvious comment that the ultrasound did nothing to change the status of a tenuous pregnancy to less than tenuous and that the D and C was in any event a totally unnecessary operation as foetal death would result in a spontaneous abortion. Why, AIMS asked, were so many doctors recommending abortion anyhow on the basis of the 'flimsy evidence' of ultrasound conducted in this way. See AIMS (1987), *AIMS Quarterly Journal*, autumn 1987, p. 3.
82. *WOMAN*, 21 March 1994, op. cit.
83. Ibid.
84. Ibid.
85. S. Reinharz, 'The social psychology of a miscarriage: an application of symbolic interaction theory and method', M. J. Deegan and M. Hill (eds.), *Women and Symbolic Interaction* (London: Allen and Unwin, 1987).
86. Ibid. The routine D and C after a spontaneous abortion, or in the case of foetal death as in Sara's case, has to be read as part of the interventionist package, 'just in case' there might be any retained 'products of conception' that might become infected. As with third-stage management, the thesis is that the physiology of the body, the bleeding that accompanies a spontaneous abortion will not totally clear out the woman's uterus. I would also suggest that the blood loss even with a first-trimester spontaneous abortion panics many women, who are reliant on medical management of their reproductive bodies and lacking the confidence and alternative readings to reject the hurried dash to hospital, the incarceration and operative procedures which obstetrics imposes.
87. M. Stacey (1988), *The Sociology of Health and Healing* (London: Unwin Hyman, 1988), p. 242.
88. E. Martin (1987), *The Woman in the Body: A Cultural Analysis of Reproduction* (Boston: Beacon Press, 1987), p.13.
89. F. Jebb, 'Of an Haemorrhage occasioned by the adhesion of the placenta to the Os Uteri' *Transactions, Medical and Philosophical Memoirs*, vol. 3, 3 December 1772, Dublin.
90. See E. Shorter (1983), *A History of Women's Bodies* (London: Allen Lane, 1983).
91. The *Guardian* reported on such a case in 1996 when a woman sued St George's Healthcare Trust for obtaining a court order to carry out a Caesarean section because of suspected pre-eclampsia. The woman was a trained medical professional, knew the parameters of her decision and stated that if their diagnosis had been correct, it could have ended in her baby's death but that she was prepared to make an informed choice about treatment. Instead the judge ruled her mentally incompetent – the only legal route open to him under English law once he was convinced of the medical arguments – and gave the hospital authorities leave to go ahead with the section against the woman's express wishes. See the *Guardian*, 'Mother vs Big Brother', 19 December 1996. In a second case in Britain in 1996, a woman who had had three previous Caesarean sections and who presented at a hospital department fully dilated and ready to deliver was also the subject of an emergency court order. See D. Brahams (1996), 'Caesarean sections by court order', the *Lancet*, no. 348, 21 September, p. 770.

92. A. Phillips and J. Rakusen, *The New Our Bodies, Ourselves*, Boston Women's Health Book Collective, British Edition (Harmondsworth: Penguin, 1989), p. 339.
93. Ibid., p. 374.
94. This process of careful reflection is integral to the business of how we now give birth and the stories that result from this reflection are often a turning point of politicisation, as Oakley and O'Connor have indicated. That deeply contested moment pushes us towards reframing our relationships with medicine and concomitantly with the notion of risk. On this, see also S. Bell, 'Becoming a political woman: the reconstruction and interpretation of experience through stories', A. Todd and S. Fisher (eds.), *Gender and Discourse: The Power of Talk* (Norwood, NJ: Ablex, 1988), on the experiences of child-bearing women affected by DES.
95. I.M. Gaskin, *Spiritual Midwifery* (Summertown, TN: The Book Publishing Company, 1977), p. 230.
96. Ibid., pp. 284–5.
97. *Evening Herald*, 28 May 1996, 'Your view, birth in the home'.
98. N. Mulvany, personal communication.
99. K. Colgan, *If It Happens to You* (Dublin: A. and A. Farmar, 1994).
100. M. Wagner (1994), op. cit., p. 113.
101. Ibid., p. 114.
102. E. Martin, 'Body narratives, body boundaries', L. Grossberg and P. Treichler (eds.), *Cultural Studies* (New York: Routledge, 1992). Susan Sherwin says that the problem for women in trying to achieve agency is that autonomy is seen as the traditional instrument whereby to exercise agency, and that it stems from a definition of the individual as separate, independent, fully rational. See S. Sherwin, *No Longer Patient: Feminist Ethics and Health Care* (Philadelphia: Temple University Press, 1992), p. 137. In the face of the now scrambled distinctions between the human, the natural and the artificial, and endlessly complicated by our relationship to the sciences, Sadie Plant suggests that the traditional concept of individual responsibility is questionable, but on the other hand, agency and intention are not removed; they become instead more complicated and perplexed. See S. Plant, 'The virtual complexity of culture', G. Robertson et al. (eds.), *FutureNatural: Nature/Science/Culture* (London: Routledge, 1996).
103. See R. Petchesky, 'Foetal images: the power of visual culture in the politics of reproduction', M. Stanworth (ed.), *Reproductive Technologies: Gender, Motherhood and Medicine* (Cambridge: Polity Press, 1987).
104. Monica Caspar writes that the status of the foetus as a 'work object' is changing for scientists and clinicians, so that the foetus can now be (overlapping and simultaneously), person, patient, research material, therapeutic technology and tissue source. See M. Caspar (1994), 'At the margins of humanity: fetal positions in science and medicine', *Technology and Human Values*, vol. 19, no. 3.
105. In one such case in 1990, a baby boy was eventually born prematurely and was being kept alive on a ventilator, after surgery on his defective heart valve at thirty-one weeks' and thirty-three weeks' gestation. He required a further operation after birth, the press release from Guy's Hospital in London stated. See *Irish Times*, 'Baby critically ill after in-womb surgery', 23 January 1990. What the press release failed to indicate was that the woman required these operations as well in which a catheter was passed though her abdominal wall and then through the wall of the uterus, twice during her pregnancy, accompanied by complete medical management of the pregnancy and then a Caesarean section to have a quick birth on the grounds that it all might save her baby's life. It also facilitated the testing of a technique which surgeons later declared had been shown to

be feasible. What can 'informed consent' mean in these circumstances? If a woman rejects this surgery, does she face an accusation of failing to care for her unborn child? Certainly, the denial of her embodiment in such concrete terms is also a denial of agency.

106. S. Bartky (1988), op. cit., pp. 76–8.
107. M. O'Brien, *Reproducing the World* (Boulder, CA: Westview Press, 1989), p. 14.
108. L. Code, *Rhetorical Spaces: Essays on Gendered Locations* (London: Routledge, 1995), p. x.
109. Ibid. Code speaks about epistemic responsibility in which 'patients' for example might rethink what they need to know in order to give informed consent.
110. E. Scarry, *The Body in Pain: The Making and Unmaking of the World* (New York: Oxford University Press, 1985), p. 169.
111. E. Scarry (1985), op. cit., p. 171.
112. L. Code (1995), op. cit., p. 21. What Code suggests is that the authority we give to experts to speak empirically could be revalued, thus valorising our own empiricism, with scope for developing our personal agency.
113. H. Rose, 'Victorian values in the test-tube: the politics of reproductive science and technology', M. Stanworth (ed.), *Reproductive Technologies: Gender, Motherhood and Medicine* (Cambridge: Polity Press, 1987), p. 157.
114. E.F. Keller (1992), op. cit., p. 76.
115. L. Fleck, *Genesis and Development of a Scientific Fact* (Chicago: University of Chicago Press, 1979), p. 22.
116. See M. Enkin et al., *A Guide to Effective Care in Pregnancy and Childbirth*, 2nd edition (Oxford: Oxford University Press, 1995).
117. E. Scarry (1985), op. cit., pp. 146–7.
118. Ironically, Fielding Ould, who first wrote about the value of episiotomy to deal with birth, also described the vagina in his preface as having the 'Appearance' and 'Texture', 'as though it were knit like a Stocking'. F. Ould, *A Treatise of Midwifry in Three Parts* (Dublin: Oli Nelson and Charles Connor, 1742). The split between observation, perception and practice is telling.
119. S. Kitzinger and R. Walters, *Some Women's Experiences of Episiotomy* (London: National Childbirth Trust, 1981), p. 1.
120. This oxytocic release mechanism created by the stretching of the perineum during the crowning of the baby's head is documented by Newton who also comments that the value of it is lost unless the perineum is allowed to fully stretch. See N. Newton, 'The role of oxytocic reflexes in three reproductive acts', *Clinical Psychoneuroendocrinology in Reproduction* (London: Academic Press, 1978), pp. 411–18.
121. C. Begley (1990), 'A comparison of "active" and "physiological" management of the third stage of labour', *Midwifery*, no. 6, 1990; 'Explaining postpartum haemorrhage – the value of a physiological third stage', P. Kennedy and J. Murphy-Lawless (eds.), *Returning Birth to Women: Challenging Policies and Practices* (Dublin: Centre for Women's Studies, TCD/WERRC, 1998).
122. I.M. Gaskin (1977), op. cit., p. 397.
123. T. Lewis and G. Chamberlain, *Obstetrics by Ten Teachers*, 15th edition (London: Edward Arnold, 1990), pp. 208–9.
124. See I.M. Gaskin (1988), 'Shoulder dystocia: controversies in management', *Birth Gazette*, vol. 5, no.1, pp. 14–17; E. Davis, *Heart and Hands: A Midwife's Guide to Pregnancy and Birth* (Berkeley, CA: Celestial Arts, 1992); M. Glynn and K. Oláh (1994), 'The management of shoulder dystocia', *British Journal of Midwifery*, vol. 2, no. 3, March 1994.

Notes to pp. 258–61 317

125. L. Fleck (1979), op. cit., p. 96.
126. Midwives have spoken in interview to me about having to 'unlearn' aspects of the obstetric regimes under which they initially trained. See J. Murphy-Lawless (1991), op. cit. Cecily Begley has now explored the reactions of midwives to their training and how they must work to make sense of the hospital regime. See C. Begley, *Midwives in the Making: a Longitudinal Study of the Experiences of Student Midwives During Their Two-Year Training in Ireland* (Unpublished Ph.D. thesis, University of Dublin, Trinity College, 1997).
127. M. Foucault, 'Two lectures', C. Gordon (ed.), *Power/Knowledge: Selected Interviews and Other Writings 1972–77* (Brighton: Harvester Wheatsheaf, 1980), pp. 80–2.
128. See M. Wagner (1994), op. cit., p. 37, on what might constitute appropriate birth technologies. These may not be able to be separated from technologies of the body. Gélis quotes Marcel Mauss that now in the West, we have lost the ability to crouch. See J. Gélis, *History of Childbirth: Fertility, Pregnancy and Birth in Early Modern Europe* (Cambridge: Polity Press, 1991), p. 288.
129. Foucault also argues that even while discourse produces power and reinforces it, discourse can undermine and expose power. See M. Foucault (1981), op. cit.
130. See B. Jordan (1989), 'Cosmopolitical obstetrics: some insights from the training of traditional midwives', *Social Science and Medicine*, vol. 28, no. 9, pp. 925–44; D. Arnold, M. Tito and J. Yapita, *Vocabulario Aymara del Parto y de la Vida Reproductiva de la Mujer* (La Paz: UNICEF, 1997); R. Davis-Floyd and C. Sargent (1996), 'Introduction: the social production of authoritative knowledge in pregnancy and childbirth', *Medical Anthropology Quarterly*, n.s., vol. 10, no. 2, June 1996, pp. 111–20
131. S. Kitzinger and R. Walters (1981), op. cit.
132. See M. Enkin et al. (1995), op. cit., p. 231.
133. C. Begley (1987), 'Episiotomy: a change in midwives' practice', *Irish Nursing Forum and Health Studies*, November–December 1987.
134. Ibid., p. 34.
135. Wagner argues that the optimum length of labour is not knowable. See M. Wagner (1994), op. cit., pp. 114–15.
136. I.M. Gaskin (1977), op. cit.; J. Balaskas, *Active Birth* (London: Unwin, 1983).
137. C. Flint, *Sensitive Midwifery* (London: Heinemann Medical Books, 1986).
138. See G. Lenstrup et al., 'Warm tub bath during delivery', *Acta Obstetrica et Gynecologia Scandinavica* vol. 66, no. 8, 1987.
139. See B.K. Rothman, *In Labour: Women and Power in the Birthplace* (New York: W.W. Norton, 1982); R. Weitz and D. Sullivan, 'Licensed lay midwifery and the medical model of childbirth' *Sociology of Health and Illness*, vol. 7, no. 1, 1985; E. Annandale, 'How midwives accomplish natural birth: managing risk and balancing expectations', *Social Problems*, vol. 35, no. 2, April 1988.
140. The extent of this threat in the Irish context was apparent in the closing months of 1997 when a County Dublin midwife, Ann O'Ceallaigh, went to the High Court seeking a judicial review after a complaint about her practice as a domiciliary midwife had been made by medical doctors of the National Maternity Hospital and the Rotunda. The complaint had resulted in Ms O'Ceallaigh's suspension by the nursing registration board, An Bord Altranais, until a full disciplinary hearing could be held. Ms O'Ceallaigh sought to have her right to practise restored so that she could assist in the births of fourteen women who had contracted her services prior to her suspension and had no alternative to Ms O'Ceallaigh's services if they wanted to give birth at

home. There are at present only four other domiciliary midwives serving the greater Dublin area with a population of over a million. Ms O'Ceallaigh also sought to have the proceedings against her heard in a public court. See *Irish Times*, 13 September 1997, 'Home births midwife is facing suspension'; 24 September 1997, 'Co. Dublin midwife seeks leave to challenge injunction'; 25 September 1997, 'Judge grants midwife right to challenge court ban'; 4 October 1997, 'Court lets midwife fulfil her contracts with 14 women'. The case was ongoing at time of writing. Ms O'Ceallaigh has had the overwhelming support of the Irish childbirth organisations, including Cuidiú and the Home Birth Association. It is striking that the complaints made against Ms O'Ceallaigh were by doctors, and not complaints from women, and that unless she had taken court actions, this disciplinary hearing would have been heard in private. Similar to instances where parents have had to go to court to get hold of medical records, including post-mortem records from maternity hospitals, Ms O'Ceallaigh has experienced the quasi-legal status of obstetric medicine to her disadvantage.

141. C. Shilling (1993), op. cit, p. 113.
142. J. Sawicki (1991), op. cit., p. 10.
143. Ibid.
144. E. Davis-Floyd, *Birth as an American Rite of Passage* (Berkeley, CA: University of California Press, 1992).
145. E. Nihell, *Treatise on the Art of Midwifery: Setting Forth Various Abuses Therein, Especially as to the Practice of Instruments* (London: Haymarket, 1760), pp. ii–iv.
146. M. Foucault (1980), op. cit., p. 83.
147. I am indebted to Dominick Jenkins for his insights on power, repetition and violence. See D. Jenkins (forthcoming), *Poison and Justice*, for his analysis of the repetition of violence in the chemical warfare industry and the wider networks of power which have sustained these operations.

Bibliography

Adam, B. E. (1990) *Time and Social Theory.* Cambridge: Polity Press.
Adam, B. E. (1992) 'Time and health implicated: a conceptual critique', R. Frankenburg (ed.) *Time, Health and Medicine.* London: Sage.
AIMS (1987) *AIMS Quarterly Journal,* autumn 1987.
Akrich, M. and Pasveer, B. (1995) 'Technologies of giving birth: comparing women's bodies and competencies during "normal" birth in France and The Netherlands', paper delivered at the international workshop 'The Mutual Shaping of Gender and Technology', October 6–8, University of Twente, The Netherlands.
Annandale, E. (1988) How Midwives Accomplish Natural Birth: Managing Risk and Balancing Expectations, *Social Problems,* Vol. 35, No. 2, April.
Arancibia, B., Nina, P. and Platt, T. (1995) *Informe sobre la Encuesta Cuantitativa de Madres Campesinas (supplementado con informacin de las entrevistas con los medicos y auxiliares de los Hospitales y Postas Sanitarias).* Sucre, Bolivia: Institute of Amerindian Studies, St Andrew's University (unpublished).
Aris, P. (1974) *Western Attitudes Towards Death: From the Middle Ages to the Present.* Baltimore: Johns Hopkins.
Arms, S. (1977) *Immaculate Deception.* Boston: Houghton Mifflin.
Armstrong, D. (1986) 'The invention of infant mortality', *Sociology of Health and Illness,* Vol. 8, No. 3, pp.211–232.
Armstrong, D. (1987) 'Bodies of knowledge: Foucault and the problem of human anatomy', G. Scambler (ed.), *Sociological Theory and Medical Sociology.* London: Tavistock.
Armstrong, D. (1993) 'Public health spaces and the fabrication of identity', *Sociology,* Vol. 27, No. 3, pp. 393–410.
Arnold, D. and Yapita, J. (1994) *Traditional Maternity in Qaqachaka, Oruro: An Outline Summary of the Existing Health Care Facilities, Practices and Beliefs Surrounding Childbirth in One Andean Ayllu,* preliminary report to the European Community. La Paz: ILCA (unpublished).
Arnold, D., Tito, M., and Yapita, J. (forthcoming) *Vocabulario Aymara del Parto y de la Vida Reproductiva de la Mujer.* La Paz: UNICEF.
Atthill, L. (1879) 'Report and clinical records of the Rotunda Hospital for the year ending 5th November, 1878', *Dublin Quarterly Journal of Medical Science,* Vol. LXVIII.
Balaskas, J. (1983) *Active Birth.* London: Unwin.

Bartky, S. (1988). 'Foucault, femininity, and the modernization of patriarchal power', I. Diamond and L. Quinby (eds.), *Feminism and Foucault: Reflections on Resistance*. Boston: Northeastern University Press.
Bauman, Z. (1992) *Mortality, Immortality and Other Life Strategies*. Cambridge: Polity Press.
Beatty, T. E. (1834) 'Contributions to midwifery', *Dublin Quarterly Journal of Medical Science*, Vol. IV.
Beatty, T. (1835) 'First report of the new lying-in hospital, Dublin for the year 1834', *Dublin Quarterly Journal of Medical Science*, Vol. VIII.
Beatty, T. E. (1842) 'Contributions to midwifery, IV: cases illustrative of the use of forceps', *Dublin Quarterly Journal of Medical Science*, Vol. XXI.
de Beauvoir, S. (1997) *The Second Sex*. London: Vintage.
Begley, C. (1987) 'Episiotomy: a change in midwives' practice', *Irish Nursing Forum and Health Studies*, November–December.
Begley, C. (1990) 'A comparison of "active" and "physiological" management of the third stage of labour', *Midwifery*, 6, pp. 3–17.
Begley, C.(1997) *Midwives in the Making: A Longitudinal Study of the Experiences of Student Midwives During their Two-Year Training in Ireland*, unpublished PhD. thesis, University of Dublin, Trinity College.
Begley, C.(1998) 'Explaining Postpartum haemorrhage – the value of a physiological third stage', P. Kennedy and J. Murphy-Lawless (eds.) *Returning Birth to Women: Challenging Policies and Practices*, Dublin: Centre for Women's Studies, TCD/WERRC.
Bell, S. (1988) 'Becoming a political woman: the reconstruction and interpretation of experience through stories', A. Todd and S. Fisher (eds.) *Gender and Discourse: The Power of Talk*. Norwood, NJ: Ablex.
Boland, E. (1995) *Object Lessons: The Life of the Woman and the Poet in Our Time*. Manchester: Carcanet Press.
Boston Women's Health Collective (1971) *Our Bodies, Ourselves*. New York: Simon and Schuster.
Botha, M. C. (1968) 'The management of the umbilical cord in labour', *South African Journal of Obstetrics and Gynecology*, Vol. 16, No. 2.
Bourne, G. (1975) *Pregnancy*. London: Pan.
Brahams, D. (1996) 'Caesarean sections by court order', *The Lancet*, Vol. 348, No. 21, p. 770.
Bronfen, E. (1992) *Over Her Dead Body: Death, Femininity and the Aesthetic*. Manchester: Manchester University Press.
Brown, J. (1986) 'Professional language: words that succeed', *Radical History Review*, 34, pp. 33–51.
Browne, T.D. O'Donel (1947) *The Rotunda Hospital, 1745–1945*. Edinburgh: E. and S. Livingstone.
Caldeyro-Barcia, R. (1960) 'Effect of position changes on the intensity and the frequency of uterine contractions during labour', *American Journal of Obstetrics and Gynecology*, 80.
Cameron, D. (1985) *Feminism and Linguistic Theory*. London: Macmillan.
Campbell, R. and Macfarlane, A. (1995) *Where to be Born?* 2nd edition. Oxford: Crown Publications for National Perinatal Epidemiology Unit.
Canguilhem, G. (1980) 'What is psychology?' *Ideology and Consciousness*, No. 7, pp. 37–50.
Canguilhem, G. (1989) *The Normal and the Pathological*. New York: Zone Books.
Cartwright, A. (1979) *The Dignity of Labour? A Study of Childbearing and Induction*. London: Tavistock.
Caspar, M. (1994) 'At the margins of humanity: fetal positions in science and medicine', *Technology and Human Values*, Vol. 19, No. 3, p. 105.

Castel, R. (1991) 'From dangerousness to risk', G. Burchell, C. Gordon, and P. Miller (eds.) *The Foucault Effect: Studies in Governmentality.* Hemel Hempstead: Harvester Wheatsheaf.
Central Statistics Office (1995) *Vital Statistics, 1994.* Cork: CSO.
Chalmers, I. (1978) 'Implications of the current debate on obstetric practice', S. Kitzinger and J. Davis (eds.) *The Place of Birth.* Oxford: Oxford University Press.
Chalmers, I. et al. (1989) *Effective Care in Pregnancy and Childbirth.* Oxford: Oxford University Press.
Chard, T. and Richards, M. (1977) *Benefits and Hazards of the New Obstetrics.* London: Heinemann.
Children's Defence Fund (1988) *A Call for Action to Make Our Nation Safe for Children: A Briefing Book on the Status of American Children in 1988.* Washington, DC: Children's Defence Fund.
Churchill, F. (1838) 'Second medical report of the western lying-in hospital and dispensary, 31 Arran Quay', *Dublin Quarterly Journal of Medical Science,* Vol. XIII.
Churchill, F. (1849) 'Epidemics of puerperal fever', F. Churchill (ed.) *Collected Essays on Puerperal Fever.* London: Sydenham Society.
Churchill, F. (1851) *Researches on Operative Midwifery.* Dublin: Martin Keene and Son.
Churchill, F. (1858) 'Obstetric Morality', *Dublin Quarterly Journal of Medical Science,* Vol. XXVI.
Clarke, J. (1817) 'Abstract of a registry kept for some years in the lying-in hospital in Dublin', *Transactions of the Association of Fellows and Licentiates of the King and Queen's College of Physicians,* Vol. 1, Dublin.
Clarke, J. (1849) 'Observations on the puerperal fever', F. Churchill (ed.) *Collected Essays on Puerperal Fever.* London: Sydenham Society.
Coakley, D. (1988) *The Irish School of Medicine: Outstanding Practitioners of the Nineteenth Century.* Dublin: Town House.
Code, L. (1995) *Rhetorical Spaces: Essays on Gendered Locations.* London: Routledge.
Cohen, N. and Estner, L. (1983) *Silent Knife: Cesarian Prevention and Vaginal Birth after Cesarian.* South Hadley, MS: Bergin and Garvey Publishers.
Colgan, J. (1992) *The Marginalisation of the Dublin Community Midwife: 1950–1973,* unpublished MA thesis, WERRC, UCD.
Colgan, K. (1994) *If It Happens to You.* Dublin: A. and A. Farmar.
Collins, R. (1836) *A Practical Treatise on Midwifery Containing the Results of Sixteen Thousand Six Hundred and Fifty-Four Births Occurring in the Dublin Lying-in hospital During a Period of Seven Years Commencing November 1826.* London: Longman, Rees, Orme, Browne, Green and Longman.
Collins, R. (1837) 'Observations on the artificial dilatation of the mouth of the womb during labour, and upon instrumental delivery'. *Dublin Quarterly Journal of Medical Science,* Vol. XI.
Collins, R. (1849) *A Short Sketch of the Life and Writings of the late Joseph Clarke.* London: Longman, Brown, Green and Longman.
Cunningham, F. et al. (1993) *Williams Obstetrics.* 19th edition. London: Prentice Hall International.
Davis, E. (1992) *Heart and Hands: A Midwife's Guide to Pregnancy and Birth.* Berkeley, CA.: Celestial Arts.
Davis-Floyd, R. (1992) *Birth as an American Rite of Passage.* Berkeley, CA: University of California Press.

Davis-Floyd, R. and Sargent, C. (1996) 'Introduction: The Social Production of Authoritative Knowledge in Pregnancy and Childbirth', *Medical Anthropology Quarterly*, New Series, Vol. 10, No. 2.

Dease, W. (1783) *Observations in Midwifery Particularly on the Different Methods of Assisting Women in Tedious and Difficult Labours*. Dublin: Williams, White, Wilson, Byrne and Cash.

Department of Health, Comhairle na n-Ospidéal (1976) *Development of Hospital Maternity Services: A Discussion Document*. Dublin: Stationery Office.

Department of Health (1984) *Vital Statistics, 1983*. Dublin: Stationery Office.

Department of Health (1991) *Vital Statistics, 1990*. Dublin: Stationery Office.

Department of Health (1994) *Report of the Maternity and Infant Care Scheme Review Group, April, 1994* (unpublished).

Department of Health (1995) *Developing a Policy for Women's Health*. Dublin: Government Stationery Office.

Department of Health (1995) *Perinatal Statistics, 1991*. Dublin: Stationery Office.

Department of Health (1996) *Perinatal Statistics, 1992*, Dublin: Stationery Office.

Department of Health (1996) *Vital Statistics, Fourth Quarter and Yearly Summary, 1995*. Dublin: Stationery Office.

Descartes, R. (1912) *A Discourse on Method*. London: J.M. Dent and Sons.

Deventer, H. (1716) *The Art of Midwifery Improv'd*. London: E. Curll, J. Pemberton and W. Taylor.

Diaz, A. G. et al. (1980) 'Vertical position during the first stage of the course of labour and neonatal outcome', *European Journal of Obstetrics and Gynaecology*, Vol. 11, No. 1.

Dick-Read, G. (1969) *Childbirth Without Fear: The Principles and Practice of Natural Childbirth*. 5th Edition. London: Pan Books.

Dingwall, R. (1977) '"Atrocity stories" and professional relationships', *Sociology of Work and Occupations*, Vol. 4, No.4.

le Doeuff, M. (1981) 'Pierre Roussel's chiasmas: from imaginary knowledge to the learned imagination', *Ideology and Consciousness*, No. 9. 1981–2, pp. 39–70.

Donegan, J. (1978) *Women and Men Midwives: Medicine, Morality and Misogyny in Early America*. Westport, CT: Greenwood Press.

Donnison, J. (1977) *Midwives and Medical Men. A History of Interprofessional Rivalries and Women's Rights*. London: Heinemann.

Douglas, M. and Wildavsky, A. (1982) *Risk and Culture: An Essay on the Selection of Technological and Environmental Dangers*. Berkeley: University of California Press.

Douglas, M. (1986) *Risk Acceptability According to the Social Sciences*. London: Routledge and Kegan Paul.

Dublin Obstetrical Society (1869) 'Proceedings: discussion on Dr. Evory Kennedy's proposal', *Dublin Quarterly Journal of Medical Science* Vol. XLVIII.

Duden, B. (1991) *The Woman Beneath the Skin: A Doctor's Patients in Eighteenth-Century Germany*. Cambridge, MA: Harvard University Press.

Dunn, P. M. (1991) 'Franois Mauriceau (1637–1709) and maternal posture for parturition', *Archives of Disease in Childhood*, Vol. 66, No.1, January, pp. 78–79.

Durward, L. and Evans, R. (1990) 'Pressure Groups and Maternity Care', J. Garcia et al. (eds.) *The Politics of Maternity Care: Services for Childbearing Women in Twentieth Century Britain*. Oxford: Oxford University Press.

Dye, N. (1991) 'The history of the relationship between women's health and technology', J. Rodin and A. Collins (eds.) *Women and New Reproductive Technologies: Medical, Psychosocial, Legal and Ethical Dilemmas*. Hillsdale, NJ: Lawrence Erlbaum Associates.

Easlea, B. (1981) *Science and Sexual Oppression: Patriarchy's Confrontation with Women and Nature*. London: Weidenfeld and Nicolson.
Eccles, A. (1982) *Obstetrics and Gynaecology in Tudor and Stuart England*. London: Croom Helm.
Ehrenreich, B. and English, D. (1976) *Complaints and Disorders: The Sexual Politics of Sickness*. London: Writers and Readers Publishing Cooperative.
Ehrenreich, B. and English, D. (1979) *For her own Good: 150 Years of the Experts' Advice to Women*. London: Pluto Press.
Elliott, J. (1867) 'Description and statistics of the Waterford lying-in hospital', *Dublin Quarterly Journal of Medical Science*, Vol. XLIV, November.
Enkin, Keirse, M., Renfrew M. and Neilson, J. (1995) *A Guide to Effective Care in Pregnancy and Childbirth*. 2nd edition. Oxford: Oxford University Press.
Enkin, M. et al. (1995) *A Guide to Effective Care in Pregnancy and Childbirth*. 2nd edition. Oxford: Oxford University Press.
Erickson, R. A. (1982) 'The "Books of Generation": some observations on the style of British midwife books, 1671–1764', P. Bouc (ed.) *Sexuality in Eighteenth-Century Britain*. Manchester: Manchester University Press.
Ewald, F. (1991) 'Insurance and risk', G. Burchell, C. Gordon, and P. Miller (eds.) *The Foucault Effect: Studies in Governmentality*. Hemel Hempstead: Harvester Wheatsheaf.
Eyer, D. (1992) *Mother-Infant Bonding: A Scientific Fiction*. Woburn, Massachusetts: Yale University Press.
Fairclough, N. (1985) 'Critical and descriptive goals in discourse analysis', *Journal of Pragmatics*, 9, pp. 739–763.
Farmar, T. (1994) *Holles Street, 1894–1994: The National Maternity Hospital – A Centenary History*. Dublin: A. and A. Farmar.
Faulkner's Dublin Journal, No. 1884, 23 to 26 March, 1745.
Feeney, J. A. (1955) 'The grand multipara: trauma of labour', *Journal of the Irish Medical Association*, January–June.
Figlio, K. (1989) 'Unconscious aspects of health in the public sphere', B. Richards (ed.) *Crises of the Self: Further Essays on Psychoanalysis and Politics*. London: Free Association Press.
Finger, A. (1987) 'Claiming all of our bodies: reproductive rights and disability', R. Arditti et al (eds.) *Test-tube Women: What Future for Motherhood?* London: Pandora Press.
Fleck, L. (1979) *Genesis and Development of a Scientific Fact*. Chicago: University of Chicago Press.
Flint, C. (1986) *Sensitive Midwifery*. London: Heinemann Medical Books.
Foucault, M. (1974) *The Archaeology of Knowledge*. London: Tavistock.
Foucault, M. (1976) *The Birth of the Clinic*. London: Tavistock.
Foucault, M. (1977) 'Neitzsche, genealogy, history', D. Bouchard (ed.) *Language, Counter-Memory, Practice, Selected Essays and Interviews*. Ithaca, NY: Cornell University Press.
Foucault, M. (1979) *Discipline and Punish: The Birth of the Prison*. Harmondsworth: Penguin.
Foucault, M. (1980) 'Two Lectures', C. Gordon (ed.) *Power/Knowledge: Selected Interviews and Other Writings, 1972–77*. Brighton: Harvester Wheatsheaf.
Foucault, M. (1980) *Power/Knowledge: Selected Interviews and Other Writings. 1972–77*. Brighton: Harvester Wheatsheaf.
Foucault, M. (1980) 'The history of sexuality', C. Gordon (ed.) *Power/Knowledge: Selected Interviews and Other Writings 1972–77*. Brighton: Harvester Wheatsheaf.
Foucault, M. (1983) 'On the genealogy of ethics: an overview of work in progress', H. Dreyfus and P. Rabinow (eds.) *Michel Foucault: Beyond Structuralism and Hermeneutics*. Chicago: University of Chicago Press.

Foucault, M. (1981) *The History of Sexuality, Volume 1: An Introduction.* Harmondsworth: Penguin.
Foucault, M. (1988) 'Critical theory/intellectual history', L. Kritzman (ed.) *Michel Foucault: Politics, Philosophy, Culture. Interviews and Other Writings, 1977–1984.* London: Routledge.
Foucault, M. (1988) 'Technologies of the self', L. Martin et al. (eds.) *Technologies of the Self: A Seminar with Michel Foucault.* London: Tavistock.
Foucault, M. (1988) 'The Dangerous Individual', L. Kritzman (ed.) *Michel Foucault: Politics, Philosophy, Culture. Interviews and Other Writings, 1977–1984.* London: Routledge.
Frankenberg, R. (1992) '"Your time or mine": temporal contradictions of biomedical practice', R. Frankenberg (ed.) *Time, Health and Medicine.* London:Sage.
Freud, S. (1991) *Introductory Lectures on Psychoanalysis.* Vol. 1. Harmondsworth: Penguin.
Friedman, E. A. (1973) 'Patterns of labour as indicators of risk' *Clinical Obstetrics and Gynecology,* 120.
Friedman, E. A. et al. (1977) 'Dysfunctional labor: long term effects on the infant', *American Journal of Obstetrics and Gynecology,* 127.
Gálvez Murillo, A. et al. (1997) *Obstetricia Práctica.* La Paz: Medicon.
Gaskin, I. (1977) *Spiritual Midwifery.* Summertown, TN: The Book Publishing Company.
Gaskin, I. M. (1988) 'Shoulder dystocia: controversies in management', *Birth Gazette,* Vol. 5, No.1, pp. 14–17.
Gélis, J. (1991) *History of Childbirth: Fertility, Pregnancy and Birth in Early Modern Europe.* Cambridge: Polity Press.
Gerth, H. and Mills, C. W. (1991) *From Max Weber's Essays in Sociology.* London: Routledge.
Glynn, M. and Oláh, K. (1994) 'The management of shoulder dystocia', *British Journal of Midwifery,* Vol. 2, No.3. 1994.
Gordon, A. (1795) *A Treatise on the Epidemic Puerperal Fever of Aberdeen.* London: G.G. and J. Robinson.
Gyte, G. M. L. (1994) 'Evaluation of the Meta-analyses on the effects, on both mother and baby, of the various components of 'active' management of the third stage of labour', *Midwifery,* 10, pp. 183–199.
Hacking, I. (1990) *The Taming of Chance.* Cambridge: Cambridge University Press.
Hacking, I. (1991) 'How Should we do the History of Statistics?' G. Burchell, C. Gordon, and P. Miller (eds.) *The Foucault Effect: Studies in Governmentality.* Hemel Hempstead: Harvester Wheatsheaf.
Hamilton, J. (1838) 'A letter from Professor Hamilton of Edinburgh in reply to the objections made to his practical precepts in midwifery by Dr. Collins', *Dublin Quarterly Journal of Medical Science,* Vol. XIII.
Harvie, J. (1935) 'Delivery of the placenta', H. Thoms (ed.) *Classical Contributions to Obstetrics and Gynecology.* Springfield, IL: Charles C. Thomas.
Hazell, L. (1976) *Commonsense Childbirth.* New York: G.P. Putnam's Sons.
Herzlich, C. and Pierret, J. (1987) *Illness and Self in Society.* Baltimore: Johns Hopkins University Press.
Hill, S. (1989) *Family.* Michael Joseph: London.
House of Commons, Social Services Committee (1980) *Second Report from the Social Services Committee, Session 1979–80, Perinatal and Neonatal Mortality.* Vol. I. London: HMSO.
House of Commons, Health Committee (1992) *Second Report, Session 1991–2, Maternity Services.* Vol. I. London: HMSO.
House of Commons, Social Services Committee (1993) *Changing Childbirth.* London: HMSO.

Hibbard, B. (1988) *Principles of Obstetrics*. London: Butterworths.
Holmes, O. W. (1935) 'The contagiousness of puerperal fever', H. Thoms (ed.) *Classical Contributions to Obstetrics and Gynecology*. Springfield, IL: Charles C. Thomas.
Hulme, N. (1849) 'On the puerperal fever' F. Churchill (ed.) *Collected Essays on Puerperal Fever*. London: Sydenham Society.
Huntingford, P. (1982) 'Foreword', S. Inch *Birthrights*, first edition. London: Hutchinson.
Huntingford, P. (1984) 'Birth right: the parent's choice', British Broadcasting Corporation.
ILCA (1995) *Maternidad Tradicional en el Altiplano Boliviano: las prcticas del parto en algunas comunidades aymaras. Informe borrador para la comunidad Europea*. La Paz: ILCA (unpublished).
Illsley, R. (1967) 'The sociological study of reproduction and its outcome', S. Richardson and A. Guttmacher (eds.) *Childbearing – Its Social and Psychological Aspects*. Baltimore: Willams and Wilkins.
Inch, S. (1989) *Birthrights: A Parent's Guide to Modern Childbirth*. 2nd edition. London: Green Print.
Instituto Nacional de Estadstica/Demographic and Health Surveys (1994) *Encuesta Nacional de Demografia y Salud, 1994*. La Paz: Instituto Nacional de Estadstica/ Demographic and Health Surveys.
International Congress of Obstetrics and Gynaecology (1947) *Transactions of the International Congress of Obstetrics and Gynaecology, Rotunda Bicentenary Congress*. Dublin: Parkside Press.
Irish Association for Improvement in the Maternity Services (n.d.) *A Consumer's Guide to the Maternity Units in Ireland*. Dublin: Health Promotion Unit, Department of Health.
Irish Office (1830) *Reports of the Commissioners on Certain Charitable Institutions in Dublin, 1830*. Appendix No. 6. London: Irish Office.
Jacob, F. (1974) *The Logic of Living Systems*. London: Allen Lane.
Jellett, H. (1900) 'The Dublin method of effecting the delivery of the placenta', *Dublin Journal of Medical Science*, Vol. CIX.
Jellett, H. (1929) *The Causes and Prevention of Maternal Mortality*. London: J. and A. Churchill.
Jebb, F. (1772) 'Of an haemorrhage occasioned by the adhesion of the placenta to the os uteri', *Transactions, Medical and Philosophical Memoirs*, Volume III, 3 December, Dublin.
Johnston, G. (1870) 'Clinical report of the Rotunda lying-in hospital for the year ending 5th November, 1869', *Dublin Quarterly Journal of Medical Science*, Vol. XLIV.
Johnston, G. (1872) 'Clinical report of the Rotunda Lying-in hospital for the Year ending 5th November, 1871', *Dublin Quarterly Journal of Medical Science*, Vol. LIII.
Johnston, G. (1873) Clinical Report of the Rotunda lying-in hospital for the year ending 5th November, 1872. In *Dublin Quarterly Journal of Medical Science*, Vol. LV.
Johnston, G. (1875) 'Clinical report of the Rotunda lying-in hospital for the year ending 5th November, 1874', *Dublin Quarterly Journal of Medical Science*, Vol. LIX.
Johnston, G. (1879) 'Clinical report of 752 cases of forceps delivery in hospital practice', *Dublin Quarterly Journal of Medical Science*. Vol. LXVIII.
Jordan, B. (1989) 'Cosmopolitical obstetrics: some insights from the training of traditional midwives', *Social Science and Medicine*, Vol. 28, No. 9, pp.925–944.
Jordanova, L. (1989) *Sexual Visions: Images of Gender in Science and Medicine Between the Eighteenth and Twentieth Centuries*. Hemel Hempstead: Harvester Wheatsheaf.
Kaufert, P. and O'Neil, J. (1993) 'Analysis of a dialogue on risks in childbirth: clinicians, epidemiologists and Inuit women', S. Lindenbaum and M. Lock (eds.) *Knowledge,*

Power and Practice: The Anthropology of Medicine and Everyday Life. Berkeley: University of California Press.

Keller, E. F. (1990) 'From secrets of life to secrets of death', M. Jacobus et al. (eds.) *Body/Politics: Women and the Discourses of Science*. London: Routledge.

Keller, E. F. (1992) *Secrets of Life, Secrets of Death: Essays on Language, Gender and Science*. London: Routledge.

Kember, S. (1996) 'Feminist figuration and the question of origin', G. Robertson et al. (eds.) *FutureNatural: Nature/Science/Culture*. London: Routledge.

Kennedy, E. (1869) 'Zymotic diseases as more especially illustrated by puerperal fever', *Dublin Quarterly Journal of Medical Science*, Vol. XLVIII.

Kennedy, P. (1998) 'Between the lines: mother and infant care in Ireland', P. Kennedy and J. Murphy-Lawless (eds.) *Returning Birth to Women: Challenging Policies and Practices*. Dublin: Centre for Women's Studies, TCD/WERRC.

Kerrigan, G. (1990) *Nothing but the Truth*. Dublin: Tomar Press.

Kirkpatrick, T. and Jellett, H. (1913) *The Book of the Rotunda Hospital*. London: Adlard and Son, Bartholomew Press.

Kitzinger, S. (1972) *The Experience of Childbirth*. Third Edition. Harmondsworth: Penguin.

Kitzinger, S. and Walters, R. (1981) *Some Women's Experiences of Episiotomy*. London: National Childbirth Trust.

Kitzinger, S. (1988) 'Why women need midwives', S. Kitzinger (ed.) *The Midwife Challenge*. London: Pandora Press.

Klaus, M. H. et al. (1994) 'The Dublin experience', *Mothering*, No. 72.

Kuhn, T. (1977) *The Essential Tension: Selected Essays in Scientific Transition and Change*. Chicago: University of Chicago Press.

Kwast, B. (1991) 'Postpartum haemorrhage: its contribution to maternal mortality', *Midwifery*, Vol. 7, pp. 64–70.

Kwast, B. (1995) 'Building a community-based maternity program', *Reproductive Health The MotherCare Experience*, supplement to *International Journal of Gynaecology and Obstetrics*,. Vol. 48, June, 1995. pp. S67–S82.

Lane, J. (1887) 'Report of the Rotunda hospital for three years ending 3rd November, 1886', *Dublin Quarterly Journal of Medical Science*, Vol. LXXXIV.

Lawson, J. (1759) *A Sermon Intended to Have Been Preached at the Publick Opening of the Chapel of the Lying-in Hospital in Great Britain Street, Dublin*. Dublin.

Latour, B. (1987) *Science in the Making: How to Follow Scientists and Engineers Through Society*. Milton Keynes: Open University Press.

Latour, B. (1988) *The Pasteurisation of France*. Cambridge, MS: Harvard University Press.

de Lauretis, T. (1987) 'The violence of rhetoric: considerations on representation and gender', *Technologies of Gender: Essays on Theory, Film, and Fiction*. Bloomington: Indiana University Press.

Lee, H., trans. (1965) *Timaeus* by Plato. Harmondsworth: Penguin.

Leap, N. and Hunter, B. (1993) *The Midwife's Tale: An Oral History from Handywoman to Professional Midwife*. London: Scarlet Press.

Leavitt, J. (1986) *Brought to Bed: Childbearing in America, 1750–1950*. New York: Oxford University Press.

de Lee, J. (1920) 'The prophylactic forceps operation', *American Journal of Obstetrics and Gynaecology*, 1.

Lenstrup, G. et al. (1987) 'Warm tub bath during delivery', *Acta Obstetrica et Gynecologia Scandinavica*, Vol. 66, No. 8.

Lévi-Strauss, C. (1963) *Structural Anthropology*. New York: Basic Books.
Lewis, T. and Chamberlain, G. (1990) *Obstetrics by Ten Teachers*. 15th edition. London: Edward Arnold.
Llewellyn-Jones, D. (1969) *Fundamentals of Obstetrics and Gynaecology*. Vol. I. London: Faber and Faber.
Londoño, M. L. (1993) 'Initial document for the study of an ethics from women and for women (Latin American and Caribbean Women's Health Network)', *IN/FIRE Ethics, Newsletter of the International Network of Feminists Interested in Reproductive Health*. Volume 2, Issue 3.
Loudon, I. (1992) *Death in Childbirth: An International Study of Maternal Care and Maternal Mortality 1800–1950*. Oxford: Clarendon Press.
Maine, D. (1991) *Safe Motherhood Programs: Options and Issues*. New York: Prevention of Maternal Mortality Program, Center for Population and Family Health, Columbia University.
Maine, D. et al. (1995) 'Risks and rights: the uses of reproductive health data', *Reproductive Health Matters*, No. 6, November.
MacCormack, C. (1980) 'Nature, culture and gender: A critique', C. MacCormack and M. Strathern (eds.) *Nature, Culture and Gender*. Cambridge: Cambridge University Press.
MacKenzie, D. (1990) *Inventing Accuracy: A Historical Sociology of Nuclear Missile Guidance*. Cambridge, MA: MIT Press.
Martin, E. (1987) *The Woman in the Body: A Cultural Analysis of Reproduction*. Boston: Beacon Press.
Martin, E. (1990) 'The ideology of reproduction: the reproduction of ideology', F. Ginsburg and A.L. Tsing (eds.) *Uncertain Terms: Negotiating Gender in American Culture*. Boston: Beacon Press.
Martin, E. (1992) 'Body narratives, body boundaries', L. Grossberg and P. Treichler (eds.) *Cultural Studies*. New York: Routledge.
Mason, M. (1998) 'Childbirth education: empowerment or indoctrination?' P. Kennedy and J. Murphy-Lawless (eds.) *Returning Birth to Women: Challenging Policies and Practices*. Dublin: Centre for Women's Studies, TCD/WERRC.
McAdam-O'Connell, B. (1998) 'Risk, responsibility and choice: the medical model of birth and alternatives', P. Kennedy and J. Murphy-Lawless (eds.) *Returning Birth to Women: Challenging Policies and Practices*. Dublin: Centre for Women's Studies, WERRC/TCD.
McDonagh, M. (1996) 'Is antenatal care effective in reducing maternal morbidity and mortality?' *Health Policy and Planning*, Vol. 11, no. 1, pp. 1–15.
McKeown, T. (1988) *The Origins of Human Disease*. Oxford: Basil Blackwell.
McNay, L. (1992) *Foucault and Feminism*. Cambridge: Polity Press.
Ministry of Social Affairs and Health (1996) *itiyskuolleisuus, 1960–1994*. Helsinki, Finland: Ministry of Social Affairs and Health.
Mitford, J. (1992) *The American Way of Birth*. London: Victor Gollancz.
Moore, W. (1978) 'Antenatal care and the choice of place of birth', S. Kitzinger and J. Davis (eds.) *The Place of Birth*. Oxford: Oxford Medical Publications.
de la Motte, G. (1746) *A General Treatise of Midwifery*, reprinted 1985. New York: Garland.
Moscucci, O. (1990) *The Science of Woman: Gynaecology and Gender in England, 1800–1929*. Cambridge: Cambridge University Press.
Murphy, E. W. (1839) 'An examination of Dr. Hamilton's letters in defence of his opinions, especially in reference to the management of the first stage of labour', *Dublin Quarterly Journal of Medical Science*, Vol. XIV.

Murphy, E. W. (1857) 'Puerperal fever', *Dublin Quarterly Journal of Medical Science*, Vol. XXIV.

Murphy-Lawless, J. (1987) 'Women and childbirth: male medical discourse and the invention of female incompetence', Ph.D. Thesis. University of Dublin, Trinity College, (unpublished).

Murphy-Lawless, J. (1988) 'The obstetric view of feminine identity: a case history of the use of forceps on unmarried women in nineteenth-century Ireland', A. Todd and S. Fisher (eds.) *Gender and Discourse: The Power of Talk*. Norwood, NJ: Ablex, pp.190–192.

Murphy-Lawless, J. (1988) 'The silencing of women in childbirth or let's hear it from Bartholomew and the boys', *International Women's Studies Forum*, Vol. 11, No. 4, pp. 293–298.

Murphy-Lawless, J. (1989) 'Male texts and female bodies: the colonisation of childbirth by men midwives', B. Torode (ed.) *Text and Talk as Social Practice: Discourse Difference and Division in Speech and Writing*. Dordrecht, Holland: Foris Publications.

Murphy-Lawless, J. (1991) 'Piggy in the Middle: The Midwife's Role in Achieving Woman-controlled Childbirth', *Irish Journal of Psychology*, Vol. 12, No. 2.

Murphy-Lawless, J. (1991) 'Images of "poor women" in the writings of Irish men midwives', M. MacCurtain and M. O'Dowd (eds.) *Women in Early Modern Ireland*. Edinburgh: Edinburgh University Press.

Murphy-Lawless, J. (1992) 'Reading birth and death through obstetric practice' *Canadian Journal of Irish Studies*, Vol. 18, No. 1, pp. 129–145.

Murphy-Lawless, J. (1993) 'Fertility, bodies and politics: the Irish case' *Reproductive Health Matters*, No. 2.

Murphy-Lawless, J. (1998) 'Women dying in childbirth: the international context of "safe motherhood"', P. Kennedy and J. Murphy-Lawless (eds.) *Returning Birth to Women: Challenging Policies and Practices*. Dublin: Centre for Women's Studies, TCD/WERRC.

Murphy-Lawless, J. (forthcoming). 'Women and Childbirth: The Institutional Experience', S. Deane (ed.) *The Field Day Anthology, Volume IV, Women in Ireland*. Field Day Publications in association with W. W. Norton.

Musgrave, J. A. (1932) The Role of the Midwife in the Public Health Service. In *Irish Journal of Medical Science*, Sixth Series, No. 77.

Newton, N. (1978) 'The role of oxytocic reflexes in three reproductive acts', *Clinical Psychoneuroendocrinology in Reproduction*. London: Academic Press.

Nihell, E. (1760) *Treatise on the Art of Midwifery: Setting Forth Various Abuses Therein, Especially as to the Practice of Instruments*. London: Haymarket.

Nijhof, G. (1989) 'On naturalisation in health care', B. Torode (ed.) *Text and Talk as Social Practice: Discourse Difference and Division in Speech and Writing*. Dordrecht, Holland: Foris Publications.

North Inner City Folklore Project (1991) *Living in the City*. Dublin: Mount Salus Press.

Oakley, A. (1976) 'Wisewoman and medicine man', J. Mitchell and A. Oakley (eds.) *The Rights and Wrongs of Women*. Harmondsworth: Penguin.

Oakley, A. (1979) *From Here to Maternity: Becoming a Mother*. Oxford: Martin Robertson.

Oakley, A. (1980) *Women Confined: Towards a Sociology of Childbirth*. Oxford: Martin Robertson.

Oakley, A. and Graham, H. (1981) 'Competing ideologies of reproduction: medical and maternal perspectives on pregnancy', H. Roberts (ed.) *Women, Health and Reproduction*. London: Routledge and Kegan Paul.

Oakley, A. (1984) *The Captured Womb: A History of the Medical Care of Pregnant Women.* Oxford: Basil Blackwell.
O'Brien, M. (1981) *The Politics of Reproduction.* London: Routledge and Kegan Paul.
O'Brien, M. (1989) *Reproducing the World.* Boulder, CO: Westview Press.
O'Connor, M. (1992) *Women and Birth: A National Study of Intentional Home Births in Ireland.* Dublin: Coombe Hospital and the Department of Health (unpublished).
O'Connor, M. (1995) *Birthtides: Turning Towards Home Birth.* London: HarperCollins.
O'Driscoll, K. (1972) 'Impact of active management on delivery unit practice', *Proceedings of the Royal Society of Medicine,* Vol. 65, August, pp. 697–698.
O'Driscoll, K. and Meagher, D. (1986) *Active Management of Labour,* second edition. London: Baillire Tindall.
O'Driscoll, K., Meagher, D. and Boylan, P. (1993) *Active Management of Labour,* third edition. Aylesbury, England: Mosby Year Book Europe Ltd.
Oudshoorn, N. (1996) 'A natural order of things? Reproductive sciences and the politics of othering', G. Robertson et al. (eds.) *FutureNatural: Nature/Science/Culture.* London: Routledge.
Ould, F. (1742) *A Treatise of Midwifry in Three Parts.* Dublin: Oli. Nelson and Charles Connor.
Petchesky, R. (1987) 'Foetal images: the power of visual culture in the politics of reproduction', M. Stanworth (ed.) *Reproductive Technologies: Gender, Motherhood and Medicine.* Cambridge: Polity Press.
Phelan, D. (1867) 'Comparative advantages of attending women in lying-in hospitals and their own homes', *Dublin Quarterly Journal of Medical Science,* Vol. XLIII.
Phillips, A. and Rakusen, J. (1989) *The New Our Bodies, Ourselves.* Boston Women's Health Book Collective. British edition. Harmondsworth: Penguin.
Pizzini, F. (1992) 'Women's time, institutional time', R. Frankenburg (ed.) *Time, Health and Medicine.* London: Sage.
Plant, S. (1996) 'The virtual complexity of culture', G. Robertson et al. (eds.) *FutureNatural: Nature/Science/Culture.* London: Routledge.
Poor Law Commission (1841) *Report of the Poor Law Commissioners on Medical Charities, Ireland Pursuant to the 46th Section of the Act 1 & 2 Victoria, C. 56.* Dublin: Alexander Thom.
Poovey, M. (1988) *Uneven Developments: The Ideological Work of Gender in Mid-Victorian England.* Chicago: University of Chicago Press.
Porter, R. (1989) 'Death and the doctors in Georgian England', R. Houlbrooke (ed.) *Death, Ritual and Bereavement.* London: Routledge.
Porter, R. (1996) *Cambridge Illustrated History of Medicine.* Cambridge: Cambridge University Press.
Rapp, R. (1985) 'XYLO: a true story', R. Arditti et al. (eds.) *Test-tube Women: What Future for Motherhood?* London: Pandora Press.
Reinharz, S. (1987) 'The social psychology of a miscarriage: an application of symbolic interaction theory and method', M. J. Deegan and M. Hill (eds.) *Women and Symbolic Interaction.* London: Allen and Unwin.
Richards, M. (1978) 'Place of safety? An examination of the risks of hospital delivery', S. Kitzinger and J. Davis (eds.) *The Place of Birth.* Oxford: Oxford Medical Publications.
Romalis, S. (1985) 'Struggle between providers and recipients: the case of birth practices', V. Olesen and E. Lewin (eds.) *Women, Health and Healing: Towards a New Perspective.* London: Tavistock.
Rose, H. (1987) 'Victorian values in the test-tube: the politics of reproductive science and technology', M. Stanworth (ed.) *Reproductive Technologies: Gender, Motherhood and Medicine.* Cambridge: Polity Press.

Ross, I. (1986) 'Midwifery', I. Ross (ed.) *Public Virtue, Public Love, The Early Years of the Dublin Lying-in Hospital.* Dublin: O'Brien Press.

Rothman, B. K. (1982) *In Labour: Women and Power in the Birthplace.* New York: W.W. Norton.

Rothman, B. K. (1986) 'Reflections: on hard work', *Qualitative Sociology,* Vol. 9, No. 1, Spring, pp. 48–53.

Rothman, B.K. (1994) *The Tentative Pregnancy: Amniocentesis and the Sexual Politics of Motherhood.* 2nd edition. London: Pandora Press.

Rotunda Hospital (1756) *A Copy of His Majesty's Royal Charter for Incorporating the governors and Guardians of the Hospital for the Relief of Poor Lying-in Women in Dublin,* 2nd December.

Ruzek, S. (1991) 'Women's Reproductive rights: the impact of technology', J. Rodin and A. Collins (eds.) *Women and New Reproductive Technologies: Medical, Psychosocial, Legal and Ethical Dilemmas.* Hillsdale, NJ: Lawrence Erlbaum Associates.

Savage, W. (1986) *A Savage Enquiry: Who Controls Childbirth.* London: Virago.

Sawicki, J. (1991) *Disciplining Foucault: Feminism, Power and the Body.* London: Routledge.

Scarry, E. (1985) *The Body in Pain: The Making and Unmaking of the World.* New York: Oxford University Press.

Schiebinger, L. (1989) *The Mind has no Sex?: Women in the Origins of Modern Science.* Cambridge, MA: Harvard University Press.

Schwarcz, R. et al. (1976) 'Influence of amniotomy and maternal position on labour', *Proceedings of the VIII World Congress of Gynaecology and Obstetrics.* Amsterdam: Excerpta Medica.

Secretaria Nacional de Salud, Secretaria Regional de Salud, Distrito de Salud Ocuri, IIAM.-UNICEF-IPTK (1994) *Plan Vida: Plan Estrategico para la Reduccin Acelerada de la Mortalidad Materna y del Menor, 1994–1997, Provincia Chayanta, Causas de mortalidad en la Provincia Chayanta.* Ocuri: authors.

Semmelweis, I. P. (1981) 'Childbed fever. Classics in infectious diseases', *Reviews of Infectious Diseases,* Vol. 3, No. 4. July–August, pp. 808–811.

Sherwin, S. (1992) *No Longer Patient: Feminist Ethics and Health Care.* Philadelphia: Temple University Press.

Shilling, C. (1991) 'Educating the body: physical capital and the production of social inequalities', *Sociology,* Vol. 25, No.4, pp. 653–672.

Shilling, C. (1993) *The Body and Social Theory.* London: Sage.

Shorter, E. (1983) *A History of Women's Bodies.* London: Allen Lane.

Silverton, L. (1993) *The Art and Science of Midwifery.* London: Prentice Hall.

Sinclair, E. and Johnston, G. (1858) *Practical Midwifery: Comprising an Account of 13,748 Deliveries which Occurred in the Dublin Lying-in Hospital During the Course of Seven Years Commencing November, 1847.* London: J. Churchill.

Smith, D. E. (1988) *The Everyday World as Problematic.* Milton Keynes: Open University Press.

Solomons, B. (1933) 'Report of the Rotunda hospital (November 1st 1931 to October 31st 1932)', *Irish Journal of Medical Science,* No. 92.

Solomons, B. (1935) 'A letter on maternal mortality', *British Medical Journal,* 11 February.

Solomons, B. and Falkiner, N. (1937) *Tweedy's Practical Obstetrics,* seventh edition. London: Oxford University Press.

Southwell, T. (1742) *Remarks on some of the Errors both in Anatomy and Practice in a late Treatise of Midwifery by Fielding Ould, Man-midwife.* Dublin: Thomas Bacon.

Spencer, H. (1927) *The History of British Midwifery from 1650 to 1800.* London: John Bales, Sons and Danielsson.

Stacey, M. (1988) *The Sociology of Health and Healing.* London: Unwin Hyman.
Starr, P. (1982) *The Social Transformation of American Medicine.* New York: Basic Books.
Stearns, J. (1935) 'The introduction of ergot', H. Thoms (ed.) *Classical Contributions to Obstetrics and Gynaecology.* Springfield, IL: Charles C. Thomas.
Stimson, G. and Webb, B. (1975) *Going to See the Doctor.* London: Routledge and Kegan Paul.
Stoppard, M. (1996) *The Breast Book.* London: Dorling Kindersley.
Supple, B. (1970) *The Royal Exchange Assurance: A History of British Assurance.* London: Cambridge University Press.
Tew, M. (1990) *Safer Childbirth? A Critical History of Maternity Care.* London: Chapman and Hall.
Tierney, G. (1932) 'Maternal mortality', *Irish Journal of Medical Science*, Sixth Series, No. 82, October.
Todd, A. (1989) *Intimate Adversaries: Cultural Conflict between Doctors and Women Patients.* Philadelphia: University of Pennsylvania Press.
Torode, B. (1989) 'Discourse analysis and everyday life', B. Torode (ed.) *Text and Talk as Social Practice: Discourse Difference and Division in Speech and Writing.* Dordrecht, Holland: Foris Publications.
Torrico, C. (1995) *Las tabues y la tecnologa del parto en una comunidad de pastores de puna. Informe Qualitativa para Proyecto Para la Reducción en Mortalidad Materna: Prácticas Apropiadas del Parto.* Sucre, Bolivia: TIFAP (unpublished).
Torrico, C. (1995) *Reading Figures.* Sucre, Bolivia: TIFAP (unpublished).
Treichler, P. (1990) 'Feminism, medicine and the meaning of childbirth', M. Jacobus et al. (eds.) *Body/Politics: Women and the Discourses of Science.* London: Routledge.
Tweedy, E. H. (1908) 'Clinical reports of the Rotunda hospital', *Dublin Journal of Medical Science,* Vol. CXXXV.
Tweedy, E. H. (1909) 'Clinical reports of the Rotunda hospital', *Dublin Journal of Medical Science,* Vol. CXXVIII.
Ulrich, L. (1991) *A Midwife's Tale: The Life of Martha Ballard, Based on Her Diary, 1785–1812.* New York: Vintage Books.
UNICEF (1996) *Progress of Nations, 1996.* New York: UNICEF.
Wagner, M. (1986) Birth and Power. In J. Phaff (ed.) *Perinatal Health Services in Europe: Searching for Better Childbirth.* London: Croom Helm.
Wagner, M. (1994) *Pursuing the Birth Machine: The Search for Appropriate Birth Technology.* Sevenoaks, Kent: ACE Graphics.
Weedon, C. (1987) *Feminist Practices and Poststructuralist Theory.* Oxford: Basil Blackwell.
Weitz, R. and Sullivan, D. (1985) Licensed Lay Midwifery and the Medical Model of Childbirth. In *Sociology of Health and Illness,* Vol. 7, No.1.
Wertz, D. and Wertz, R. (1977) *Lying In: A History of Childbirth in America.* New York: Free Press.
White, C. (1849) 'A treatise on pregnant and lying-in women', F. Churchill (ed.) *Collected Essays on Puerperal Fever.* London: Sydenham Society.
WHO (1985) *Having a Baby in Europe, Public Health in Europe, Number 26.* Copenhagen: WHO.
WHO (1990) *The Prevention and Management of Postpartum Haemorrhage. Report of a Technical Working Group, Geneva, 3–6 July, 1989.* Geneva: WHO.
WHO (1994) *Mother-Baby Package: Implementing Safe Motherhood in Countries.* Geneva: WHO.

WHO/UNICEF (1996) *Estimates of Maternal Mortality: A New Approach by WHO and UNICEF.* Geneva: WHO.

Wilde, W. (1849) 'A short account of the superstitions and popular practices relating to midwifery, and some of the diseases of women and children, in Ireland', *The Monthly Journal of Medical Science*, New Series, No. XXXV, May, pp. 711–729.

Willughby, P. (1972) *Observations in Midwifery.* Reprint. East Ardsley: S. R. Publishers.

Wright, P. and Treacher, A. (1982) 'Introduction', P. Wright and A. Treacher (eds.) *The Problem of Medical Knowledge: Examining the Social Construction of Medicine.* Edinburgh: Edinburgh University Press.

Wright, P. (1988) 'Babyhood: the social construction of infant care as a medical problem in the years around 1900', M. Lock and D. Gordon (eds.) *Biomedicine Examined.* Dordrecht, Netherlands: Kluwer Academic Publishers.

Index

Aberdeen, 116, 118, 131, 133
abortion, 26, 155, 192, 237
    foetal material, 254
    illegal, 193
active birth, 260–1
active management of labour, 14, 25, 59
    accountability of women, 213–14
    Dunne case, 215–23
    early forms of, 172–3
    from induction to acceleration, 204–14
    Irish development of, 205–14
    post-partum haemorrhage, 185–90
    statistics, 212–13, 223–5
    woman's response, 245
Active Management of Labour (O'Driscoll), 197, 205–14, 223–4, 233
actuarial tables, 160
afterbirth. *see* placenta
agency
    cognitive authority denied, 196
    decision-making power, 238
    demand for, 4, 26–9
    exercise of, 250
    loss of, 6–7, 17–22, 156 (*see also* induction of labour)
    reclaiming, 249–56
    understanding loss of, 22–5
    usurpation of, 9–10, 25–31
    women's horror stories, 244–9
Allen, Isabel, 130
Allgemeines Krankenhaus, Vienna, 122
anaemia, 191, 192
anatomy
    gendered, 36
    normal *vs* pathological, 167–8
    science of, 142–3
antenatal clinic, 12
anthropometry, 168

antibiotics, 101, 192
antisepsis, 100, 101
    acceptance of, 152–7
Appropriate Technology for Birth, conference on, 253
Armstrong, David, 35
Arneth, Professor D.F.H., 25
asepsis, 100, 101, 124, 148, 192
atrocity stories, 236
Atthill, Lombe, 185, 201
auscultation, 93, 216, 218
Australia, 205
Austria, 134
Avicenna, 106

bacteraemia, 111
barber-surgeons, 53, 90, 92
Bartky, Sandra, 208–9, 254
Bauman, Zygmunt, 46, 47
Beatty, Thomas, 126–7, 145, 177, 182
Begley, Cecily, 189, 191–2, 257, 260
binders, 182, 183
biomedicine, 4, 24, 33
bio-social medicine, 64–5
birth. *see* childbirth; labour
Birth of mankinde, The (Rhodion), 107
Birth of the Clinic (Foucault), 33
birthing pool, 39
birthing stool, 37
Birthrights Rally, 1982, 18–19, 20, 21
birth-weight, 225, 226, 232
'black box,' 79–82, 103, 167, 228
    error/truth, 82–8
Blake, Mrs, 131
blood pressure, high, 188
blood-letting, 123–4, 125, 126, 132–3
bodily integrity, 26
Boland, Eavan, 25

333

bonding, 208
'born before arrival' (BBA), 242–3
Boston Women's Health Collective, 34
bougies, 201
Bourne, Gordon, 60
brain damage, 232
breast cancer, 13
breech birth, 9, 14, 55, 75, 175
    perception of, 256–7
British Medical Association, 23
Bronfen, Elaine, 48
Broussais, 116–17, 118, 168
Brown, Joan, 51, 52
Browne, 99–100
buildings, renovation of, 121–2
Burns, Professor, 85

Caesarean sections, 9, 14, 39, 100, 175, 237, 258
    under active management of labour, 206–7, 213
    and epidurals, 41
    maternal mortality, 97–9, 100
    statistics, 101, 193, 223
calomel, 124, 126, 127
Cameron, Deborah, 32
Campbell, Dr, 134–5
Canada, 40, 192, 241–2
Canguilhem, Georges, 112, 168, 191
Cardiff Infusion Unit, 202
cardio-vascular risks, 188
Cartwright, Ann, 203
'cascade of intervention,' 204
Castel, Robert, 212
castor oil, 126, 201
Catherine, 243
causality, 170–1
cellulitis, 127
Census Office, 147
cerebral palsy, 207, 232, 245–6
    Dunne case, 217–20
cervix
    artificial dilatation of, 82–3, 200, 209
    dilatation of, 209–12, 260–1
    'sweeping' of, 73, 200–1
Chalmers, Iain, 198
Chamberlen family, 93
Changing Childbirth (UK), 239
Chicago Lying-In Hospital, 172
childbed fever. *see* puerperal fever
childbirth
    classifications of, 82–8
    corporeal feminisms for, 262–4
    as critical moment, 40–1

models and approaches, 256–62
natural or medical, 39
norm and risk, 11–13
normality in, 8–9, 253
problematising, 38–45
recording of history of, 31–2
scientific control of, 19–20
women's evaluation of risk, 144–5
women's horror stories, 244–9
childbirth movement, 14, 38, 256, 259
chloroform, 42, 165
Churchill, Fleetwood, 91, 100, 139, 174
    on post-partum haemorrhage, 183
    on puerperal fever, 106–7, 121
        contagion, 134–5
        treatment, 123
    on removal of placenta, 185
cintura, 3, 6, 7
Clarke, Joseph, 81, 82, 87, 90, 102, 132, 140, 207, 259
    assessment of, 103
    classification system, 79–80
    clinical reports, 76–9, 144–5
    on dissections, 128–9
    importance of observation, 49–50
    on midwives, 53
    on natural birth, 82
    on post-partum haemorrhage, 181
    on puerperal fever, 113–16, 137–8, 151
        causation, 118–19
        treatment, 121, 123, 125
    removal of placenta, 185
    on tedious labours, 166, 207
    use of instruments, 95–6
    vaginal lacerations, 103–4, 165
    violent practices, 96–7
    'watchful waiting,' 82, 83, 85, 171
class distinction. *see* social class
cleidotomy, 258
Code, Lorraine, 196, 197, 254–5
Colgan, Karina, 252
Collins, Robert, 90, 103, 114, 119, 162–3, 206, 207, 250
    assessment of, 103
    dispute with Hamilton, 82–8, 95, 161, 167
    on post-partum haemorrhage, 182
    on puerperal fever, 126, 130–1, 137–8, 144, 145
    statistics, 158, 159, 224–5
    tedious labours, 166
    watchful waiting, 171
Comhairle na n-Ospidéal, 203–4, 238
communication, lack of, 235

Comte, Auguste, 36
congenital abnormality, 225
constipation, 119
consultant units, 203–4
contraceptive pill, 13
Coombe Women's Hospital, 126, 145, 148
    BBAs, 243
    epidurals, 41
    grand multiparity, 190–1
    international comparisons, 140–1
    post-partum haemorrhage, 182
    use of episiotomy, 260
Cooper, Davina, 60
Copland, Dr, 135
cordials, 123
Craft, Professor Ian, 18, 19, 21, 197
Cranbrook Committee, 1959, 203
craniotomy, 57, 95, 100
Crede, Dr, 183–4
crotchet, use of, 55, 85–6, 91–3, 96, 99
cuckolds, 9
Cuna Indians, 9
cyanosis, 217

Davis-Floyd, Robbie, 262
de la Motte, Guillaume, 178–9, 218
de Lauretis, Teresa, 103
de Lee, Joseph, 172, 256
Dease, William, 76, 81, 92
    assessment of, 103
    on Caesareans, 98
    on natural labour, 74–5
    on symphyiotomies, 98, 99
    use of forceps, 93
death
    avoidable death, 167–76
    causes of, 242
    Dunne case, 220–3
    at home, 251–3
    loss of productivity, 19–20, 58
    problem of, 45–50
    risk of, 14–15, 21–2, 25–31, 40
    role of, 235
    shift in medical reaction to, 143–5
    use of statistics, 158–67, 223–8
Denham, 136
Denmark, 40, 81
depression, 204
DES, 24
Descartes, R, 83
Development of Hospital Maternity Services, Discussion Document on, 203–4
Deventer, Henrik, 37, 52, 54, 63, 66–7, 81, 84, 198
    on labour induction, 201
    on natural birth, 68–9
    removal of placenta, 179–80
    on vaginal examination, 70–1
diarrhoea, 124–5
Dick-Read, Grantly, 42–3, 198
dilatation
    artificial, 82–3, 200, 209
    encouragement of, 260–1
    Friedman curve, 209
    rates of, 209–12
Dingwall, 236
Discourse on Method (Descartes), 83
disease, theories of
    causation models, 109–10
    local irritation, 116–17
    periodicity, 118–19
disinfectant, 133, 155
dissection, clinical, 46, 78, 86, 140, 159
    Dunne case, 218, 219
    invasiveness, 97
    relatives' permission, 128
    source of infection, 59, 128–37, 133–4, 152–3, 156
Donally, Mary, 98
donated ovarian material, 23
Douglas, Dr, 104
Douglas, Mary, 175–6, 221
Doulcet, 125
drugs, use of, 172
Dublin Journal of Medical Science, 82, 84
Dublin Obstetrical Society, 146, 147–8, 159
    discussion on forceps delivery, 163–7
Dublin Quarterly Journal of Medical Studies, 136
Dublin School of Midwifery, 25
Duden, Barbara, 33
Dunne, Catherine, 30, 31, 59, 215–23, 236–7, 262–3
Dunne, William, 30, 215–23, 263
dural puncture, 41
Durkheim, Emile, 167
dystocia, 49

Eccles, Audrey, 115
eclampsia, 188, 193
Edinburgh, 83, 87, 119, 121, 134–5, 138
'E.F.', 96, 104
Effective Care in Pregnancy and Childcare, 198
Ehrenreich, 27
Elliott, John, 139–40

emotional lability, 208, 210–11, 213–14, 231
  Dunne case, 220–1
empowerment, 250
England, 50, 81, 146, 185, 198
  active management of labour, 205
  dialogue, 238–9
  hospital delivery, 203, 204
  induction, 202
  maternal mortality, 193
  midwifery, 53
  perinatal mortality, 226
  puerperal fever, 108
  statistics, 40
English, 27
Enlightenment, 20, 28, 31
  rescue of women, 33–4, 36
epidural anaesthesia, 39, 47, 203, 204, 231, 235, 261
  reasons for use, 42
  staffing hazards, 244–5
  statistics, 41
episiotomy, 39, 53, 91, 204
  Ould on, 62–3, 73
  perception of, 256
  reasons for, 259–60
ergometrine, 185, 187, 188
ergot, 185, 201, 202
error/truth dyad, 58–9, 82–8
erysipelas, 111, 116, 120, 123, 135
essentialism, 29, 42, 103
Evening Herald, 251–2
Evory, Dr, 96
Ewald, Francois, 170

face masks, 155
Farr, William, 160
Feeney, J.K., 190–1
female body
  model of, 97
  naturalist thesis, 38–9
  studies of, 34–7
  'syndromes,' 24–5
  ways of 'seeing,' 142–3
female frailty, 29–30, 59, 72–3, 80, 87, 156, 174
  active management of labour, 206
  assumption of, 93–4
  and contagion, 134–5
  Dunne case, 218, 220–3
  and puerperal fever, 109–10, 142–52
femininity, 48
feminism, 103, 230, 253
  challenge of obstetric science, 263–4
  and childbirth, 21, 22
  and choice, 26–7
  corporeal feminisms for birth, 262–4
  influence on health, 233
  natural female body, 38–9
  reclaiming power, 60–1, 261–2
  silencing of women, 31–4
fertility control, 192, 193, 195, 213, 233, 248
fertility rate, Irish, 25
fever hospitals, 139
fillet, 92–3
Finger, Anne, 27
Finland, 40, 240
Fitzgerald Report on General Hospital Services, 203
Fleck, Ludwig, 60, 64–5, 74, 81, 102, 110, 112, 120–1, 136, 137, 223, 258
Flint, Caroline, 204, 260–1
foetal-heart monitor, 199, 200, 216, 217
  twins, 219, 222
foetus. *see also* perinatal mortality
  disability in, 27
  dismembering, 92–3
  personification of, 253–4
forceps
  invention of, 93
  use of, 18, 39, 77, 78, 81, 172, 204, 228
    under active management of labour, 206–7, 213
    Johnston paper on, 163–7
    mortality rates, 150–1
    risks of, 91
    speeding labour, 83, 85–6, 90, 200
    statistics, 101, 223
Forster, Dr, 114, 129
Foucault, Michel, 10, 20, 23, 60, 123, 169, 195, 208, 234
  biopolitics of population, 159, 160
  Birth of the Clinic, 34, 45
  constitution of the subject, 31
  on dissection, 129–30
  epidemics, 108–9
  exploration of self, 43
  'gazing,' 115, 142
  on Hippocrates, 128
  power, 65, 235, 245, 262
  rationality, 112
  subjugated knowledges, 259
  truth and error, 222
France, 50, 73, 81, 97–9, 125, 177, 178, 198
Franco-Prussian war, 152
Frankenberg, Ronald, 88

Freud, Sigmund, 65, 230–1, 259
Friedman curve, 209, 261

Garrow, Mrs James, 131
Gaskin, Ina May, 22, 251, 258
Gelis, Jacques, 36–7, 73, 107, 115, 120, 155
General Board of Health, Dublin, 109
General Medical Council, 156
genetic tests, 13
geography
    and puerperal fever, 137–42
Germany, 40, 50, 81, 250
Gigli, 99
Glasgow, 85
Gordon, Alexander, 114, 140
    and approaching death, 143, 144
    on dissections, 128, 129
    on puerperal fever, 115, 116–17, 138
        causation, 118–19
        contagion, 131–4, 152
        treatment, 123–4, 127
Gordon, John, 130
Gordon, Yehudi, 18
Graham, Hilary, 200
Grant, Margaret, 126–7
Grave, Robert, 46
Greece, 178, 226–7
Gregory, Lady, 9
Grudzinskas, Gedis, 197

Hacking, Ian, 60, 160, 161–2, 166, 240
    normality, 167, 168–9
    risk assessment, 176–7
Hamilton, James, 90, 104, 119, 161, 164, 206, 207, 210
    assessment of, 103
    avoidable death, 171
    dispute with Collins, 82–8, 95, 161, 163, 167
hand-washing, 132, 133, 136, 152, 153, 155
Harvard Medical School, 135
Harvey, Mr, 130
Harvie, John, 54, 180–1, 185
Health, Department of, 195, 232
Hill, Susan, 225–6
Hippocrates, 106, 118, 128, 178
Holmes, Oliver Wendell, 134, 135–6, 136, 152, 153
home attendance scheme, 146
Home Birth Centre, 236
home births, 14, 39, 241
    and death, 251–3
    emergency only, 21

Irish discussion, 19, 20
    mortality rates, 227–8, 239–40
    O'Connor study, 234–5, 245
    and puerperal fever, 141–2, 155
    statistics, 40
hormonal infusions, 39
'horror stories,' 60
hospitals
    BBAs, 242–3
    consultant units, 203–4
    dominance of, 39–40, 239–41
    hierarchy, 95
    importance of timing, 88
    lack of communication, 240–1
    mortality rates, 47, 227–8
    no proof safest place, 193, 198
    official policy on, 203–4
    puerperal fever in, 59, 107–8, 109, 137–42, 145–52
    role of, 24–5, 28
    staff, 210–11
    throughput, 42
    women's horror stories, 244–9
    women's voices lost, 238
Hotel-Dieu, Paris, 28, 52
    dissections, 128
    mortality rates, 122
    puerperal fever epidemics, 107, 117, 125
Houghton, Dr, 126–7
House of Commons Committee on Dublin Hospitals, 145–6
House of Commons Committee on Maternity Services, 226
HRT, 24
Hulme, Dr, 105, 106, 109, 114, 118
humoral medicine, 115, 124–5
Hunter, William, 94, 99
Huntingford, Peter, 198
hypertension, 11, 188
hypoxia, 225
hysteria, 34, 64–5, 123, 143
hysteritis, 121

If It Happens to You (Colgan), 252–3
Illsley, Raymond, 226
Inch, Sally, 174, 188
    'cascade of intervention,' 204
induction of labour, 197–204, 230
    under active management of labour, 213
    movement to acceleration, 204–14
    social reasons, 203
infections, 91, 111
    statistics, 101
    treatment of epidemics, 108–9

Innuit women, 241–2
instruments, use of, 28–9, 55, 68, 75
   choosing between lives, 91–101
   controversies, 81–2
   'heroic rescues,' 95–6
   premature, 70
insurance, 170
intercranial haemorrhage, 188, 246
internal version, 92
inverted uterus, 6
ipecacuanha, 125, 126
Ireland, 11, 44
   fertility control, 233
   foetal mortality, 226, 231–2
   home births, 234–5
   hospital dominance, 203–4, 239–41
   labour girdle, 7
   labour induction, 203
   lack of midwives, 50
   maternal mortality, 100–1
   midwives' practices, 6, 9, 53
   obstetric science in, 24–5, 34
   puerperal fever, 108
   statistics, 40
Irish Free State, 101
Irish Times, 234, 245
iron supplements, 192
IVF programme, 245–6

Jackson, Dr, 30, 216–17, 237
Jacob, 112
jalap, 124
Jebb, Frederick, 25–6, 63–4, 66–7, 250
Jellett, Henry, 99, 156–7, 162–3, 184, 223–8
Johnson, Charles, 166
Johnston, G. and Sinclair, E., 162–3, 181–2
Johnston, George, 91, 120
   avoidable death, 171
   intervention policy, 171–2, 173
   paper on forceps delivery, 163–7
   Practical Midwifery, 162–3
   on puerperal fever, 105–6, 148–51
   risk system, 171
Jordanova, Ludie, 24, 33, 35, 51, 94, 96
Journal of the Irish Medical Association, 190–1
journal science, 81, 115–16

Keller, Evelyn Fox, 230, 256
Kennedy, Dr H., 105–6
Kennedy, Evory, 135, 142, 151, 159
   open letter to governors, 146–8, 152
   statistics, 161

Kennedy, Patricia, 41, 239
Kidd, Dr, 166, 167
Kierkegaard, S., 10, 14–15
Kirkland, 132
Kitzinger, Sheila, 18, 204, 231
Klaus and Kinnell, 208
Kuhn, Thomas, 17, 161

Labatt, 138, 145
labile hypertension, 11
labour, 6–7, 40. *see also* active management of labour; induction of labour; position of labour
   attendance of partner, 231
   classification of, 79–82
   drive towards intervention, 171–3
   'heroic rescues,' 95–6
   knowledge claims of women, 254–6
   'normal' length of, 82–8, 84–6, 174–5, 206, 208–12, 223–4, 260–1
   norms and risks, 31–4
   obstetric horror stories, 235–43
   overriding woman's responses, 149–51
   risk factors, 174–5, 177
   'seeing' the body, 173–4
   tedious labour, 72, 166, 207
   theories of natural labour, 68–79
   walking during, 150, 216, 224, 261
labour belt, 3
labour girdle, 7
Lancet, 152
Lane, 151, 154
language, medical, 32, 50–1, 53–6
Latour, Bruno, 60, 65, 82, 84, 102, 153–4, 155, 198
le Doeuff, Michèle, 35–36, 38
Lee, Dr, 134–5
leeches, 126
legal action, 214, 245–6, 263
   Dunne case, 214–23
lever, invention of, 93
Levi-Strauss, 9
Lister, J., 152, 155
Liverpool, 140–1
London, 138, 140–1
London Medical Gazette, 84
Londoño, M.L., 026
Loudon, Irvine, 155, 194–5
Louth County Hospital, 244
Low, Mrs John, 118

McAdam-O'Connell, Bridget, 234
Macan, Arthur V., 152
MacDonald, Dermot, 219–20

maceration, 217, 218, 219
MacKenzie, Donald, 224
McKeown, Thomas, 192, 231, 233
McMahon, Louise, 236
McNay, Lois, 38–9, 45
male midwives, 27–9
   attitude to female midwives, 50–7
   birth positions, 36–7
   dissension among, 66
   eroticised violence, 94
   female death objectified, 47–50
   heroic rescues, 95–6
   Nihell on, 55–6
   private practices, 139, 146–7
   reading of Nature, 73–4
   theories of femininity, 48–50
   treatises by, 51–2, 62–8
      natural/preternatural labour, 68–79
Manchester, 119, 121
mania, 151
manteo, 8–9, 260
Martin, Emily, 20, 24, 249–50, 262
masculine discourse, 33, 230–1, 261–2
maternal mortality, 13–14, 147, 156–7, 239
   and asepsis, 154–5
   avoidable death, 190–6
   Caesarean sections, 41
   forceps deliveries, 150–1
   historical, 25–31, 45–50
   non-obstetric improvements, 191–3, 233
   post-partum haemorrhage, 185
   statistics, 89–90, 100–1, 122
   types of statistics, 162–3
maternity units, closure of, 203–4
Mauriceau, 37, 81, 92, 93
meconium, 216, 217, 230–1
medical journals, 81
medical students, 154, 156
medoag, 53
Meigs, 42, 136
menarche, age of, 57
menopause, 24
menstruation, 35, 65
mercury, 124–5, 126
miasmic disease, 112, 132, 139, 145, 148
microbiology, 124
micro-organisms, 111, 136–7, 155
Middlesex lying-in hospital, 116
midwifery movement, 60
midwives, 3, 9, 40, 155, 156, 231
   alternative readings, 256
   Caesarean sections, 98
   carrying infection, 131

community midwives, 195, 198, 242
definition of normal labour, 199–200, 260–1
and episiotomy, 260
and mortality rates, 227–8
Nihell's *Treatise*, 27–9
seen as incompetent, 50–7, 77, 78, 81–2, 199
tethering umbilical cord, 6
use of ergot, 185
women's aptitude as, 67–8
miscarriage, 27, 248–9
Mosse, Bartholomew, 25
mother/foetus dyad, 58, 88–101, 253–4
   balance of interests, 90–1
   techniques for saving one life, 91–101
M'Rae, Joseph, 130
Murphy, Edward, 136
Murphy, E.W., 86–7, 88
Musgrave, J.A., 156, 157
Muu, song of, 9

Napoleonic Wars, 117, 168
National Maternity Hospital, Holles St, 25, 30, 234, 236, 245
   active management of labour, 59, 205–14
   Dunne case, 30, 214–20, 236–7
   epidurals, 41, 44
   statistics, 223–5
   symphysiotomy, 99
National Perinatal Epidemiology Unit, 198
Nationalist, 245
naturalist thesis, 32–4, 38–9
   different models, 256–62
natural/preternatural dyad, 58, 68–79, 82
Netherlands, The, 40, 50, 81, 227
   home births, 239–40
Niamh, 251–2
Nightingale, Florence, 139
Nihell, Elisabeth, 60, 61, 82, 88, 97, 103, 263
   birth position, 80
   classification of labour, 79, 80
   critical of male midwives, 37, 53, 74, 84
   on labour induction, 201
   on natural labour, 63, 69–70, 75, 256
   non-scientific, 104
   on post-partum haemorrhage, 178, 180, 181
   references cited by, 81
   saving foetus, 90–1
   Treatise, 27–9, 33
   umbilical cord, 102

    on use of instruments, 95
    on vaginal examination, 70–1
    walking during labour, 150
    women as midwives, 50, 54–6, 66–8
    women seen as weak, 51
non-marital pregnancy, 105–6
normality, 11–13, 59
    avoidable death, 167–76
    concept of, 168–9
    construction of, 31–4
    definition of normal labour, 199–200
nosometry, 160
nurses, 155, 206, 207–8
nutrition, 101, 192, 193, 213, 233

Oakley, Ann, 10, 22, 200–2, 204, 233
    labour induction, 203
O'Brien, Mary, 254
Observations on Midwifery (Hamilton), 82
Observations on Midwifery (Dease), 74–5
obstetric science, 2, 4–5, 9–10, 10–11. *see also* puerperal fever; risk assessment
    alternative readings to, 256–62
    avoidable maternal death, 190–6
    classifications of labour, 79–82
    as continuous history, 223–8
    controversies, 115–16
    definitions of natural labour, 66–79
    failures of, 13–14
    heroic practices, 95–6, 258, 259–60
    horror stories, 235–43
    immortality strategy, 47–8
    jeopardising knowledge, 220–3
    knowledge claims of women, 254–6
    limitations of, 7–8, 171
    maintaining discourse on risk, 229–35
    male discourse, 23–5
    problematic construct, 194–6
    rationality, 17–22, 57–61
    sustaining knowledges, 101–4
    theoretical development, 62–8, 81–2
    theory and practice, 62–8
    use of statistics, 223–8
    women's relationship with, 30–1, 262–3
O'Connor, Marie, 234–5, 237, 238, 241, 245
Odent, Michel, 198
O'Driscoll, Kieran, 197, 199, 227, 232
    active management of labour, 205–14
    Dunne testimony, 222
    statistics, 223–5
'old wives' tales,' 60, 231, 236
omentum, inflammation of, 120, 121

O'Neal, Alice, 98
opiates, 77, 92, 125, 126, 127, 144
O'Sullivan, Dr Donal, 19
Ould, Fielding, 55, 66, 79, 81, 89, 96, 102
    assessment of, 103
    on Caesareans, 97–8
    description of episiotomy, 62–3
    episiotomy, 259
    labour induction, 200–1
    left lateral side position, 37, 80
    on natural labour, 71–4, 75
    removal of placenta, 179–80, 183, 184
    treatise, 51, 52
    use of instruments, 93–5
Our Bodies, Ourselves, 34, 250–1
ovary donation, 23
oxytocic drugs, 41, 42, 187, 188, 189, 235
    acceleration of labour, 213
    and analgesics, 204
    evaluation of, 191–2
    labour induction, 201–2
    physiological production, 257, 260
    replaced by active management of labour, 205

pain relief, 39, 41–4, 47
    transferral of pain, 9
palpation, 261
Panama Republic, 9
partner, role of, 39, 40–1, 231
partogram, 207, 209–10, 211, 212, 213
    multigravid labour, 215
Pasteur, Louis, 153–4
patriarchy, 20–1, 31–4, 102, 233–4, 235, 254
Peel Committee, 1970, 203
pelvic cellulitis, 111
pelvis
    contracted, 97, 193
    deformation of, 78, 101
    disproportion, 95–6
perinatal mortality, 14, 19, 26, 49, 226
    avoidable death, 197–204
    labour induction, 197–204
    statistics, 89–90, 224–8, 231–2
    in utero, 68, 85, 217, 218
peritonitis, 86, 107, 111, 114, 118, 120, 121, 129
Petchesky, Rosalind, 254
Peu, M., 107, 117, 152
pharmacology, 185, 187, 195, 207, 230
Phelan, Denis, 140–1
phlebitis, 121, 193
pituitary extract, 201

placenta, 5–6, 15, 177–8, 183. *see also* post-partum haemorrhage
  retention of, 26, 53
  terms for, 54
plague, 136–7
Pluto, 178
PMT, 24
Pomme, Dr, 34, 142
Poovey, Mary, 42, 123
Porter, Roy, 143, 144
position of labour, 36–7, 80, 258–9
  and episiotomy, 62–3
  left lateral side position, 37, 80
  supine position, 6–7, 8, 32, 37, 87
postnatal depression, 24
post-partum haemorrhage, 2, 5–6, 15, 76, 90, 91, 102, 193, 228, 230
  avoidable death, 176–85
  measurement of blood loss, 186
  mortality rates, 185
  moving towards active management, 185–90
  perception of, 256
  risk factors, 177, 186–7
  scientific evaluation of treatment, 191–2
  unpredictability, 7–8
Potter's syndrome, 251–2
poverty
  and difficult labour, 75–6, 77
  and foetal mortality, 226
  and puerperal fever, 112, 120, 138
Practical Midwifery (Johnston and Sinclair), 162–3, 181–2
Practical Treatise on Midwifery, A (Collins), 82, 137–42, 158, 159
pregnancy
  after puerperal fever, 128
  fear of infant death, 232–3
  'normal' length of, 202–3
  and risk, 13
private practices, 139, 146–7
pro-choice movement, 26
prostaglandin, 260
pubiotomy, 99–100
public health, 153–4, 157, 160
  statistics, 239–40
puerperal fever, 2, 25, 57, 86, 90, 91, 96, 183, 185
  acceptance of asepsis, 152–7
  after-effects, 128
  Caesarean sections, 100
  causation theories, 118–28
  classification, 111–12
  contagion, 131–4, 131–7, 146, 152–3
  definitions, 110–11
  descriptions of, 113–17
  epidemics, 107–8, 109, 113–14
  and forceps deliveries, 164–5
  in hospitals, 59, 107–9, 137–42, 145–52
  international comparisons, 140–1
  local irritation, 168
  prior health of mother, 119–20
  risk assessment, 159–60
  social class and geography, 137–42
  statistics, 107–8
  struggle against, 105–57
  symptoms, 120
  treatments of, 121–8
  use of dissections, 128–37
  women's fear of, 144–5
  women's responsibility for, 142–52
pulmonary oedema, 188
Purefoy, 101
purgatives, 124–5
purging, 123–5, 126, 132–3
pyaemia, 111, 151, 154

quarantine, 138–9
Quechua Indians, 1–4, 11, 15, 260
  birth blanket, 8–9
  childbirth practices, 1–4
  expulsion of placenta, 177–8
  infant mortality, 2
Quetelet, 168
quinine, 201

Raidió na Gaeltachta, 19
Raynalde, Thomas, 106–7
Reinharz, Shulamith, 247–8
Report of the Maternity and Infant Care Scheme Review Group, 238, 239
Rhodion, Eucharius, 107
rickets, 95
risk assessment, 12–13, 14, 21–2, 199
  anthropological perspective, 175–6
  avoidable death, 170–6, 190–6
  coercion, 176
  Dunne case, 220–3
  hospital *vs.* home, 40–1, 234
  maintaining discourse on, 229–35
  post-partum haemorrhage, 176–85, 186–7
  removal of agency, 249–56
  use of statistics, 158–67
  by women, 144–5
risk/death dyad, 158–96
Rochford, Judith, 24
Roonhausen, 93

Rose, Hilary, 255–6
Rotunda Maternity Hospital, 24–5, 37, 49, 53, 63–4, 82, 136
  asepsis, 152, 153, 154–5
  Caesarean sections, 98–9, 101
  charter, 50, 58
  clinical reports, 76–9, 83, 100
  criticisms of, 85–7
  details of babies, 91
  epidurals, 41
  forceps deliveries, 163–7
  international comparisons, 140–1
  labour induction, 201
  maternal mortality, 122, 142, 147, 154–5
  midwife training, 50
  open admissions policy, 145–6
  position of labour, 37, 80
  post-partum haemorrhage, 181, 182, 184, 185
  puerperal fever, 105–6, 109, 137–8, 144–5, 154
    causation, 119
    different approaches to, 145–52
    statistics, 158
    treatment of, 121, 125, 126
  role of, 54, 88–9
  'shroud-waving,' 239–40
  statistics, 89–90
  threatened with closure, 137–8
Rousseau, Jean Jacques, 36
Roussel, Pierre, 33, 35, 36, 51, 65, 164–5
Royal Free Hospital, London, 18–19, 20, 21, 197
Royal Medical Society, Paris, 125
rubber gloves, 155
Rusek, Sheryl, 242

St Catherine's hospital, Dublin, 74
St Nicholas's hospital, Dublin, 74
St Petersburg, 140–1
Savage, Wendy, 197, 198
Sawicki, Jana, 60, 234–5, 262
scarlatina, 91
Scarry, Elaine, 43, 44, 165, 255
Schiebinger, Londa, 36
Scotland, 108
Second Commission on the Status of Women, 238
Second World War, 193
self-definition, 245, 262
Semmelweis, Ignaz, 134, 135–6, 144, 152, 153
sensory perception, 256

sepsis, 96, 101, 133, 193
septicaemia, 151, 154
sexual activity, 52
sexual organs, 35, 164–5
  mutilation of, 99–100
Sherwin, Susan, 4
Shilling, Chris, 39, 46, 261
Short Committee, 1980, 203
Shorter, Edward, 26–7, 40, 84, 90, 128, 194–5, 250
  concern for foetus, 197
  foetal mortality, 202
  post-partum haemorrhage, 182
  on puerperal fever, 111, 155
shoulder dystocia, 258–9
Sigault, 99
Silverton, Louise, 199, 211–12
Simon, John, 140–2
Simpson, 42, 43
Sinclair, Edward
  Practical Midwifery, 162–3, 181–2
Sir Patrick Dun's hospital, 126–7
Sligo General Hospital, 244
smallpox, 91
Smellie, William, 28, 71, 81, 180, 181
  labour induction, 201
  removal of placenta, 184–5, 188
Smith, Dorothy, 31–4
Smith, Mrs James, 131
social class, 29, 33
  difficult labours, 75–6, 77
  grand multiparity, 190–1
  maternal mortality, 193
  perinatal mortality, 226, 232
  puerperal fever, 120, 137–42, 143, 147
Solomons, Bethel, 156, 201–2, 237–8
Southwell, Thomas, 98, 180
Stacey, Margaret, 249
stapholococci, 111
State of the World's Children Report (UNICEF), 239
statistics
  avoidable death, 167–76
  use of, 158–67, 223–8
stays, 119
stethoscope, 85
Stimson and Webb, 236
streptococci, 111, 155
stuping, 126
sulphonamides, 155, 193
Sunday Tribune, 246
superstition, 5, 10
surface irritation, 125
suturing, 99

Switzerland, 185, 250
symphysiotomy, 98, 99, 100, 258
synochus, 132
Syntocinon, 187, 202
Syntometrine, 188
syphilis, 110, 132
Systeme physique et moral de la femme (Roussel), 33, 35

technology, role of, 236, 238, 246–8, 261
terebra occulta, 94–5
Tew, Marjorie, 192–3, 194, 227
thalidomide, 24
thrombophlebitis, septic, 111
tire-tête, 92, 93–4
Todd, Alexandra, 24
toxaemia, 193
Transition to Motherhood (Oakley), 204
transverse lie, 76, 77, 96, 245
Treatise of Midwifry in Three Parts, A (Ould), 71–3
Treatise on the Art of Midwifery, A (Nihell). see under Nihell
Treichler, Paula, 22
turpentine, oil of, 126
Tweedy, 99, 154–5
    assessment of, 103
    clinical report, 100
    post-partum haemorrhage, 186
twins, 214–15
    Dunne case, 215–20
typhus fever, 105, 106, 132, 140, 151
    and puerperal fever, 120–1

ultrasound, 175, 218, 246–8, 252, 254, 256, 261
umbilical cord
    pulling on, 178–80
    tethering of, 5–6, 178
    time of cutting, 102, 187–8, 189
UNICEF, 239
United States of America, 39, 40, 50, 134, 185, 192
    active management of labour, 172, 205
    Caesarean sections, 193, 207
    perinatal mortality, 226
unmarried mothers, 145–6
    forceps deliveries, 164–5, 173
    puerperal fever, 148–9, 150

vaginal examination, 70–1
vaginal lacerations, 14, 103–4, 165
ventilation, 121–2
ventouse, 39
Vienna Krankenhaus, 144, 153
Vienna Lying-In Hospital, 25, 122, 136, 140–1
violence, 103, 183–4, 264. *see also* instruments, use of
visibility, principle of, 34–5

Wagner, Marsden, 14, 21, 59, 176, 193, 194, 198–9, 235–6, 238
Wales, 40, 146, 202
    maternal mortality, 193
    perinatal mortality, 226
Wassermann test, 110, 132
Waterford Lying-In Hospital, 139–40
Weber, Max, 11
Weedon, Chris, 23, 67
Western Lying-In Hospital, 139, 183
Westminster lying-in hospital, 116
White, Charles, 81, 119–20, 121, 122
'white leg,' 111
whitewashing, 121–2
Wildavsky, Aaron, 175–6
Wilde, Sir William, 6, 7, 9, 53–4
Winterton Parliamentary Report, 238, 239
Woman, 246–7
Woman's Way, 243
women
    accountable for own behaviour, 213–14
    categorisation of, 174–5
    emotionalism of, 208.210–11, 213–14, 220–1, 231
    weakness of (*see* female frailty)
women's health care movement, 14
workhouses, 139–40, 142
World Health Organisation, 193, 198, 226, 240
    Conference on Appropriate Technology for Birth, 253

Young, Dr, 121

Zavanelli manoeuvre, 258
zymotic disease, 139, 145, 146, 148, 159